Setting Nutritional Standards

Rochester Studies in Medical History

Senior Editor: Theodore M. Brown
Professor of History and Preventive Medicine
University of Rochester

Additional Titles of Interest

Stress, Shock, and Adaptation in the Twentieth Century
Edited by David Cantor and Edmund Ramsden

Female Circumcision and Clitoridectomy in the United States: A History of a Medical Treatment
Sarah B. Rodriguez

The Spanish Influenza Pandemic of 1918–1919: Perspectives from the Iberian Peninsula and the Americas
Edited by María-Isabel Porras-Gallo and Ryan A. Davis

Infections, Chronic Disease, and the Epidemiological Transition: A New Perspective
Alexander Mercer

Save the Babies: American Public Health Reform and the Prevention of Infant Mortality, 1850–1929
Richard A. Meckel

Intrusive Interventions: Public Health, Domestic Space, and Infectious Disease Surveillance in England, 1840–1914
Graham Mooney

The Antivaccine Heresy: "Jacobson v. Massachusetts" and the Troubled History of Compulsory Vaccination in the United States
Karen L. Walloch

Healthy Boundaries: Property, Law, and Public Health in England and Wales, 1815–1872
James G. Hanley

Psychiatry and Racial Liberalism in Harlem, 1936–1968
Dennis A. Doyle

Childbirth, Maternity, and Medical Pluralism in French Colonial Vietnam, 1880–1945
Thuy Linh Nguyen

A complete list of titles in the Rochester Studies in Medical History series may be found on our website, www.urpress.com.

Setting Nutritional Standards

Theory, Policies, Practices

Edited by Elizabeth Neswald,
David F. Smith, and Ulrike Thoms

University of Rochester Press

The University of Rochester Press gratefully acknowledges the Brock University Advancement Fund and the Humanities Research Institute of Brock University for their generous support of this publication.

First published 2017

University of Rochester Press
668 Mt. Hope Avenue, Rochester, NY 14620, USA
www.urpress.com
and Boydell & Brewer Limited
PO Box 9, Woodbridge, Suffolk IP12 3DF, UK
www.boydellandbrewer.com

ISBN-13: 978-1-58046-576-2
ISSN: 1526-2715

Library of Congress Cataloging-in-Publication Data

Names: Setting Standards: The History and Politics of Nutritional Theories and Practices, 1890–1950 (2010 : Brock University), author. | Neswald, Elizabeth, editor. | Smith, David F., 1954– editor. | Thoms, Ulrike, 1962– editor.
Title: Setting nutritional standards : theory, policies, practices / edited by Elizabeth Neswald, David F. Smith, and Ulrike Thoms.
Other titles: Rochester studies in medical history ; v. 38. 1526-2715
Description: Rochester, NY : University of Rochester Press, 2017. | Series: Rochester studies in medical history, ISSN 1526-2715 ; v. 38 | The essays in this volume emerged from the symposium Setting Standards: The History and Politics of Nutritional Theories and Practices, 1890–1950, held in 2010 at Brock University in Ontario. | Includes bibliographical references and index.
Identifiers: LCCN 2016037839 | ISBN 9781580465762 (hardcover : alk. paper)
Subjects: | MESH: Food—standards | Diet—standards | Nutrition Policy—history | Nutritional Sciences—history | History, 19th Century | History, 20th Century | Congresses
Classification: LCC QP141 | NLM QU 11.1 | DDC 363.802/18—dc23 LC record available at https://lccn.loc.gov/2016037839

A catalogue record for this title is available from the British Library.

This publication is printed on acid-free paper.
Printed in the United States of America.

Contents

Acknowledgments

In 2010, the Institute of Nutrition, Metabolism, and Diabetes of the Canadian Institutes of Health Research (CIHR) generously funded an international symposium on "Setting Standards: The History and Politics of Nutritional Theories and Practices, 1890–1950," which was held at Brock University in Ontario. The essays in this volume emerged from that symposium and the discussions that followed in its wake. The editors would like to thank the CIHR for making the symposium and this volume possible and the Faculty of Humanities at Brock University for its infrastructural support. Additional thanks go to Dinah Martin and Monika Pries-Klassen for their assistance with the symposium organization.

Introduction

ELIZABETH NESWALD AND DAVID F. SMITH
IN COLLABORATION WITH ULRIKE THOMS

"Nutrition is not a discipline, it is an agenda." This declaration, made by the French American nutrition scientist Jean Mayer has been adopted as the mission statement of the Friedman School of Nutrition Science and Policy at Tufts University in Massachusetts.[1] As the title of the school indicates, it offers a program that is explicitly socially engaged, but the statement also demonstrates that the disciplinary status of nutrition as a university program is not a matter of consensus. This has long been the case. In the United Kingdom after the Second World War, for example, one nutrition scientist, John Yudkin, returning from his military service to a chair of physiology, set about constructing a university discipline and degree in nutrition, combining biochemical, physiological, and social scientific approaches. In response, Robert Garry, president of the British Nutrition Society, declared in 1953 that nutrition should be regarded not as a science or discipline but as a "meeting place of the sciences and of scientists."[2] Yet nutrition scientists interact not only with scientists but also with many others: professionals such as doctors and veterinarians, politicians, administrators, policymakers, representatives of funding bodies, industrialists, agriculturalists, campaigners, lay and alternative experts, and media representatives. They meet members of the general public and their families. And all those they meet eat and have views on nutrition.

Around the world and throughout history, one of the commonest subjects of everyday domestic discourse has been food, and food has likewise been a persistent topic in public and political discourse. Historically, this discourse has often been shaped by concern about hunger and food scarcity and insecurity. In more recent times, such concerns have been joined by worries about overabundance, overeating, and the seeming inscrutability of world food systems.[3] During the last two centuries, these discourses have been increasingly shaped by the sciences of food and nutrition, as scientific and medical actors participated in public health, social welfare, and political policy debates surrounding food and diet. From the early days of the field, scientific nutritional knowledge became the basis for advertising copy and product innovation in the food and pharmaceutical industries. It was embraced by campaigners pursuing a wide variety of causes and by publics interested in maintaining and improving health. But although physicians traditionally dispensed dietary advice as part of clinical medicine, their response to the advent of nutrition science has varied from enthusiasm to scepticism. Today, the electronic and print media frequently report the research findings and views of nutrition scientists and self-declared nutrition experts, and in the media limelight nutrition has become a contested field populated by numerous actors with different agendas and expertise, manufactured controversies, and overstated claims.[4] In short, Jean Mayer's and Robert Garry's statements underestimate the multifaceted, porous, and "leaky" nature of nutrition science. The theoretical concepts of "boundary work" and "boundary objects," used in Science Studies to analyze the movement of scientific ideas and products, as well as scientists, through society, hardly do justice to the cultural resonances and indistinct and variable borders of nutrition science.[5] Combining Mayer and Garry, we might say that, in and through nutrition science, multiple and variable agendas meet and are played out by a diversity of actors.

The current collection of essays brings together scholars from the history of science and medicine, and social, political, and administrative history. As a collection on the history of nutrition science, of which there have been several,[6] it is the first to appear since the upsurge of interest in food among scholars in the social sciences and humanities, which has been described as "the burgeoning field of food studies."[7] In particular, it seeks to develop historical perspectives on a theme that has recently become of concern to food studies scholars, social historians, historians of science and medicine, and others: the history of dietary and nutritional standards.

A historical assessment of such standards is particularly relevant in the current situation in which there is not only widespread anxiety about the so-called obesity epidemic of the developed world, and about the health and environmental costs of industrial food production, but also attacks on nutrition science from both popular and academic commentators. In the light of the rise of specialized journalism and food activism, and interchange between the activist and academic arenas, it is not surprising that academic and journalistic analyses of food issues have much in common, as several recent works that focus on dietary and nutritional standards and their impacts show.[8] Although criticism of the food industry, its influence on the formulation of nutritional guidelines, and the unwillingness of governments to make guidelines that offend the food and agricultural industry is not new,[9] in the last decade three authors—the American journalist Michael Pollan, the Canadian science communication writer Jessica Mudry, and the Australian philosopher Gyorgy Scrinis—have mobilized history to bolster their positions against "reductionist" and "quantitative" approaches to nutrition and to advocate alternative "qualitative" standards for food and diet.[10] All three consider their historically based arguments as a contribution toward solving the great nutritional issues of the day, and in particular the much discussed "obesity epidemic."

In essence, Pollan, Scrinis, and Mudry challenge nutrition science's entire project of defining food in terms of nutrients and calculating the levels of nutrients required in diets. Pollan especially condemns the provision of health advice in terms of the need to increase or decrease intakes of certain nutrients. The seeming impotence of this approach in the face of the advancing "obesity epidemic" is, in his view, just one example of the failure of the contemporary nutrition science paradigm. Instead, Pollan advocates an alternative approach following qualitative "food rules" such as, "Do not eat anything that your grandmother would not recognise as food."[11] Mudry and Scrinis likewise criticize the focus on quantities of nutrients rather than food, a position that Scrinis sums up as "nutritionism." Like Pollan, they argue for the substitution of alternative criteria for assessing diets, such as traditional sensory means of judging food quality. Both of these authors base their analyses on historical material. In Mudry's case, the history is narrowly focused on successive American government documents formulating dietary advice for the general public. Her case for now discarding past approaches is based on the premise that they have failed to change nutritional behavior in the past and are unlikely to have any impact on current nutritional problems.

More comprehensive, in contrast, is Scrinis's historical purview. He selects from a range of sources in order to construct a framework involving three periods of nutrition science. As he describes it, in the era of "quantifying nutritionism," which lasted from the mid-nineteenth to the mid-twentieth century, the main concern was attaining an adequate supply of nutrients and the primary actors were nutrition scientists. Scrinis's second era of "good and bad nutritionism" lasted from the mid-1960s until the mid-1990s. During this time nutrients were differentiated into "good" and "bad" types that could protect against or lead to chronic degenerative "diseases of civilisation," principally coronary heart disease and diabetes. According to Scrinis, during this period government agencies and public health institutions were the primary actors. Finally, during Scrinis's current period of "functional nutritionism" since the mid-1990s, some nutrients and foods are represented as health enhancing and able to modify biomarkers such as blood cholesterol. In this phase, food corporations are the primary actors.

Scrinis's attempt to define periods in the history of nutrition science is, however, problematic and oversimplified. There are numerous cases of nutrition scientists leading initiatives beyond the mid-twentieth century,[12] and the tendency toward quantification outlived the "quantifying era." If the latter were not the case, Scrinis's call for "qualitative standards" would make little sense. Likewise, perceptions of good and bad foods and nutrients can be found prior to the "good and bad nutritionism" era. Edward Mellanby's classification of foods into those preventing and tending to cause rickets can serve as an example.[13] In addition, biomarkers were present in the late nineteenth and early twentieth century, as shown by the theory of Alexander Haig and his followers regarding levels of uric acid in the body and the impacts of various foods in raising or lowering it.[14] The bacteria-containing bonbons, soda, tablets, yoghurt pills, and "scientifically fermented milk" inspired by the claims of Elie Metchnikoff in the early twentieth century provide an early example of "functional foods,"[15] and the food industry exploited nutrition science long before the late twentieth century.[16] But it is hardly news that history is usually much more complex than the schemata set up by journalists, sociologists, philosophers, activists, and some historians.

As the growing literature on the history and philosophy of standards and standardization shows, not only standards themselves, but also the methods of determining them, are constantly changing and often contested.[17] In this volume, we define dietary and nutritional standards broadly, looking at standards in terms of foodstuffs, quantities of nutrients, and dietary needs, and accepting the particularly fluid nature of definitions, as nutrition science and the contexts in which it was discussed and applied shifted. We regard the history of all such standards to involve more than the efforts of scientists to devise quantitative measures of desirable intakes and of subsequent attempts to use such standards to guide the feeding or eating habits of individuals and populations. Rather, we take it to include any endeavor to devise and propagate new ways of eating, wherever the initiative originates. Historically, attempts to change the way people eat have consistently involved invoking scientific principles, co-opting scientific actors, and generating new scientific knowledge, even when they originate outside of professional scientific circles and begin, for example, with ethical or religious principles. Vegetarians, for example, opposed to eating animals for ethical reasons, have often sought scientific support for their dietary choices, and the studies they initiated led to the generation of new scientific knowledge.[18] The standards in question may be qualitative as well as quantitative, covering not only amounts of foods and nutrients but also types of foods. The "standard bread" campaign in Britain in the early 1910s, which encouraged the consumption of brown bread of specified composition, analyzed by Mark Weatherall, was largely a lay movement promoted by a newspaper, but it drew support from prominent scientists, including the vitamin pioneer F. G. Hopkins.[19] Dietary and nutritional standards may even involve ways of eating, as Margaret Barnet has discussed elsewhere in regard to the American businessman and dietary reformer Horace Fletcher, who popularized the practice of extensive chewing.[20] It should also be noted that the distinction between quantitative and qualitative standards is not clear-cut: any standard that entreats eaters to eat more or less of something (such as unrefined or refined foodstuffs) must be regarded as at least semiquantitative.

Even when new standards, quantitative or qualitative, appear to arise directly from scientific research, the route from research to policymaking and implementation has rarely been straightforward, for a variety of reasons. There is no simple linear process in which the generation of scientific knowledge leads to the formulation of new standards and then their application. Nutrition scientists frequently advocate changing food habits on the basis of knowledge that is still very much "in the making," and complete consensus in this field is, in any case, frequently elusive. Personal, professional, and institutional interests and contextual factors may encourage either activism or reclusiveness among scientists.

Public health professionals, medical practitioners, administrators, politicians, industry, and the public, who are cast as the transmitters, appliers, and consumers of scientific nutritional knowledge, have all often been resistant to or ambivalent about the messages received from nutrition scientists. Politics, culture, customs, and economic interests frequently explain such reactions, but questions of economics and national security have also often facilitated applications. The rapid and enthusiastic uptake of vitamins by the food and pharmaceutical industries, as described elsewhere by Sally Horrocks and Rima Apple, serves as an example.[21] Summing this up, we can say that the generation and application of nutritional knowledge takes place at the intersection of diverse and often conflicting interests and frequently involves a wide range of negotiations.

For those less familiar with the field we will now provide a brief outline of the early history of nutrition science before turning to the history and historiography of dietary and nutritional standards and the essays in this volume. In conclusion we will offer some reflections on the question of what contributions the history of nutrition in general and the essays in this volume in particular can make to current debates and action.

Nutrition Science Takes Shape

Beleaguered nutrition scientists, caught up in media-fuelled controversies and seemingly impotent in the face of nutrition-related public health problems, frequently claim, by way of explanation, that nutrition is a "young science."[22] This is a useful position, implying that increased and continued public investment in the field will allow it to mature to a time when definitive results will be obtained, controversy will abate, and the public will comply with the scientists' prescriptions. But characterizing nutrition science as "young" is not strictly accurate, since the field began to acquire some of the usual attributes of a scientific discipline, such as specialized research institutes, professional societies, and dedicated journals, by the early twentieth century. Admittedly, the process of institutionalization of nutrition came later than for physiology, of which nutrition was regarded by some as a subdiscipline, but it overlapped with that for biochemistry, endocrinology, genetics, and other such biomedical research fields. A closer look at the history of nutrition science reveals that nutrition can hardly be accurately described as any "younger" than most modern biomedical disciplines. Moreover, many of the problems and controversies faced by earlier nutrition scientists are similar to those faced by today's nutrition professionals.

However the emergence of nutrition science is located historically, governments and public institutions appreciated the utility of scientific approaches to food and feeding long before nutrition acquired any of the features of an institutionalized science. Scientists in postrevolutionary France developed schemes for alleviating food shortages, in part as a means to stabilize the new government.[23] The repression of urban begging lay behind the Bavarian king's engagement of the American adventurer Benjamin Thomson, later known as Count Rumford. Presented as a humanitarian endeavour, Rumford devised a Foucauldian disciplinary system of coercive, "improving" institutions to house the indigent poor, and a barley and legume-based gruel to feed them. Given the popular name of "Rumford soup," it was designed to be both inexpensive and, at least according to Rumford, satisfying, nutritiously sufficient, and palatable.[24]

Similarly, in the 1830s, the pioneering physiologist François Magendie was recruited by the French Academy of Science to investigate a pragmatic and socially sensitive question in the so-called gelatine commission, a project that in many ways reflects the particular intersection of interests that would shape and strain the emerging science of nutrition, combining physiology, medicine, and social welfare with economic interests.[25] Magendie's reputation and expertise were based on his foundational laboratory studies of 1816, in which he established that food was the source of nitrogen (protein) in the body.[26] He brought a similar precise experimental approach to the task of assessing whether gelatine, derived from animal bones, a waste product, was a nourishing substance suitable as a supplement or replacement for the more expensive meat and meat broth in hospitals and institutional feeding regimes.[27] The commission effectively sought to apply the emerging science of nutrition to a recurrent problem: how could states economically feed those members of society for whom they were responsible?

The mixture of experimental approaches with public health concerns, institutional populations, perceptions of state responsibility, and economic interests that were manifest in the gelatine commission and Rumford's workhouse and feeding regimes configured the landscape in which future nutrition researchers situated their research, structured their experiments, appealed for support and funding, and presented themselves in the public arena. Although the specific focus of individual nutrition scientists varied, maintaining the health and vitality of individuals and populations has always been among their stated aims. Even laboratory scientists investigating fundamental metabolic processes did not hesitate to refer to such potential practical outcomes.

The interest in public health and populations, as well as a focus on what the historian of biochemistry Frederic Holmes has termed the "intake-output" model,[28] differentiated the emerging field of nutritional physiology from studies of digestion, the chemical breakdown of food in the alimentary canal, and the older tradition of dietetics, which focused on individual constitution and health. The intake-output approach interpreted metabolism as an accounting problem, one of weights and balances. The idea of balances and equilibrium—that what went into a process needed to be accounted for at its end—structured not only approaches to metabolism but also more broadly fundamental scientific and social assumptions.[29] Since Antoine Lavoisier at the end of the eighteenth century, chemists assumed that matter was conserved in chemical processes and was neither created nor destroyed. In the 1840s, a similar proposal was made in physics that force or energy was conserved in natural processes and could also be neither generated nor annihilated.

The assumptions of balanced chemical accounts and of the conservation of matter formed the basis of Justus Liebig's approach to physiological chemistry and nutrition in the 1840s.[30] Calculating through chemical equations the various forms of intake and output in the body, Liebig explained the sources and maintenance mechanisms of both animal heat and muscular work. Animal heat was, in Liebig's theory, a process of combustion, in which the carbon in food combined with the oxygen of respiration and burned like the oil of a candle to produce the heat of life.[31] Muscular action, in contrast, came from the consumption of muscular tissue, which required regular replacement through an intake of nitrogen, that is, protein-containing foods, in amounts commensurate with physical activity.

As counterintuitive as Liebig's theory might seem, given the low protein diets of the hardest laborers, it guided nutrition research over the next few decades. The early research of the Munich professors Theodor Bischoff, Carl Voit, and Max Pettenkofer, which laid the methodological, experimental, and instrumental foundations for nutritional physiology, was developed within a Liebigian framework. They were quickly forced to modify and continuously revise this framework, until it was finally rejected entirely. Careful experimentation had proven Liebig's balance between intake and output of matter, but contradicted his two-function division.

Physiologists increasingly assumed that the energy conservation law applied to physiological processes and that energy transformations formed a fundamental part of nutrition and metabolism. It was not until the 1880s, however, that Max Rubner, a former pupil of Voit, was able to prove energy conservation in the living body and to formulate a coherent energy-based nutrition theory. Food became fuel with an energy value; the nutritional calorie was born. Forthwith, casual analogies between physical labor and machine labor received potent structural support. From the point of view of the energy laws and the industrialist, the manual laborer and the steam engine were both apparatus to transform carbon-based fuel into heat and mechanical work.

Between the 1900s and 1920s, much research interest turned toward the links between certain diseases and organic micronutrients, termed "accessory food factors," and later "vitamins." The idea that certain foods were valuable in maintaining health and curing particular maladies was hardly new and had formed a part of practical medical knowledge since ancient Greece.[32] Around 1900 diseases such as scurvy, rickets, and beriberi remained controversial in terms of both theory and therapy, despite some partially successful preventative strategies, for example, scurvy prevention and cures in the British Navy. Physicians and physiologists debated whether these diseases were caused by contagions, environmental toxins, general hygienic conditions, or the absence of some significant substance in the diet, and whether they had a single cause or arose from a combination of factors that increased susceptibility.[33]

In the nutritional theories of Liebig and the early energeticists there had been no place for organic nutrients other than the macronutrients protein, carbohydrate, and fat, but the vitamin concept quickly took shape as physiologists found animal models for the study of deficiency diseases. Contributions came from various corners and international actors. In 1906, the British biochemist Frederick Gowland Hopkins speculated that scurvy and rickets might be caused by missing "minimal qualitative factors," discussing the failure of animals to thrive on purified diets.[34] In 1912 he reported experiments in which rats on purified diets failed to grow unless a small quantity of milk was added to the ration, and suggested that the milk contained essential nutrients that he dubbed "accessory food factors."[35] Research on scurvy was boosted in 1907 when the Norwegians Axel Holst and Theodor Fröhlich discovered that the guinea pig could serve as an animal model for this disease.[36] In 1899 in Jakarta, part of the Dutch colonial empire, the physician Christiaan Eijkmann noticed that laboratory poultry fed white rice developed the neurodegenerative condition polyneuritis, but remained free of the disease on brown rice.[37] Eijkmann developed a complex multicausal theory of human beriberi that included roles for bacteria and toxins, as well as protective food factors. Following up on Eijkmann's observations, in 1912 the Polish chemist Casimir Funk of the Lister Institute of London attempted to isolate the antiberiberi factor in the outer layers of rice and introduced the term "vitamine."[38] Funk's term denoted "vital amine," reflecting his view of the chemical nature of the antiberiberi factor. It became the accepted term for referring to organic micronutrients but was shorted to "vitamin" when it became clear that vitamins were not amines.

Although the focus of nutrition research prior to the advent of the "vitamin" concept had been on energy and macronutrients, physicians and physiologists knew that certain minerals were essential for life and health. Calcium and phosphorus were known components of bone, iron had been used for the treatment of anaemia for centuries, and iodine had first been prescribed for goiter as early as 1820, nine years after its discovery as an element, although it had fallen out of favor owing to toxic effects. Interest in goiter and iodine revived in the early twentieth century after it was shown that the thyroid is relatively rich in iodine. By the 1920s the essential nature of additional trace elements had been demonstrated.[39] Thus by the end of the first quarter of the twentieth century, the key elements of modern nutrition science were in place.

This core nutritional knowledge was produced at a variety of sites, including various institutions focusing on health and the life sciences, such as medical schools and their constituent departments and associated institutes, as well as agricultural experiment stations, home economics departments, colonial outposts, and pharmaceutical laboratories. Research questions and approaches varied with these diverse sites and actors, and they left their mark on perceptions of what the study of nutrition entailed and what it ought to achieve. Chemists, home economists, and hospital clinicians, for example, investigated very different problems when they studied nutrition.

Much research on nutrition took place outside of the universities, supported by governments, medical foundations, and private initiatives. In Germany, the Landwirtschaftliche Hochschule, founded in Berlin in 1881, was primarily a veterinary and agricultural college, but included some research on human nutrition in its program. Similarly, the United States Department of Agriculture Experiment Stations, modeled on the experiment stations of Germany, focused on agricultural research and animal feeding but supported a significant human nutrition research program from 1887 to 1902. In the United Kingdom, dedicated animal nutrition laboratories were established in 1913 at Cambridge and Aberdeen. The latter became the Rowett Institute, which covered human nutrition as well during the interwar period.[40] In the United States, human nutrition found a place at the privately funded Carnegie Nutrition Laboratory from 1907 to 1947, the first laboratory dedicated solely to the study of human nutrition. Hospitals and pharmaceutical laboratories also supported human nutrition research, the former often in collaboration with universities and with a focus on diagnostics and pathologies, the later particularly well-suited to the biochemical aspects of nutrition studies.

The experience of food shortages and malnutrition during the First World War, the growing interest in vitamins, and the economic depression of the 1930s catalyzed many European governments and official bodies into the foundation of national institutions for the study of nutrition and assessment of national nutritional status during the interwar period. For example, the Dutch Institute for Nutrition Research, a small government-sponsored institute with a practical orientation housed within the University of Amsterdam's Department of Tropical Medicine and later Hygiene, was founded in 1919.[41] With the intention of pursuing basic research on vitamins, the British Medical Research Council opened a nutrition laboratory in Cambridge in 1927.[42] In the wake of the League of Nations reports of 1935–36 on "The Problem of Nutrition" and its call for the establishment of national bodies for the formulation of nutrition policy, most European governments established institutions for nutrition research to assess the nutritional state of the population and to promote the League's new dietary and nutritional standards.[43] Nutrition councils and national research institutes were established not only in Europe but also in countries as wideranging as Canada and Australia, Japan, and colonial India.[44] Despite its leading role in the study of nutrition in the late nineteenth and early twentieth centuries, central institutes were not established in Germany until after the Second World War (in 1946 and 1953 for East and West Germany, respectively), a period that saw a second flurry of national nutrition institute foundations.[45]

Similar tendencies can be found in the development of professional societies and publications, many of which were concerned with the role of nutrition in public health. In France, the Société scientifique d'hygiène alimentaire (Scientific Society for Alimentary Hygiene), was created in 1904.[46] An alliance of doctors, scientists, and activists, it originally focused as much on food reform as on research. It survives today as an agency offering training and analytical services. The clinically orientated Société de nutrition et de diététique de langue française (Society of Nutrition and Dietetics of the French Language) was not founded until 1966, whereas the Association française de nutrition (French

Nutrition Association), which focused on laboratory research, was established even later. Both eventually merged to form the current Société française de nutrition (French Nutrition Society).

In Germany, the public-health-oriented Reichsverein für Volksernährung (Imperial Society for Public Nutrition) traces its history back to 1928. It was replaced during National Socialism by the Deutsche Gesellschaft für Ernährung (German Society for Nutrition) in 1936, which was reestablished after the war in 1953. The American Institute of Nutrition was, from its origins in 1928, a conventional scientific society modeled on those of other biomedical disciplines. Its *Journal of Nutrition* began in the same year. In the United Kingdom the Nutrition Society was founded in 1941, after the secretary of the Medical Research Council felt that some nutrition workers who sought to influence wartime food policy were becoming too politicized.[47] In the past, as now, nutrition researchers also participated in a wide range of national and international conferences and congresses in allied fields such as physiology, hygiene, medicine, and home economics.

While much nutrition research took place outside of universities, there were also numerous university-based researchers and research groups. Much nutrition research from the mid-nineteenth century was undertaken at, or in connection with, departments of physiology, "hygiene" (public health), and chemistry. In the early twentieth century, home economics departments played an increasingly significant role in the study of dietaries, infant feeding, and the effect of cooking on the nutrient content and digestibility of food. Such departments provided employment to women with degrees in chemistry, medicine, and physiology. Since home economists rarely had the laboratory facilities and funding to conduct elaborate experiments, their work tended to focus on the applications of nutritional knowledge.[48]

Although by the 1920s individual researchers and their research groups at a large number of universities studied nutrition from a variety of disciplinary perspectives, it was not until the Second World War that universities began to establish nutrition departments. In the United States, the Department of Nutrition at the Harvard School of Public Health was founded in 1942 with funds from the Rockefeller Foundation. Soon after the war, two nutrition departments were set up in Britain, both in London—one at the School of Hygiene and Tropical Medicine and one at the College of Household and Social Science. It was at the latter that the undergraduate degree course mentioned at the beginning of this introduction was established. But university departments, dedicated chairs, and undergraduate degrees in nutrition were rare for decades. It was only with the expansion of higher education and the development of what John Pickstone termed "consumerist medicine"[49] that degrees in nutrition proliferated, many combined with, for example, sports or exercise science but also "football studies" and dance.[50] As this brief outline shows, nutrition can hardly be described as an especially young science. It can, perhaps, be more accurately described as fragmented, fluid, and unevenly developed.

Toward a History of Dietary and Nutritional Standards

The preceding outline of the institutionalization of nutrition science and the emergence and development of scientific nutritional knowledge can only offer some background for the focus of this book. Dietary and nutritional standards were posited as part of an applied and reformist dimension of nutrition science. They were strongly context dependent, subjects of consensus building, and frequently contested and revised. They were initially generated at an intersection of concerns and interests that arose in the nineteenth century, and were transformed with the scientific, social, and political changes that unfolded in the following century.

The construction of dietary and nutritional standards must be interpreted within the context of broader tendencies in the second half of the nineteenth century toward standards and standardization. Supraregional and international trade, precision industries, and mass production became increasingly economically important. Standards were conventions that allowed parts, products, and knowledge to move across industries and countries into completely different areas of application, transcending the specific context of their development. Scientists, politicians, and industrialists discussed standard units that could replace local and idiosyncratic measures to regulate diversity and enable communication across regional and national boundaries. Weights and measures, electrical units, telegraphic communication, machine parts, and even time were made uniform. As an article of commerce, food was affected by trade laws, and food safety and purity were increasingly legislated and controlled.[51] Improved transportation routes deregionalized food supplies and markets, enabling supraregional, national, and international brands to become established, thus requiring standardization of food production, labeling, and packaging. The impetus could come from a wide range of actors including scientists, doctors, politicians, lawyers, administrators, the press, and consumers, especially women.

Dietary and nutritional standards, although not drafted within the context of trade and exchange, were nonetheless a product of this drive to reduce diversity to exchangeable numerical expressions. They provided a set of norms against which variable diets could be assessed and measured. These standards combined impulses from anthropometrics and medical statistics, both developing in the middle decades of the nineteenth century, with thermodynamics, the new science of heat. Anthropometrics and medical statistics determined bodily norms and averages, setting up a standard body, whereas thermodynamics offered the concept of "calories," units of heat, which could be applied to foods and physical needs in energetic theories of nutrition. The "calorie" concept focused a new, rigorously quantitative approach to nutrition. Although vitamin researchers often represented their field as a turn away from quantitative and back to qualitative approaches in the assessment of dietary adequacy, they nevertheless quickly attempted to put numbers to the vitamin content of foods and the vitamin needs of population groups. When industrially produced vitamin concentrates and synthetic vitamins became available, manufacturers, scientists, and medical professionals sought to define their biological potency, reinforcing the quantitative dimension of vitamin science.[52]

With the nutritional calorie, food became fuel, a source of energy, and the human body was perceived as a motor that transformed this fuel into economically productive labor under the primate of efficiency.[53] The integration of thermodynamics into nutritional theory and the development of calorie and protein-based dietary norms reflected deeper concerns about dietary sufficiency and industrial society in general. These concerns grew in the wake of urbanization, increasing factory labor, and the demographic changes wrought by population shifts to larger settlements, declining birth rates, and immigration. Governments were anxious about their ability to compete with their rivals industrially and militarily and worried that food insecurity would increase the potential for political radicalism in the working classes. Fears about the possible "degeneration" of the population and a decline in the health and fitness of military recruits were widespread. "Efficiency" became the watchword in debates about social reform, the physical and economic health of the nation, factory management, and, as a number of authors have explored for the American and European cases, diet.[54]

Such concerns went hand in hand with the emergence of the "interventionist" or "providential" state and the introduction, spread, and modernization of social welfare programs such as school lunch programs and medical check-ups for children.[55] Public health professionals also began to take more interest in personal behavior,[56] for example, introducing new programs directed at mothers to improve housewifery skills such as the purchase and preparation of food and advice on childcare and breast-feeding.[57] In the words of John Pickstone, in public discussion medicine became "productionist." It connected to the broader societal debates on human, economic, and industrial efficiency, in that its potential for improving efficiency was emphasized.[58]

Nutrition science was allied to this movement. Nutritional physiologists and food chemists correlated nutritional content with the market prices of foods in order to supply persons of limited financial means with guidelines for financially and nutritionally economical food purchases and consumption. At the same time, dietary surveyors viewed efficiency in food consumption as a means to ameliorate the problem of working-class poverty. If workers learned to eat according to principles of physiological efficiency, they could reduce their food expenditure, leaving a larger portion of their income for other purposes, thus increasing general standards of living and satisfaction. Labor unrest could be avoided without raising wages, if nutrition was viewed as an accounting problem that balanced calorie and protein consumption with physical activity, physiology, and finances.

Connections between nutrition and sociomedical concerns only increased with the discovery of vitamins. The "vitamin" concept did not capture the public imagination or become the subject of well-funded research programs until after the First World War.[59] This new approach to nutrition, however, encountered skepticism from some physicians, medical administrators, and physiologists.

With vitamin knowledge still very much in the making, it was unclear what quantities were necessary and what the health benefits of vitamins were, and vitamin enthusiasts frequently made overstated claims about vitamin requirements and the range of diseases and conditions that vitamins could cure.[60]

The strongest claims of vitamin science were limited in scope. Several deficiency diseases were endemic among the poor in particular regions, but most were absent or uncommon in the general populations of Western countries. Rickets was relatively common in the cities of Northern Europe and North America, although its status as a vitamin-deficiency disease remained under challenge until the mid-1920s.[61] Pellagra was also suspected to be a vitamin deficiency and had long been a problem in parts of Southern Europe and in the Southern United States, where impoverished populations relied on maize for much of their food intake. In such cases, the amounts of "protective foods" required to cure the disease could be experimentally tested within rough parameters. But with true deficiencies rare in most of Europe and North America, ideas of improving efficiency widespread, and the amount of vitamins needed to maintain optimal health unknown, vitamin proponents developed hypotheses of "partial deficiencies," that is, suboptimal levels of vitamins that impaired health short of outright deficiency, including general malaise, lack of vitality, and increased susceptibility to infectious diseases, in short—the inability to perform to potential. Furthermore, the status of vitamins had political implications. Since vitamin-rich foods were expensive and therefore lacking in the diet of the poor, the new knowledge could form the basis for radical political demands, much as had been the case for the earlier protein and energy standards. Dietary and nutritional standards, and, indeed, nutritional needs and knowledge in general, were highly contested, owing not only to the relatively new and still insecure status of this knowledge but also too variable and often incompatible political, social, economic, and professional agendas.

Although the essays in this volume focus on Germany, the United States, France, and Great Britain, central countries for nutrition research owing in part to their leading positions in science in general, similar interests motivated nutrition studies in numerous other countries. Concerns about connections between nutrition and public health, working-class wages and political unrest, and military and economic capacity were international. Physiologists, philanthropists, civil servants, physicians, and governments in countries as varied as Finland, Mexico, Switzerland, Hungary, Australia, and India applied the approaches and methods of German and American nutrition research and dietary surveys to their own populations. In the period between the 1880s and the First World War, dietary studies spread throughout North America and Europe to Scandinavia and Russia, often following the paths of German-educated physiologists. Japan was an early adopter, less surprising than it seems at first glance, given the scientific exchange between German and Japanese medicine in this period and the Meiji Emperor Mutsuhito's interest in integrating Western knowledge to strengthen Japan's economic and industrial position, as well as concern with the possible dietary origins of beriberi.[62] Studies of national and ethnic diets and nutrition were, regardless of their results, open to ambiguous and conflicting conclusions and could be used both to underline the fundamental similarity of human physiology across cultures and populations and to support racist and chauvinist assumptions about the relationship between diet and national strength and character.

A number of scholars have analyzed how colonial powers came to use nutrition science and dietary studies to evaluate and assess colonized peoples and their traditional diets. Definitions of malnutrition and food emergencies became integral parts of imperial government, the administration of food resources, and debates about development and the responsibilities of humanitarianism.[63] Just as American nutrition researchers often found the diets of immigrants to the United States wanting, due in part to their limited incomes but to a large degree also to the "ethnic" character of the consumed foods,[64] the diets of non-European peoples were often viewed as inherently deficient. In particular, the traditionally low meat consumption in South and East Asian and many African diets was viewed as directly connected to their subordinate status. Their diets supposedly made them physically and intellectually weak and inferior to Europeans, whose natural superiority was expressed through their protein-rich diet.[65]

Food policy and new definitions of dietary needs during the First World War demonstrated the degree to which dietary and nutritional standards were conventional, malleable, and political. With nutrition science so intertwined with diverse interests and concerns, it is not surprising that it proved useful in a variety of situations. Nutrition researchers had long advised governments on the feeding of armies and navies, and since the later nineteenth century attempted to achieve broader influence as food policy advisers and "public scientists." The First World War provided an unprecedented opportunity for them to garner state support, actively intervene in public policy, and establish the importance of their field.[66] Nutrition scientists advised governments and became directly involved in managing food supplies in all combatant countries.[67] Calorie counting came into its own, not in the contemporary sense of self-limitation, but as a means to assess wartime food supply, the adequacy of rations, and the basic needs of the military and civilian populations. Working with the existing dietary and nutritional standards, German nutrition scientists struggled to balance the estimated dietary needs of the German population with the estimated food supplies of a blockaded country and to formulate rationing and food policy recommendations. In the Inter-Allied Scientific Food Commission, set up in 1917, nutrition researchers from the allied countries negotiated calorie and protein requirements in order to employ these standards in calculations and decision making surrounding food aid, especially from the United States to Europe.[68] In both cases, nutritional needs proved to be a moving goalpost: the standards set in peacetime and for situations of abundance no longer held in situations of scarcity and limited food resources. Although opinions differed as to what could be considered adequate nutrition in a given situation, experience nonetheless showed that there were limits beyond which standards could not be reduced without affecting health, performance, and morale.

The question of nutritional needs and standards continued in the interwar period. The war had painfully revealed the vulnerability of modern states to disruptions in food trade, and the immediate and lingering effects of inadequate nutrition and malnutrition during war were the subject of extensive study throughout the 1920s, for example, by the private Carnegie Endowment for International Peace. In the 1930s the widespread financial hardship due to global economic depression again led to increasing problems with suboptimal and inadequate nutrition in regions no longer routinely affected by them. In several countries, government and nongovernment organizations attempted to establish dietary and nutritional standards, adding to debates and controversies about the impacts of the depression on nutrition and health. In 1934 the British Medical Association appointed a committee to assess the minimum cost of an adequate diet. By adopting energy and protein standards more generous than those of the government's Advisory Committee on Nutrition, they generated a short-lived but intense public controversy.[69] *Food, Health and Income* by John Boyd Orr, director of the Rowett Institute, used American quantitative standards for an extended range of nutrients, provoking prolonged debate. The standards he deployed—which covered some vitamins and minerals as well as energy and protein—were supposed to represent optimum rather than minimum intake. Orr claimed that over half the British population was deficient in one nutrient or another.[70] The "qualitative turn" had become quantified, and Orr's report was influential worldwide.

These British initiatives were not unique. The League of Nations had been investigating what it called "the problem of nutrition" since the mid-1920s. Committees of scientists working for the League revived the project of devising international dietary and nutritional standards, publishing a series of reports from the early 1930s.[71] In contrast to most governments, however, in their comprehensive report of 1935 they presented standards that claimed to represent optimal intake, as Orr did in his report mentioned above, not average or minimum requirements.[72] The League of Nations standards were the first wide-ranging, consensual international dietary and nutritional standards, and predecessors of the current ones.[73]

After the Second World War, the British government, in an attempt to depoliticize nutrition, invited the British Medical Association to produce a revised comprehensive set of standards, which were used to assess annual food consumption surveys, among other purposes, over subsequent decades.[74] In the United States, the National Research Council established the Food and Nutrition Board, which set the US Recommended Dietary Allowance (RDA), one of the most widely known dietary and nutritional standards. These standards were derived by surveying existing literature and formulating tentative standards, soliciting the opinions of fifty nutrition scientists on whether they agreed with them all or in part, then engaging in a process of revision and resubmission until relative consensus was reached, a process that Lydia Roberts describes as the "democratic approach."[75] Other countries produced their own diverging figures, more or less generous for particular nutrients, while the League of Nations successor organizations, the United Nation's World Health Organization and Food and Agricultural Organization, produced and revised tables of requirements, which guided development programs. What became known famously as the "great protein fiasco" was one result: decades of attempts to develop animal production and high-protein weaning foods were eventually deemed wasteful and unproductive when protein requirements were revised downward in the 1970s.[76]

In this section we have sought to provide a partial outline history of dietary and nutritional standards based on relevant work in the history of nutrition science that has been published to date. There are undoubtedly numerous opportunities for further research and numerous gaps in this history. Our collection of essays, which we outline in the next section, is a step toward filling these gaps.

The Essays

The essays in this volume weave together threads of the history of dietary and nutritional standards with social and political history and the history of science and medicine, covering elements of the generation and deployment of knowledge, controversy, and impacts. In the first essay, Elizabeth Neswald analyzes the dual emergence of dietary norms and standards in laboratory experiments and field surveys. As Neswald shows, while incorporating the physicochemical and experimental methods that characterized late nineteenth-century physiology, nutritional physiology also had an application orientation that forced it to look outside the laboratory for its sources of knowledge. The conditions of the lab differed greatly from the conditions of daily life, to the extent that it was uncertain to what degree laboratory knowledge applied to the external world. The search for dietary and nutritional standards meant that physiologists needed to leave the lab and head out into the field to gather large amounts of data through observation and surveys of dietary practices.

The history of nutrition science clearly reaches both into social history and into the history of social control, and several authors have written about nutrition using the concepts of Michel Foucault. Bryan Turner considers that the advent of nutrition science eliminated the moral dimensions of the "discourse of diet," a notion that has now been amply demonstrated to be erroneous, notably by Charlotte Biltekoff and Helen Zoe Veit, whereas John Coveney emphasizes the positive dimensions of Foucaudian discipline as applied to nutrition."[77] In the second essay Corinna Treitel shows that the generation and modification of biopolitical knowledge is not necessarily a simple top-down process initiated by social elites. Instead, Treitel shows, using the example of debate and disagreement about protein standards in late nineteenth- and early twentieth-century Germany, how heterogeneous actors, including self-experimenting physiologists, German vegetarians, and Japanese researchers, collaboratively and independently questioned established protein standards. The simple top-down diffusionist models of biopolitics, she concludes, must be replaced by more flexible ones that allow for lateral and reverse hierarchical, rather than simple hierarchical, influences. Nutrition science and the making and unmaking of the protein standard can thus function as a case study for a more differentiated approach to the generation of biopolitical knowledge.

Chapter 3, by Deborah Neill, connects the discourses of diet, nationalism, and colonialism in late nineteenth- and early twentieth-century France. As Neill shows, the culturally multivalent category "food," with its thick layers of consumption traditions and assumptions, could not be fully replaced by the new quantitatively expressed physicomedical category of "nutrition." Meat emerges again as the central controversial and socially sensitive food in the European diet, tied not only to working power but also to concepts of "masculinity," "status," "military strength," and "aggression." Like Treitel's physiologists, Neill's alimentary hygienists were intrigued by the confluence of a high level of worker productivity and a low level of meat consumption in Japan, but they struggled with the idea that a diet without meat could maintain the health of male European bodies. Neill's essay traces shifts in French debates about meat in this period, demonstrating how debates on diet were as much about political contexts and concerns as they were about food consumption.

Institutional feeding perhaps offers the greatest opportunities for those who aspire to standardize the food intake of eaters, but even here there are limitations arising from cultural expectations. The application of dietary and nutritional standards in institutional feeding is covered in the essay by Ulrike Thoms, who charts debates surrounding military provisioning in Germany from the mid-nineteenth to the mid-twentieth century. As Thoms shows, standards for military rations developed out of the collaboration and competition of a diverse set of actors, including physicians and physiologists, army administrators, food chemists, and food processors. The feeding regimes of the army incorporated many different kinds of standards, ranging from dietary and nutritional standards to standards for food manufacturing. Far from representing a unique food environment, army feeding was both a product of and a model for civilian diet.

Despite strong connections to medical research establishments, nutrition scientists retained a certain "outsider" status after the First World War and were under challenge to demonstrate the widespread importance and relevance of their work to health and medical practice. In the fifth essay, David Smith provides an account of rival British research programs that sought to demonstrate the role of nutrition in resistance to infection during the interwar period. Edward Mellanby, a former student and colleague of F. G. Hopkins, was enthusiastic about vitamins, whereas John Boyd Orr was skeptical, but enthusiastic, instead, about minerals. Despite their differences, their work marks a common qualitative turn in nutrition, and both imagined new standards of nutrition that would go beyond alleviating the effects of malnutrition, as ordinarily understood, to defeat common infections that were responsible for widespread disability and mortality. These scientists' strategies, Smith suggests, must be understood in the context of broader medical, scientific, and social concerns, as well as professional, disciplinary, and institutional interests.

The course and outcome of a controversy about the relative healthfulness of white and brown bread in the United Kingdom was also linked to the controversy over the practical importance of vitamins, as analyzed in chapter 6 by Ina Zweiniger-Bargielowska. Zweiniger-Bargielowska's essay discusses an interwar campaign launched by the New Health Society of the maverick surgeon Sir William Arbuthnot Lane in a newspaper in 1927. Prominent in the campaign and following debate was the lower vitamin B content of white bread, demonstrated by recent research. With white bread a dietary staple of the working and poorest classes, the question of brown or white touched on issues of class entitlement, education, income, and individual and public health. As with Treitel's discussion of the protein standard, this debate illustrates the continuous public controversy that has been associated with nutrition science and its recommendations, as well as the friction between medical and lay actors, as different groups engaged with nutrition topics and aimed to create a niche for themselves as experts in the field.

Zweiniger-Bargielowska's essay amply demonstrates the kind of problems that generally confront actors who seek to impose new dietary and nutritional standards when the changes involve the population changing their food habits, and when there is also scientific and medical discord regarding the need for the change. Even when scientific and medical consensus is almost complete, changing food habits is never a simple matter. One barrier to change identified by the interested parties has been lack of knowledge of the nutritional composition of foods, which has led to the development of the modern food label. The origins of the modern food label, however, lies not in hopes to educate the public and change dietary habits, but in consumer protection regulations dating from the early twentieth century. These origins are explored in the seventh essay by Suzanne Junod, who examines the advent of net weight regulations in the United States. She provides instructive points of comparison with the kinds of standards discussed in the other chapters. Junod's focus, the Gould Net Weight Amendment, which standardized the weight labels on packaged foods, followed the better-known 1906 Pure Foods Act and intersected with a variety of Progressive-era initiatives designed to manage and control social, demographic, and economic change through regulation and standardization. The kind of standards discussed by Junod involved establishing laws and regulations that could be enforced to a degree unknown with most dietary and nutritional standards.

Returning to dietary and nutritional standards, in the final essay Nick Cullather analyzes their role in the politics of famine relief during the Cold War. This affair is much less well-known than the "great protein fiasco," another international episode involving dietary and nutritional standards during the same period. Building on his previous work,[78] Cullather shows how the politics of famine changed during this period, with the transition from local reporting to statistical prediction models based on abstract comparisons of the calories produced in a region and the assumed caloric needs of the population. Analysts began to generate predictions months or even years ahead of crises, allowing shortages to be managed and even choreographed for political effect. Analyzing the rhetoric of and reactions to the Indian Bihar Famine of 1967–68, an episode of widespread suffering and social and political turmoil but, officially at least, no starvation deaths, Cullather shows how Indira Gandhi and Lyndon Johnson staged the famine as a global spectacle of administrative prowess to divert attention from Vietnam and secure Gandhi's election. Far from introducing objective measurement criteria in the place of subjective qualitative assessments, the use of statistics and standards intensified the political dimensions of nutritional knowledge in the definition of famine and the means for its alleviation.

Taking History into the Present

One contemporary food reformer has turned to the academic study of history in order to better understand the food movement of which she was part. Charlotte Biltekoff is a former vegetarian restaurant cook and currently Professor of American Studies and Food Studies at the University of California, Davis. Her book, *Eating Right in America* (2013), explores the programs and agendas of a number of twentieth-century American initiatives related to food and diet, including the home economics movement, the US national food program during the Second World War, and the alternative food movements and antiobesity campaigns of the late twentieth century.[79] Biltekoff concludes that these food reform movements have much in common: they all sought to impose standards that were infused with middle-class assumptions and ideals on others. She advises food reformers and nutrition scientists to be aware of the social and cultural dimensions and implications of whatever they are trying to achieve. These are important but rather unsurprising general conclusions. The essays in this collection reinforce and extend them, by covering a wider range of countries, episodes, and topics than does Biltekoff. But can history in general, and this collection of essays in particular, offer any prospect of more specific conclusions of interest and value to today's participants in the generation and application of nutritional knowledge? The minimum we hope for is that this book will help readers to better appreciate the complexity of this field, which we referred to at the opening of the introduction, in connection with our comments on the work of Pollan, Mudry, and Scrinis. But besides encouraging greater emphasis on contingency and complexity are there any more specific lessons from history than we can offer? First, can we offer any insights of value to the situation in which one current of opinion considers that the foundational concepts of nutrition science—quantitative dietary and nutritional standards—should be abandoned?

One response to some of the examples that we provide, such as that of the deployment of nutritional calories in the service of postcolonial politics, might be that authors such as Pollan, Mudry, and Scrinis have been too soft on nutrition science and that nutrition science has been even more damaging than they make it out to be. But this is not our intention. Although the calorie may have been pressed into service in the postwar period in pursuit of Cold War political manoeuvring, as described by Nick Cullather, quantitative standards of nutrition have also regularly been deployed to highlight inequalities and support genuine progressive reform campaigns. An income-based analysis of food consumption conducted in the United Kingdom in the 1960s resulted in the rediscovery of food poverty and led to the foundation of the still-active Child Poverty Action Group.[80] Likewise, in the 1980s, several political movements focused on food issues, including food safety and sustainability, as well as food poverty and nutrition, and combined quantitative and qualitative analyses in their campaigns.[81]

Clearly, a division into "progressive" qualitative analyses and "retrogressive" quantitative approaches, such as that proclaimed by Pollan, Mudry, and Scrinis and other authors, is untenable. However, we also suggest that the roles that the wide range of actors have played in the generation and deployment of dietary and nutritional standards in the past offers hope to current-day campaigners. Nutrition science was never a simple top-down endeavor. As Corinna Treitel's essay shows, nutrition science has, from its early years, been shaped and informed by alternative actors and their interventions. This suggests not the condemnation and alienation of scientists, but rather attempts to engage with them. But whereas Treital demonstrates the role of outsiders in stimulating a downward revision of the protein standard in the early twentieth century, Deborah Neill's chapter demonstrates the cultural stereotyping that conditioned nutrition studies in France and tended to keep standards for meat consumption high—once again emphasising the complexity of the links between nutritional knowledge and practical outcomes. Likewise, for the nutrition campaigner and nutrition professional alike, Ina Zwieneger-Bargiolowska's chapter demonstrates the damaging impact that lack of scientific and medical consensus can have on attempts to overturn long-established eating habits. And both Ulrike Thom's and Suzanne Junod's chapters show, in different ways, the long-term developments that can arise from a focus on areas where greater control is possible. Changes made to the institutional feeding of limited sectors of society can lead to innovations and new habits with wider impact; and once food laws and regulations are in place, whatever their initial intention, they may be extendable to other purposes, including nutrition.

We hope that those currently professionally engaged in the generation and application of nutritional knowledge will find in our case studies numerous helpful points of comparison with their own practice. Since many of the problems seem to be perennial, much can be learned from the strategies, successes, and failures of nutrition professionals in the past for both professionals and publics today. The challenge of extrapolating from laboratory experimental results to everyday life, the problem faced by Elizabeth Neswald's actors, continues to trouble nutrition scientists. And David Smith's account of Orr and Mellanby's work on nutrition and infection may lead to reflection on how research programs are chosen and unfold at the present time. In the wake of the success of the human genome project, nutrition scientists are busy formulating new approaches based on combining nutrition and genetics and promising revolutionary changes to the ways health is maintained.[82] But even if the fate of Orr and Mellanby's programs give pause for thought, scientists might also observe that climbing aboard a new scientific bandwagon may not necessarily damage career prospects, even if it later grinds to a halt. The lesson for the lay campaigner may be that they should be wary of scientists' latest enthusiasms.

It could, of course, be argued that it is not the role of historians to point out the lessons of history. Nevertheless, it is our hope that that by deepening understanding of how a variety of standards and claims around food and nutrition have been imagined, formulated, revised, discarded, and applied in science, campaigning, and politics in the past, those engaged in such issues in the present as activists, journalists, food studies scholars, or nutrition scientists may gain insights allowing more reflective and effective scholarship, and action, in the present. Our hope, then, is that this book will not only be read by historians and encourage further historical research in this field, but that it will also be read and discussed by those currently engaged in the generation and application of nutritional knowledge.

Notes

1. Tufts University, Office of Corporate and Foundation Relations, Friedman School of Nutrition Science and Policy, http://cfr.tufts.edu/discover-tufts/schools-at-tufts/friedman-school-of-nutrition-science-and-policy (accessed October 2, 2013).

2. Alice M. Copping, "The New Degree in Nutrition," *Proceedings of the Nutrition Society* 12 (1953): 177–78; Robert C. Garry, "Presidential Address: The Nutrition Society of Britain, the First 12 Years," *Proceedings of the Nutrition Society* 12 (1953): 270–73.

3. Contrary to common perceptions, concern about obesity as a widespread public health problem is not a late twentieth-century phenomenon, but can already be found early in the century. See Sabine Merta, *Wege und Irrwege zum modernen Schlankheitskult: Diätkost und Körperkultur als Suche nach neuen Lebensstilformen 1880–1930* (Wiesbaden: Franz Steiner Verlag, 2003); Derek J. Oddy, Peter J. Atkins, and Virginie Amilien, eds., *The Rise of Obesity in Europe: A Twentieth-Century Food History* (Aldershot: Ashgate, 2009).

4. These sensitivities are illustrated by a recent spat in which the Harvard nutrition scientist Walter Willet attacked an epidemiologist who suggested being slightly overweight may be beneficial to health. Virginia Hughes, "The Big Fat Truth," *Nature* 497 (2013): 428–30.

5. For "boundary objects" see: Thomas F. Gieryn, "Boundary-Work and the Demarcation of Science from Non-science: Strains and Interests in Professional Ideologies of Scientists," *American Sociological Review* 48 (1983): 781–95; Susan Star and James Griesemer, "Institutional Ecology, 'Translations' and Boundary Objects: Amateurs and Professionals in Berkeley's Museum of Vertebrate Zoology, 1907–39," *Social Studies of Science* 19 (1989): 387–420.

6. Edith Heischkel-Artelt, ed., *Ernährung und Ernährungslehre im 19. Jahrhundert* (Göttingen: Vandenhoeck & Ruprecht, 1976); Harmke Kamminga and Andrew Cunningham, eds., *The Science and Culture of Nutrition, 1840s–1940s* (Amsterdam: Rodopi, 1995), David F. Smith, *Nutrition in Britain: Science, Scientists and Politics in the*

Twentieth Century (London: Routledge, 1997); David F. Smith and Jim Phillips, eds., *Food, Science, Policy and Regulation in the Twentieth Century: International and Comparative Perspectives* (London: Routledge, 2000).

7. Anne Murcott, "A Burgeoning Field: Introduction to *The Handbook of Food Research*," in *The Handbook of Food Research*, ed. Anne Murcott, Warren Belasco, and Peter Jackson (London: Bloomsbury, 2013), 1–25.

8. The proliferation and popularity of publications claiming a dietary basis and simple dietary solution to numerous and diffuse health, psychological, and behavioral conditions can be taken as evidence for widespread uneasiness and insecurity about potential connections between dietary practices and nutritional advice, individual and public health, and industrial food production. Examples of this genre include William David, *Wheat Belly: Lose the Wheat, Lose the Weight, and Find Your Path Back to Health* (Emmaus: PA Rodale, 2011); David Gillespie, *Sweet Poison: Why Sugar Makes Us Fat* (London: Penguin, 2013); Robert H. Lustig, *Fat Chance: Beating the Odds against Sugar, Processed Food, Obesity and Disease* (New York: Hudson Street Press, 2011); David Perlmutter, *Grain Brain: The Surprising Truth about Wheat, Carbs, and Sugar—Your Brain's Silent Killers* (New York: Little, Brown, 2013); Nina Teicholz, *The Big Fat Surprise: Why Butter, Meat, and Cheese Belong in a Healthy Diet* (New York: Simon and Schuster, 2014).

9. See, for example, Geoffrey Cannon, *The Politics of Food* (London: Edbury Press, 1987); Marion Nestle, *Food Politics: How the Food Industry Influences Nutrition and Health* (Berkeley: University of California Press, 2002).

10. Michael Pollan, *Omnivore's Dilemma: A Natural History of Four Meals* (New York: Penguin Press, 2006); Jessica Mudry, *Measured Meals: Nutrition in America* (Albany: State University of New York Press, 2009). Gyorgy Scrinis, *Nutritionism: The Science and Politics of Dietary Advice* (New York: Columbia University Press, 2013).

11. Michael Pollan, *Food Rules: An Eater's Manual* (New York: Penguin Press, 2009).

12. Walter Willet is an example of such an actor. See note 3.

13. Edward Mellanby, *Experimental Rickets: The Effects of Cereals and Their Interaction with Other Factors of Diet and Environment in Producing Rickets*, Medical Research Council Special Reports 93 (London: HMSO, 1925).

14. L. Margaret Barnett, "'Every Man His Own Physician': Dietetic Fads, 1890–1914," in Kamminga and Cunningham, *Science and Culture of Nutrition*, 155–78.

15. Harvey Levenstein, *Fear of Food: A History of Why We Worry about What We Eat* (Chicago: University of Chicago Press, 2012), 32.

16. Mark R. Finlay, "Early Marketing of the Theory of Nutrition: The Science and Culture of Liebig's Extract of Meat," in Kamminga and Cunningham, *Science and Culture of Nutrition*, 48–74; Sally Horrocks, "Nutrition Science and the Food and Pharmaceutical Industries in Inter-war Britain," in Smith, *Nutrition in Britain*, 53–74; Uwe Spiekermann, "Functional Food: Zur Vorgeschichte einer 'modernen' Produktgruppe," *Ernährungs-Umschau* 49 (2002): 182–88.

17. Oliver Schlaudt and Lara Huber, eds., *Standardization in Measurement* (London: Pickering & Chatto, 2015).

18. Detlef Briese, *Das gesunde Leben: Ernährung und Gesundheit seit dem 18. Jahrhundert* (Frankfurt: Campus, 2010); James Gregory, *Of Victorians and Vegetarians: The Vegetarian Movement in Nineteenth-Century Britain* (London: Taurus Academic Studies, 2007).

19. Mark W. Weatherall, "'A Revolution in the Science of Food': How 'Standard Bread' Sold Newspapers," in Kamminga and Cunningham, *Science and Culture of Nutrition*, 179–212.

20. Barnett, "'Every Man His Own Physician.'"

21. Rima D. Apple, *Vitamania: Vitamins in American Culture* (New Brunswick: Rutgers University Press, 1996); Beat Bächi, *Vitamin C für alle! Pharmazeutische Produktion, Vermarktung und Gesundheitspolitik (1933–1953)* (Zürich: Chronos, 2009); Horrocks, "Nutrition Science."

22. For this assertion see, for example, Elisabet Helsing, "On the Clear Need to Meet and Learn to Speak Clearly: Statement from the World Health Organization," *American Journal of Clinical Nutrition* 65 supp. (1997): 1098S–9S, http://ajcn.nutrition.org/content/65/4/1098S.full.pdf (accessed June 9, 2015).

23. Emma Spary, *Feeding France: New Sciences of Food, 1760–1815* (Cambridge: Cambridge University Press, 2014).

24. Benjamin Thompson Count Rumford, "Of Food; and Particularly of Feeding the Poor," in Benjamin Thomson, *The Complete Works of Count Rumford*, vol. 4 (Boston, 1875), 397–490; Benjamin Thompson, Count Rumford, "Instruction für die Kochfrauen über die Zubereitung der Rumfordschen Suppe," *Nachrichten von der Einrichtung und dem Fortgange der Braunschweigischen Armen-Anstalt* 28 (Mai 1803): 273–75.

25. For the gelatine question in France, see Spary, *Feeding France*, chap. 6.

26. François Magendie, "Mémoire sur les propriétés nutritives des substances qui ne contiennent pas d'azote," *Annales de Chimie et de Physique* 3 (1816): 66–77.

27. François Magendie, et al., "Rapport fait à l'Académie des Sciences au nom de la Commission dite de la gélatine," *Comte Rendu des Séances de l'Académie des Science* 13, no. 5, 2 (1841): 237–95.

28. Frederic L. Holmes, "The Intake-Output Method in Physiology," *Historical Studies in the Physical and Biological Sciences* 17 (1987): 245–70.

29. Johann Daniel Achelis, "Die Ernährungsphysiologie des 17. Jahrhunderts," *Sitzungsberichte der Heidelberger Akademie der Wissenschaften, Math.-naturwiss, Klasse* 3 (1938): 3–22; M. Norton Wise, "Mediations: Enlightenment Balancing Acts, or the Technologies of Rationalism," in *Thomas Kuhn and the Nature of Science*, ed. Paul Horwich (Cambridge, MA: MIT Press, 1993), 207–56.

30. Johannes Büttner, "Von der oeconomia animalis zu Liebigs Stoffwechselbegriff," in *Stoffwechsel im tierischen Organismus: Historische Studien zu Liebigs, "Thier-Chemie,"* ed. Johannes Büttner and Wilhlem Lewicki (Seesen: HisChymia Buchverlag, 2001), 61–94; Frederic L. Holmes, "Introduction," in Justus Liebig, *Animal Chemistry or Organic Chemistry in Its Application to Physiology and Pathology*, ed. William Gregory and John W. Webster (New York: Johnson Reprint Corporation, 1964), vii–cxvi.

31. Justus Liebig, *Die Thier-Chemie oder die organische Chemie in ihrer Anwendung auf Physiologie und Pathologie* (Braunschweig: Vieweg & Sohn, 1843); Everett Mendelsohn, *Heat and Life* (Cambridge, MA: Harvard University Press, 1964).

32. Since the fifteenth century fresh fruit had been used to cure scurvy, and cod liver oil was cited in German medical literature as a remedy for rickets as early as 1824. The possible role of food in beriberi was also a subject of much debate and data collection when it became a serious problem among servicemen and others

in colonial East Asia after the introduction of steam-powered milling. Kenneth J. Carpenter, *Beriberi, White Rice, and Vitamin B: A Disease, a Cause, and a Cure* (Berkeley: University of California Press, 2000); Kenneth J. Carpenter, *The History of Scurvy and Vitamin C* (Cambridge: Cambridge University Press, 1986); Ruth A. Guy, "The History of Cod Liver Oil as a Remedy," *American Journal of Diseases of Children* 26 (1923): 112–16; Kumaravel Rajakumar, "Vitamin D, Cod-Liver Oil, Sunlight, and Rickets: A Historical Perspective," *Pediatrics* 112 (2003): 132–35.

33. Aaron Ihde and Stanley Becker, "Conflict of Concepts in Early Vitamin Studies," *Journal of the History of* Biology 4 (1971): 1–33.

34. Frederick G. Hopkins, "The Analyst and the Medical Man," *Analyst* 31 (1906): 385–97.

35. Frederick G. Hopkins, "Feeding Experiments Illustrating the Importance of Accessory Food Factors in Normal Dietaries," *Journal of Physiology* 44 (1912): 425–60.

36. Carpenter, *History of Scurvy*, 177.

37. Carpenter, *Beriberi*, 38.

38. Casimir Funk, "On the Chemical Nature of the Substance Which Cures Polyneuritis in Birds Induced by a Diet of Polished Rice," *Journal of Physiology* 43 (1911): 395–400; Benjamin Harow, *Casimir Funk—Pioneer in Vitamins and Hormones* (New York: Dodd, Mead, 1955).

39. Elmer Verner McCollum, *A History of Nutrition: The Sequence of Ideas in Nutrition Investigations* (Boston: Houghton Mifflin, 1957), 106–7, 310–58, 384–404.

40. David F. Smith, "The Agricultural Research Association, the Development Fund, and the origins of the Rowett Research Institute," *Agricultural History Review* 46 (1998): 47–63.

41. Francis Gano Benedict, *Reports of Visits to Foreign Laboratories, 1926*, 286, GA 7, series 2, box 7, Countway Library of Medicine, Harvard University Archives, http://vlp.mpiwg-berlin.mpg.de/library/data/lit39750 (accessed May 30, 2015); Pim Huijnin, "De belofte van vitamines: Voedingsonderzoek tussen universiteit, industrie en overheid 1918–1945" (PhD thesis, Instituut voor Cultuur en Geschiedenis, University of Amsterdam 2011), 155, http://hdl.handle.net/11245/2.92919 (accessed May 30, 2015).

42. Mark Weatherall, "The Foundation and Early Years of the Dunn Nutritional Laboratory," in Smith, *Nutrition in Britain*, 429–52.

43. League of Nations Mixed Committee on the Problem of Nutrition, *The Problem of Nutrition*, vol. 1 (Geneva: League of Nations Publications Department, 1936), 27–28; Susan Levine, *School Lunch Politics: The Surprising History of America's Favorite Welfare Program* (Princeton, NJ: Princeton University Press, 2008), 61.

44. Anon, "Obituary: Robert McCarrison, C.I.E., M.D., D.Sc. LL.D., F.R.C.P.," *British Medical Journal* (May 28, 1960): 1663–64; Alexander R. Bay, *Beriberi in Modern Japan: The Making of a National Disease* (Rochester, NY: University of Rochester Press, 2012); Frederick W. Clements, *A History of Human Nutrition in Australia* (Melbourne: Longman Cheshire, 1986); Alec Samuel Ostry, *Nutrition Policy in Canada, 1870–1939* (Vancouver: UBC Press, 2006).

45. Ulrike Thoms, "Learning from America? The Travels of German Nutritional Scientists to the USA in the Context of the Technical Assistance Program of the

Mutual Security Agency and Its Consequences of the West German Nutritional Policy," *Food & History* 2 (2004): 117–52.

46. Alain Drouard, "Reforming Diet at the End of the Nineteenth Century in Europe," in *Food and the City in Europe to 1800*, ed. Peter J. Atkins, Peter Lummel, and Derek J. Oddy (Aldershot: Ashgate, 2007), 216.

47. Smith, "Nutrition Science and the Two World Wars," in Smith, *Nutrition in Britain*, 142–66; David F. Smith, "Nutrition in Britain in the Twentieth Century" (PhD diss., University of Edinburgh, 1986).

48. See Rima Apple, "Science Gendered: Nutrition in the United States, 1840–1940," in Kamminga and Cunningham, *Science and Culture of Nutrition*, 129–54; Maresi Nerad, *The Academic Kitchen: A Social History of Gender Stratification at the University of California, Berkeley* (Albany: State University of New York Press, 1999); Deanna L. Pucciarelli, "Early History and Evolution of Nutrition Science in the United States of America," *Family & Consumer Sciences Research Journal* 38 (2009): 106–22; Helen Zoe Veit, *Modern Food, Moral Food: Self-Control, Science, and the Rise of Modern American Eating in the Early Twentieth Century* (Chapel Hill: University of North Carolina Press, 2013).

49. John Pickstone, "Production, Community and Consumption: The Political Economy of Twentieth-Century Medicine," in *Companion to Medicine in the Twentieth Century*, ed. Roger Cooter and John Pickstone (London: Routledge, 2003), 3.

50. The number of universities in the United Kingdom offering undergraduate degrees in nutrition and the possibilities for joint degrees with other subjects can be assessed by searching the Universities and Colleges Admissions Service website, http://www.ucas.com/ (accessed March 6, 2014).

51. Janet Brian, *The Local Implementation of the Sale of Food and Drugs Act, 1875*, PhD thesis, Open University, Milton Keynes, United Kingdom, 2006; Lawrence Busch, *Standards: Recipes for Reality* (Cambridge, MA: MIT Press, 2011), 105; Michael French and Jim Phillips, *Cheated Not Poisoned? Food Regulation in the United Kingdom, 1875–1938* (Manchester: Manchester University Press, 2000).

52. See, for example, for the Netherlands: Pim Huijnen, "The Science of Measuring Vitamins: Quality Control and Competition in the Dutch Vitamin Industry before the Second World War," in *Biologics: A History of Agents Made from Living Organisms in the Twentieth Century*, ed. Alexander von Schwerin, Heiko Stoff, and Bettina Wahrig (London: Pickering & Chatto, 2013), 139–50.

53. Anson Rabinbach, *The Human Motor: Energy, Fatigue, and the Origins of Modernity* (Berkeley: University of California Press, 1992).

54. Jennifer Karns Alexander, *The Mantra of Efficiency: From Waterwheel to Social Control* (Baltimore, MD: Johns Hopkins University Press, 2008); Naomi Aronson, "Social Definitions of Entitlement: Food Needs, 1885–1920," *Media, Culture, and Society* 4 (1982): 51–61; Harvey Levenstein, *Revolution at the Table: The Transformation of the American Diet* (Berkeley: University of California Press, 2003); G. R. Searle, *The Quest for National Efficiency: A Study in British Politics and Political Thought, 1899–1914* (Oxford: Blackwell, 1971); Bernard Semmel, *Imperialism and Social Reform: English Social-Imperial Thought, 1894–1914* (London: Allen & Unwin, 1960); Jakob Tanner, *Fabrikmahlzeit: Ernährungswissenschaft, Industriearbeit and Volksernährung in der Schweiz 1890–1950* (Zürich: Chronos, 1999); Katherine Leonard Turner, *How the Other Half*

Ate: A History of Working-Class Meals at the Turn of the Century (Berkeley: University of California Press, 2014); Veit, *Modern Food.*

55. Bernard Harris, *Health of the Schoolchild: History of the School Medical Service in England and Wales, 1908–74* (Buckingham, England: Open University Press, 1995); Levine, *School Lunch Politics*; James Vernon, "The Ethics of Hunger and the Assembly of Society: The Techno-Politics of the School Meal in Modern Britain," *The American Historical Review* 110 (2005): 693–725.

56. Dorothy Porter, *Health, Civilization, and the State: A History of Public Health from Ancient to Modern Times* (Amsterdam: Rodopi, 1994).

57. Rima Apple, *Perfect Motherhood: Science and Childrearing in America* (New Brunswick, NJ: Rutgers University Press, 2006); Cynthia Comacchio, *"Nations Are Built of Babies": Saving Ontario's Mothers and Children, 1900–1940* (Montreal: McGill-Queen's, 1993).

58. Pickstone, "Production, Community and Consumption," 2.

59. Smith, "Nutrition Science"; Robyn Smith, "The Emergence of Vitamins as Bio-Political Objects during World War I," *Studies in History and Philosophy of Biological and Biomedical Sciences* 40 (2009): 179–89; Heiko Stoff, *Wirkstoffe: Eine Wissenschaftsgeschichte der Hormone, Vitamine und Enzyme, 1920–1970* (Stuttgart: Steiner, 2012); Ulrike Thoms, "'Vitaminfragen—kein Vitaminrummel?' Die deutsche Vitaminforschung in der ersten Hälfte des 20. Jahrhunderts und ihr Verhältnis zur Öffentlichkeit," in *Wissenschaft und Öffentlichkeit als Ressource füreinander*, ed. Sybilla Nikolow and Arne Schirrmacher (Bielefeld: Transcript 2007), 75–96.

60. Apple, *Vitamania*, 26, 39; Bächi, *Vitamin C für alle!*, 101–22; Peter Bartrip, *Mirror of Medicine: The BMJ, 1840–1990* (Oxford: Clarendon Press, 1990), 195.

61. David Smith and Malcolm Nicolson, "The 'Glasgow School' of Paton, Findlay and Cathcart: Conservative Thought in Chemical Physiology, Nutrition and Public Health," *Social Studies of Science* 19 (1989): 195–238.

62. Bay, *Beriberi*; Ernst Kraas, *300 Jahre deutsch-japanische Beziehungen in der Medizin* (Tokyo: Springer, 1992).

63. David Arnold, "The 'Discovery' of Malnutrition in Colonial India," *Indian Economic and Social History Review* 31 (1994): 1–26; Peter Gray, *Famine, Land, and Politics: British Government and Irish Society, 1843–50* (Dublin: Irish Academic Press, 1999); David Hall-Matthews, "Inaccurate Conceptions: Disputed Measures of Nutritional Needs and Famine Deaths in Colonial India," *Modern Asian Studies* 42 (2008): 1189–212; Deborah Neill, "Finding the 'Ideal Diet': Nutrition, Culture and Dietary Practices in France and French Equatorial Africa, c. 1890s to 1920s," *Food and Foodways* 17 (2009): 1–28; James Vernon, *Hunger: A Modern History* (Cambridge, MA: Belknap Press, 2007); Michael Worboys, "The Discovery of Colonial Malnutrition between the Wars," in *Imperial Medicine and Indigenous Societies*, ed. David Arnold (Manchester: Manchester University Press, 1988), 208–55.

64. Levenstein, *Revolution at the Table*, 98–108; Veit, *Modern Food*, 123–56.

65. Francesco S. Nitti, "Food and the Labour-Power of Nations," *Economic Journal* 6 (1896): 30–63.

66. For nutrition scientists' aspirations to be public scientists in the United States, see Mark T. Hamin, "Tables Turned, Palates Curbed: Elements of Energy, Economy and Equilibrium in American Nutrition Science, 1880–1930" (PhD diss., University

of Pennsylvania, 1999). For "public scientists" in the United Kingdom, see Frank M. Turner, "Public Science in Britain, 1880–1918," *Isis* 71 (1980): 589–608.

67. Smith, "Nutrition Science"; Mikuláš Teich, "Science and Food during the Great War: Britain and Germany," in Kamminga and Cunningham, *Science and Culture of Nutrition*, 213–34; Ina Zweiniger-Bargielowska, Rachel Duffett, and Alain Drouard, eds., *Food and War in Twentieth-Century Europe* (Farnham, England: Ashgate, 2011).

68. L. Margaret Barnett, *British Food Policy during the First World War* (Boston: Allen and Unwin, 1985).

69. David F. Smith, "The Social Construction of Dietary Standards: The British Medical Association—Ministry of Health Advisory Committee on Nutrition Report of 1934," in *Food, Eating, and Nutrition as a Social Problems: Constructivist Perspectives*, ed. D. Maurer and J. Sobal (New York: Aldine de Gruyter, 1995), 279–304.

70. David F. Smith, "The Carnegie Survey: Background and Intended Impact," in *Order and Disorder: The Health Implications of Eating and Drinking in the Nineteenth and Twentieth Centuries*, ed. Alexander Fenton (Edinburgh: Tuckwell Press, 2000), 64–80.

71. Josep Barona, *The Problem of Nutrition: Experimental Science, Public Health and Economy in Europe, 1914–1945* (Brussels: Peter Lang, 2010). See also Josep Barona, "Nutrition and Health: The International Context during the Inter-War Crisis," *Social History of Medicine* 21 (2008): 87–105; Iris Borowy, *Coming to Terms with World Health: The League of Nations Health Organisation, 1921–1946* (Frankfurt: Peter Lang, 2009).

72. League of Nations, *Report on the Physiological Basis of Nutrition* (Geneva: League of Nations Publications Department, 1935).

73. U. Hauber and M. Neuhäuser-Berthold, "Historisch Entwicklung von Empfehlungen zur Nährstoffzufuhr," *Zeitschrift für Ernährungswissenschaft* 35 (1996): 157–62.

74. David Smith and Mark Bufton, "A Case of *parturiunt montes, nascetur ridiculus mus?* The BMA Nutrition Committee 1947–50 and the Political Disengagement of Nutrition Science," *Journal of the History of Medicine and Allied Sciences* 59 (2004): 240–72.

75. Lydia J. Roberts, "Beginnings of the Recommended Dietary Allowances," *Journal of the American Dietetic Association* 34 (1958): 907.

76. Joshua Ruxin, "The United Nations Protein Advisory Group," in Smith and Phillips, *Food, Science*, 151–66.

77. Bryan S. Turner, "The Government of the Body: Medical Regimens and the Rationalization of Diet," *British Journal of Sociology* 33 (1982): 254–69; Charlotte Biltekoff, *Eating Right in America: The Cultural Politics of Food and Health* (Durham, NC: Duke University Press, 2013); Veit, *Modern Food*; John Coveney, *Food, Morals and Meaning: The Pleasure and* Anxiety of Eating (New York: Routledge, 2000).

78. Nick Cullather, *The Hungry World: America's Cold War Battle against Poverty in Asia* (Cambridge, MA: Harvard University Press, 2010).

79. Biltekoff, *Eating Right*.

80. Royston Lambert, *Nutrition in Britain, 1950–1960: A Critical Discussion of the Standards and Findings of the National Food Survey* (Welwyn,. England: Coldicote Press, 1964). For the Child Poverty Action Group, see *Family Poverty Memorandum*, http://www.cpag.org.uk/content/family-poverty-memorandum (accessed March 14, 2014). For similar discussions in Germany, see Eva Barlösius, ed., *Ernährung in der Armut:*

Gesundheitliche, soziale und kulturelle Folgen in der Bundesrepublik Deutschland (Berlin: edition sigma, 2009).

81. Tim Lang, "Going Public: Food Campaigns during the 1980s and Early 1990s," in Smith, *Nutrition in Britain,* 214–37; Jerrell B. Whitehead, "The UK Food Movement, c. 1976–96," PhD thesis, University of Cambridge, 2011.

82. For a critical perspective on nutritional epigenetics, see Hannah Landecker, "Food as Exposure: Nutritional Epigenetics and the New Metabolism," *BioSocieties* 6 (2011): 167–94.

Chapter One

Nutritional Knowledge between the Lab and the Field

The Search for Dietary Norms in the Late Nineteenth and Early Twentieth Centuries

Elizabeth Neswald

Introduction

Late nineteenth-century nutrition science occupied an ambiguous space. It emerged in the same decades as the development of quantitative, precision, and apparatus-based methods in physiology and the spread of statistical thinking, and it combined these two very different approaches in unique ways. Nutrition science connected theory with practice, studies of individuals with studies of populations, methods from the natural sciences with methods from the social sciences. It was an experimental science and an applied science. Its information sources were found in the lab, in the verbal accounts of experimental subjects, in markets, institutions, private homes, hospitals, shops, and workplaces. It aimed for the precision of physics and chemistry, but was confronted with the enormous variability of its subjects, objects, and external circumstances, and with discrepancies between the artificially controlled conditions of the lab and the variable conditions of human life.

The early history of nutrition science has been explored from a variety of perspectives. Most studies focus on Germany and the United States, the two countries that led in the development of its theories, methods, and applications in the later nineteenth and early twentieth centuries. Kenneth Carpenter, Frederic L. Holmes, and Nicolas Mani have described this history from a largely internal perspective, delineating the main figures and theoretical development of nutritional physiology.[1] Studies that approach it from a social historical perspective have also not been lacking. In particular, Harvey Levenstein and Naomi Aronson have shown how research on nutrition in the United States was intimately connected to social concerns and, in Aronson's case, to questions of social control and biopolitics.[2] Similar interactions between laboratory research and social context have been confirmed in studies on a number of countries.[3]

Studies focused primarily on physiological theory pay homage to the social context of their application, and social historical works frequently describe the theories on which nutrition policies and reform initiatives were based, but the impression can arise that the laboratory was the site for the production of nutritional knowledge, and the apparatus of the exact sciences—experiments, instruments, and precision techniques—the means of its generation. Although laboratory studies were crucial in the history of nutrition science, their methods and results were not uncontested. Dietary knowledge, the knowledge of how and whether nutritional needs were met in practice, could only be acquired through extensive studies in the field, using methods developed by the emerging social sciences, and through the activities of a diverse group of actors, including physiologists and physicians, social reformers, statisticians, and women working in home economics departments, industrial schools, teacher training programs, and philanthropic organizations.

This essay explores laboratory and field approaches in the search for dietary norms and standards in early studies of nutrition. Nutrition researchers reacted to social concerns and cultural change. The historical and national contexts of the later nineteenth and early twentieth century form the implicit background for the following study, which focuses on the question of how nutritional knowledge and norms emerged from the interaction of laboratory experiments and dietary surveys, studies on individuals and studies on groups, and experimental methods and statistical methods.

Physiology, Thermodynamics, and Statistics

Although isolated studies of nutrition and the chemistry of foods had been undertaken prior to the 1830s,[4] nutritional physiology as a specialized research field had to wait for the development of organic chemistry and strongly quantitative approaches in physiology in the middle decades of the century. The early history of nutritional physiology is inseparable from the organic chemist Justus Liebig. Liebig contributed both methods for the chemical analysis of foodstuffs and excretia and a two-part theory of nutrition that was to remain influential for several decades.[5] The theory was based on the assumption that fats and carbohydrates provided the body's heat, whereas protein was the fuel for muscular labor.[6] Protein foods, primarily meat, were required in amounts proportionate to physical activity, and physical endurance depended on their abundant presence in the diet.

A second set of influences came from physics and, especially, the energy conservation law. The conservation law was embraced in the late 1840s by a group of young German physiologists on a successful mission to establish physiology as an exact quantitative science and to explain all physiological phenomena through chemical and physical laws.[7] By the 1860s, most physiologists assumed that life processes depended on energy transformations, although they were unable to prove that energy input equalled energy output. When in the 1880s the nutritional physiologist Max Rubner demonstrated in exacting experiments on dogs in a respiration calorimeter that there was a near full equivalence between the various forms of energetic intake and output in the animal body, this was widely considered proof that the conservation law applied to animal nutrition and physiological processes in general. In the 1890s, the American physiological chemist Wilbur Olin Atwater confirmed that the conservation law also applied to the human animal. Liebig's two-substance two-function theory, under attack since the 1860s, was replaced by nutritional theories based on energy transformations.[8]

This early history of nutrition science coincided with the rise of statistical approaches in social, political, and scientific thought in the second half of the nineteenth century.[9] Governments had been collecting data on populations, agricultural production, mortality, birth, and death rates for much longer, but the "avalanche of printed numbers" gained momentum from the early decades of the century onward.[10] Not only did governments and other agencies expand the amounts and kinds of data they collected and the categories they used for classification, but what was understood under the term "statistics" also changed. The "political arithmetic" of the seventeenth century, with its qualitative modes of description, and the accounting methods of eighteenth-century government administrations, were replaced by tabular enumeration, averages, and probability in scientific disciplines, medicine, politics, and social theory.[11] Increasing use of quantitative methods and instruments of precision in the sciences had a counterpart in the increasing quantification of social data according to statistical instruments such as the law of large numbers, averages, and distribution curves.

At various stages in their studies, nutrition scientists used existing statistical data or used statistical methods to generate their own data and to manage and interpret the variability and complexity of their results. They relied on the biometric studies of the Belgian statistician Adolphe Quetelet and others to determine representative body sizes, and they turned to government statistics on slaughterhouses and populations to estimate regional meat consumption. They compiled standard tables for the chemical composition of foods so that they did not need to do an analysis for every experiment, and they summarized the results of their nutrition experiments and dietary surveys as general averages. The development of nutrition science in the laboratory and the field was intricately intertwined with the development and use of statistical methods in the social and the natural sciences. In turn, it helped establish approaches to human biological and social diversity that depended on norms and averages, quantification, and statistics as a means to express the general regularities of populations in the face of incomplete knowledge about each individual.

The "Normal" Man and the "Average" Worker

Although physicians, physiologists, and social reformers had conducted occasional studies of human food consumption and dietary needs since the earlier decades of the nineteenth century, systematic quantitative studies of human nutrition and metabolism in the laboratory did not begin until the 1860s in Germany. The newly focused interest in human nutrition was the result of a number of scientific, institutional, and social developments. In addition to the new methods and approaches of organic chemistry and physiology mentioned above, in the mid-decades of the nineteenth century, the status of physiology changed. Previously subordinate to medical studies and taught along with anatomy, it established itself as an independent field of study with its own university chairs, departments, and methods. Furthermore, in this period, Germany experienced rapid industrialization and the migration of rural laborers to the cities. Urbanization led in Germany, as in other countries, to an increase in urban poverty and its diseases and, with them, a growing concern for public health that found its expression in reform movements and numerous municipal and voluntary public health-related commissions and associations, as well as in the foundation of university chairs in public health (hygiene).[12] Human nutrition and metabolism were thus of interest from both the point of view of research physiology, which sought to investigate the processes of life, and from that of public health researchers and advocates, who were concerned with mitigating the ill effects of industrialization and urbanization on the large financially stressed sector of the population.

Early laboratory studies on nutritional physiology could look to a number of past attempts to assess food consumption and nutritional needs primarily by observing and analyzing the dietaries of individuals in institutions such as the military and prisons.[13] Liebig's investigation of the dietary needs of soldiers provided a model for the kind of input-output experiment that the following generation of physiologists later translated into a laboratory setting. In the 1840s, Liebig conducted an observational experiment in which he analyzed the food consumption of a corps of soldiers. He gathered information on the amount of food purchased for the company and divided its total food supply by the number of men in the corps to derive the rations provided to each solider. In the next step, he compared the estimated carbon content of the ration with that of the urine and excrement of individual soldiers. Although he had no means to measure respiration, he assumed that the deficit between the carbon consumed and the carbon found in the excreta had been exhaled as carbon dioxide, as his theory would predict. Since the study also did not establish how much of the ration a soldier actually consumed, how much additional food he may have purchased, or what effect individual differences had on metabolism, it could only provide a very rough estimate of dietary needs, as Liebig himself admitted.

Within the context of Liebig's study, the lack of precision was not considered a significant deficit, since his primary aim had been to find evidence for his nutritional theory.[14] More precise results required a move to the laboratory and its controlled environment, as well as the development of adequate experimental procedures and apparatus. In the early 1860s, the physiologist Carl Voit and the hygiene professor Max Pettenkofer constructed a human respiration apparatus that allowed them to conduct experiments on individual human metabolism. Voit, who had trained in Liebig's laboratory as a student, had already conducted highly successful experiments on the protein metabolism of dogs and had introduced new standards of precision to nutrition and metabolism experimentation. The experiments of Pettenkofer and Voit carried the characteristics of the new physiological approaches, in that they were precise, quantitative, apparatus-based laboratory experiments. Pettenkofer and Voit acknowledged energy conservation as the broader framework of physiological processes, but they stood closer to chemistry than physics, and Liebig's work provided the theoretical and methodological framework for their experiments.

New in their experiments was the large respiration chamber, which allowed them to directly measure the metabolism of fats and carbohydrates over a full digestive period by measuring carbon dioxide production over twenty-four hours. Unlike the face masks that had previously been used for this purpose, and which could be worn for only short periods, the chamber was the size of a small room, and thus large enough to contain a bed, chair, and table. The experimental subject could, if the experiment required, spend several days inside it in relative comfort. During an experiment, air flow into and out of the chamber was carefully controlled and the carbon content of incoming and outgoing air compared. The difference between the two revealed the amount of carbon dioxide produced by the body during the period in the chamber. With this apparatus, Pettenkofer and Voit aimed to confirm the balanced equation that Liebig and, indeed, most nutrition researchers assumed.

In 1866 they published the results of several experiments in a longer paper on "The Metabolism of the Normal Man," the first attempt to simultaneously measure nitrogen and carbon metabolism in a human being.[15] For the bulk of the experiments, Pettenkofer and Voit selected a worker, a watchmaker of average physical size,[16] who remained in the controlled environment of the respiration apparatus for twenty-four hours in each experiment, so that his metabolism could be measured in both waking and sleeping states. In some experiments the worker rested, in others he engaged in moderate activity. Food intake varied. Experiments were conducted in the fasting state, with high- and nonprotein meals. In some the worker was fed what Pettenkofer and Voit described as a normal mixed diet, which was intended to mimic the food consumption of soldiers and adult working men.[17] They determined that their worker needed 137 grams of protein, 173 grams of fat, and 352 grams of carbohydrates daily to maintain his body in intake-outgo equilibrium while at labor. Their two main conclusions were, first, that normal metabolism had a twenty-four-hour cycle, with strongly differing diurnal and nocturnal phases, and, second, that the worker metabolized the same amount of protein whether he was hard at work or quietly reading. Contrary to Liebig's theory, protein consumption did not increase with physical activity.

This paper is frequently cited, not without reason, as the foundational study for the embryonic field of nutrition science, and it was interpreted by some contemporaries as the first experimental demonstration of normal dietary requirements. Nonetheless, this was not Pettenkofer and Voit's primary intention. These first human experiments were motivated by a medical question. As the authors candidly explained in their introductory paragraph, they had interrupted their ongoing series of respiration experiments on dogs to take advantage of an unexpected opportunity to study the metabolism of two individuals with chronic illnesses, one with diabetes and the other with leukemia.[18] They hoped to discover what was different about the metabolism of a sick individual. Once they had their data, however, they realized that they had no control data and thus had no means of assessing the deviance of the pathological from the normal. Their study of the "normal man" began as an attempt to determine the characteristics of healthy metabolism. Only once the regularities of health were known could the irregularities of disease be identified and assessed.

The further development of metabolism measurement as a clinical tool and studies on the relationships between disease, metabolism, and diet cannot be elaborated here. Nonetheless, it is important to note the original question behind Pettenkofer and Voit's study and the way their interests evolved in the course of experimentation in order to understand some of the confusion that arose in later discussions about definitions and terminology. Pettenkofer and Voit's study began with the problem of differentiating the pathological from the normal, that is, determining metabolic regularity to recognize irregularity, but in the course of the experiments the focus shifted increasingly to the question of normal dietary needs, that is, the dietary needs of a man considered "normal." As Georges Canguilhem and others have noted, in the history of medicine ideas of norms and the normal have taken on different meanings, sometimes several simultaneously.[19] They can be normative and can also become synonymous with the idea of the "average." In addition, they can be interpreted in the sense of the "optimal," that is, as the ideal outcome, with the status quo or "average" demoted to a state of mediocrity in need of improvement.[20] As will be shown, these different senses of "normal" and "average" reverberated through the work of nutritional physiologists and researchers in the following decades.[21]

Although differentiating "normal" and "pathological" metabolism was of potential use for medical practitioners, and the tools of nutritional physiologists found their way into clinical medicine, Voit and his associates presented their research, not least in the hope of increased state funding, as basic physiological research with broad areas of application, especially for public health. Applying this new knowledge to assess the nutritional conditions and dietary needs of broadly conceived population groups and to develop dietary norms required modifications to the laboratory methods. Laboratory experiments could determine the specific nutritional needs of an individual, but dietary norms needed to be based on the average needs of populations. These averages could only be derived by assessing larger numbers of people than could be done in the lab.

Finding them required the cooperation of groups of individuals and of institutions such as the military, prisons, workhouses, and poorhouses.

Voit's study of human metabolism began with a laboratory orientation, but by the mid-1870s, influenced in part by Pettenkofer, who had been promoted from his position as medical chemist to one of Germany's first professorships in public health (hygiene) in 1865, he had become increasingly interested in how the new knowledge of nutritional physiology could be applied to assess the adequacy of institutional dietaries. Attention to institutionalized groups was not novel. As Ulrike Thoms has shown, the dietaries of prisoners and soldiers had long been a subject of interest for German governments, and similar concerns are reflected in other countries as well.[22] Healthy populations meant both military and economic power: strong soldiers won wars and incarcerated prisoners were future free laborers. Voit had already advised the Bavarian government on military rations, and, with the encouragement of the Verein für öffentliche Gesundheitspflege (Association for Public Health), he and his collaborators extended their research to include studies of the diets in public kitchens, prisons, poorhouses, orphanages, and hospitals.[23] Public administrative bodies, Voit declared, had to balance the necessity of financial restraint with their responsibility to provide appropriate care to the residents of their institutions.[24] The way to achieve both goals was through a rational approach to nutrition that considered the dietary needs of these institutional populations along with the costs of the various food combinations that could fulfill them.

Institutional dietary studies adopted the basic intake-outgo experimental structure that had been introduced in Liebig's soldier study and refined in the physiological laboratories. Researchers registered the amount of food purchased by the institution and divided this total by the number of inhabitants to derive individual rations. Food samples were chemically analyzed to find their macronutrient content, and these results were extrapolated to the rations. Nutrition researchers assessed the adequacy of the diet by comparing it to the observational dietary norm for an adult working man proposed by Voit in the early 1870s and by making rough judgements on whether the institutional residents seemed healthy for their particular circumstances. Such institutional studies had a dual purpose. Investigators made recommendations to directors, state officials, and budgeting bodies on achieving an acceptable compromise between humanitarian needs and the financial costs of feeding resident populations. At the same time, they collected data on the dietary needs of different groups of individuals, such as children in orphanages or pensioners in old-age homes.

Institutions thus formed a transitional space between the lab and the field. They provided a setting for translating nutritional knowledge into practices and, as Voit noted, contributed to this knowledge by supplying a greater number of study subjects than was possible through laboratory experiments alone.[25] They were a favored location for early nutrition studies, since they held a captive population fed from a common source. Neither the residents of such institutions nor the composition of their food could be measured and controlled to the same extent as in laboratory experiments, but the individuals tended to be more homogeneous and their diets less varied than in the general population. Studying the diet of an institutional population and the effects this diet had on the health of the residents thus revealed the longer-term effects of dietary practices under semicontrolled conditions. Simultaneously, it enabled nutritional physiologists to position themselves as expert advisers in questions of public health and institutional administration.

While physiological interest in institutions was based in part on humanitarian concerns, in part on their potential as large-scale quasi-experimental sites, physiologists reserved a special interest for "wild" nutritional practices, especially those of manual laborers, an economically crucial but often financially and nutritionally stressed population. Industrialization had changed the demographic structure of the country, with a population shift from the countryside to the cities and urban centers. Former agricultural laborers and small farmers, who had grown their own food, became factory workers purchasing goods with their wages in the marketplace. The rural social structure had provided a framework for traditional forms of food consumption, but models for this new kind of working-class life and the physically and financially appropriate diet did not yet exist.[26] Social reformers and trade unions conducted surveys of workers' expenses and budgets to determine whether income was sufficient to cover needs, to argue for higher wages and to counter employers' claims that working-class poverty was a product of financial irresponsibility. In 1857 the Prussian statistician Ernst Engel postulated a general law, based on extensive data for Belgium and the Kingdom of Saxony, that there was a geometric ratio between a worker`s income and the percentage of that income that was spent on food.[27] The lower the income, the greater the proportion of it had to be spent on fulfilling this basic need, and the less was available for other necessary expenses such as shelter, clothing, heating, and education.

In this context of industrialization, social reform movements, and political and economic interests, Voit proposed that an average worker (*mittlerer Arbeiter*) required 118 grams of protein and 328 grams of carbon a day to remain healthy and productive. Voit was vague about the sources of his information, stating only that he derived these norms "from a great number of observations,"[28] primarily of what average workingmen, left to their own devises and without undue financial restraint, ate. As an observational norm, it did not differ greatly from the proposals of previous nutrition researchers such as Liebig's contemporary Jakob Moleschott or the British scientist and social reformer Lyon Playfair, who had both recorded what a number of workingmen ate and presented it as a sufficient diet based on their apparent physical health and well-being.[29] Such observational norms were based on the assumption that, unless their choices were unduly constrained by financial circumstances, people naturally consumed the foods that their bodies physiologically required. Consequently, whereas laboratory studies could demonstrate different means of establishing intake-outgo equilibrium and different levels of chemical balance, observing nutritional practices produced knowledge about physiological needs.

Although Voit intended his norms to introduce clarity to the exploration of dietary needs, they instead revealed how problematic such an endeavor would be. Researchers who observed different dietary practices or found that the workers they studied consumed different quantities of foods and foodstuffs disputed his numbers, and, in addition, it was unclear what exactly characterized an "average worker." In the 1830s, Quetelet combined a broad range of biometric and social data to create his *homme moyenne*, or average man. Biometric data seemed to make sense as a basis for physiological norms; however, using such physical characteristics as height and weight to determine dietary needs led to conflicting, ambiguous, or anomalous results.[30] Similar bodies seemed to have widely variable needs, which put to question whether there was enough regularity in human nutritional needs to determine a general dietary norm at all. In addition, Voit's "average worker" had very different needs than the "normal man" of his first laboratory study, and this discrepancy demanded explanation.

In 1879 Hamilton Bowie, a student of Voit's, clarified this confusion. The word "average" in this context, he explained, was not biometrically defined. Instead of referring to body size, as many physiologists had assumed, it referred to the amount of physical labor this worker performed. An average worker was a worker who performed an average amount of work for an average working day of nine or ten hours. He worked more than a tailor, but less than a smith. He was the equivalent of a mason, a carpenter, or a soldier in the garrison.[31] His function determined his dietary needs. The normal man was defined within medical discourses of health and disease; the average worker was defined according to socioeconomic conventions. By choosing the male manual laborer as the standard-setter for dietary norms, Voit, like his predecessors, revealed the economic interests and concerns behind early nutrition research.

Although Voit claimed that studying the needs of this "average worker" would lead to knowledge about the needs of the "average man,"[32] it was, in addition, unclear to whom these norms should apply and thus what their potential applications were. As Bowie noted, numerous studies had already shown that "in regard to a rational nutrition, every human being is a special case."[33] Only rarely would two people be so similar at all levels that their nutritional needs and digestion would be exactly the same, and individual differences showed such a broad spectrum of variability that an average value offered few useful guidelines for assessing the needs of any randomly selected person, even one of the defined group. The "average worker" was an abstraction with no real counterpart, and the dietary norms for this person had a tenuous relationship to the needs of real individuals. Dietary norms were a rough estimate of needs and a concession to the limits of knowledge in regard to individual diversity. They were useful, he explained, in situations in which the ability to take this diversity into consideration was equally limited. Dietary norms provided orientation for feeding groups in institutions where individual needs could not be considered, but they applied to populations, not to individuals.

Surveying Nutrition in the Field

The search for dietary norms led nutrition researchers out of the lab and from the institutions into the field, aware that their experimental conditions and controlled institutional environments differed greatly from real-life situations and that the true test of an adequate diet was how well it stood up to the demands of daily life. Studying the food consumption of groups of humans in more "natural" settings offered the possibility of gathering large amounts of information and of assessing the effects of dietary practices on the health and well-being of the subjects. Studies of institutional dietaries increased rapidly in in the 1870s and 1880s, particularly in Germany, but studies of the dietary practices of non-institutionalized population groups remained piecemeal and unsystematic, due less to a lack of interest than to a lack of methods.

Since Ernst Engel's household budget studies of the late 1850s, statisticians and social reformers had collected data on the income and consumption patterns of wage laborers to establish their general standard of living, assess the adequacy of wages, and evaluate the effects of precarious employment on living standards. These surveys often included lists of purchased foodstuffs. Although these consumption studies did not address the nutritional adequacy of the diets, their survey methods provided a basis for the development of methods for the study of nutrition in the field.

In 1885, Carroll D. Wright, a statistician for the Massachusetts Bureau of Statistics of Labor, commissioned Wilbur Olin Atwater to collaborate on a study of the nutrition and diets of wage laborers in Massachusetts.[34] Wright, who had already led several consumption and budget studies of American laborers and their families, sent agents into the field to collect data on the food consumption of American and French Canadian working-class families and boarding house residents in a Massachusetts town and further surveys of French Canadians in Quebec. The aim of these surveys was to study the diet of American workers and assess the effects of American working conditions and wages on the dietary practices of the country's rapidly growing immigrant population. Economics, labor, wages, and immigration were the key concerns and context of this first and many following American dietary surveys.[35]

Atwater, a professor of physiological chemistry and food chemistry at Wesleyan University, had trained in Voit's laboratory a few years earlier. In his analysis of the survey information, presented in tabular format, he combined elements of laboratory experiments and physiological knowledge with household budget survey methods. His tables listed, first, food items purchased, amounts, and cost, as was customary for household budgets. Second, he treated the boarding house or family as a single experimental intake-outgo subject, similar to an institution, and, finally, he reduced the diversity of foods to their basic nutritional components of fat, protein, and carbohydrates, much as his laboratory colleagues had done. His tables revealed at a glance the nutritional and economic consequences of the surveyed dietary practices.

Assessing the consumption of the families and boarding house populations confronted Atwater with a problem that had long plagued compilers of household budgets: The families they surveyed were too diverse to allow for useful comparison or more than descriptive generalizations. Much as nutritional physiologists constructed the "average worker" to deal with diversity, social surveyors created an average family, the "normal family" (man, woman, two preadolescent children), as a means to standardize their data.[36] This method, however, could deal with consumption only at the unit level of the household, not the individual. The boarding house and family units that Atwater studied consisted, like the units of the workers' budget studies, of groups of people who, like Liebig's soldiers or the residents of institutions, partook of a common meal. Since institutional groups were fairly homogenous, researchers assumed they had similar needs and divided the food supply equally among them. Atwater could not make this assumption for his household populations of men, women, and children. In order to establish whether the household food consumption was nutritionally adequate for its members, Atwater needed to quantify these diverse individuals in relation to a general standard or equivalent. He chose the "average worker" of Voit's dietary standards, the healthy male manual laborer.[37]

In 1885, when Rubner proposed that the primary role of foodstuffs was to supply energy and that their value to the organism be quantified as units of heat or calories, he also determined the heat value of the three macronutrients.[38] Atwater was familiar with Rubner's research, but did not convert the surveyed dietaries into calories in his studies of 1886, presumably because the standardized food tables on which he relied did not yet include caloric value.[39] Nonetheless, the calorie concept was useful to him in another way. By the 1880s, European researchers and social reformers had collected laboratory and survey data on the average protein, fat, and carbohydrate consumption of men at heavy, severe, and light work, as well as for women, children of various ages, and the elderly.[40] Atwater converted these numbers into calories and then, setting the presumed nutritional needs of the "average worker" as his norm, quantified the other consumption groups as fractions of this norm, that is, as parts of man, from the housewife at eight-tenths of a man down to the toddler at two-and-a-half tenths. Although he later acknowledged that this breakdown was only partially based on experience and was partially arbitrary,[41] with these calculations he created an artificial homogeneity in his study population by reducing a diverse population to its equivalent in male manual laborers. The household consumption was divided by the number of "average workers" to derive individual consumption measured in the unit of "per man per day."[42] The "man" of the "per man per day" unit was as much a statistical fiction as Voit's "average worker."

Atwater's survey data showed that the Americans in his study had by far the most generous diet, followed by the Canadian immigrants, whereas the diet of French Canadians in Canada was the least nutritious and most restricted. He ascribed these differences to the higher wages workers earned in the United States, which translated into a higher standard of living.[43] Although he at first found that, in comparison with European consumption and the Voit norms, Americans consumed a shocking, excessive, and potentially unhealthy amount of food, especially of meats, sweets, and fats,[44] when he revisited these studies in 1891, his position had changed. He had become convinced that the American diet was not overabundant, but, in contrast, that the European norms were inadequate.[45] Americans ate more because they worked harder and enjoyed a higher standard of living:

> The kernel of the whole question is found in the fact that the European standards are based upon the food consumption of people whose plane of living is low in comparison with that of the people in the United States. . . . To make the most out of a man, to bring him to live as a man ought to live, he must be better fed than he would by these standards.[46]

According to Atwater, the European norms reproduced the status quo. It was a maintenance minimum that allowed humans to live and work, but not to thrive or achieve their potential. American dietary standards needed to be set higher to reflect American circumstances. Atwater's standards expressed the norm not as a status quo but as an optimum that would maximize human potential through a more abundant diet. Heavier labor required more food, more food enabled increased productivity, and both would lead to an even higher standard of living, as well as to increased ambition, hope, and improved morals. When Atwater set 125 grams of protein and 3,500 calories as the American standard for the average worker, he had even less of a laboratory experimental basis than Voit had for his. The standards arose out of a combination of his observations on American dietary practices and his belief in the superiority of the American way of life.[47]

Atwater's "per man per day" reduction and his combination of laboratory and social science methods were adopted internationally for dietary surveys and quickly became standard procedure for the study of nutrition in the field. Like nutrition experimenters, dietary surveyors relied on basic intake-outgo models, asked what kinds and amounts of foodstuffs a body needed to maintain health and productivity, and made assumptions about the functions of foodstuffs based on physiological knowledge.

Dietary surveys were frequently collaborative studies, bringing together researchers and skills from organic chemistry, physiology, and the social sciences, since the two sides of these studies, the physiological and the social, required very different sets of skills. Whereas chemical analysis demanded one kind of expertise, successful survey work depended on soft skills and social strategies that would enable surveyors to foster a sense of trust and to solicit cooperation from groups that were often suspicious about such intrusions into their personal lives. Owing to the sensitive nature of this interaction as well as to concerns about the nutritional state of financially stressed population groups, surveyors frequently had connections to industrial schools, home economics programs, and other institutions that allowed them to build on existing relationships with their target survey groups of immigrants, poor families, unskilled laborers, and female-headed households. Since food and diet were considered to be appropriate areas for women's activities, dietary studies opened up research fields for woman chemists, physiologists, and physicians, both within and outside of home economics programs, and numerous surveyors had connections to residential and settlement house programs, like Hill House, and to schools for the vocational instruction of lower-class girls and women.

To conduct a survey, an investigator had to establish contact with and gain the trust of a family, the proprietor of a boarding house, or the kitchen personnel at an institution, enlist their cooperation for weeks or even months, and make sensitive inquiries into income, purchasing habits, and the contents of pantries and waste buckets. Surveyors took inventory of stocks, weighed all purchased food, tracked expenditures, and deducted food waste. At the conclusion of the study, they again took inventory to derive the amount of food that had been consumed by the household unit, if not necessarily physically consumed by its inhabitants.[48] These surveys aimed to collect data on actual consumption in order to assess how and whether people of different income classes and ethnic backgrounds covered their nutritional needs in practice. They assumed, as Voit had done, that in the absence of severe deprivation, people would naturally gravitate to an adequate diet and eat what they physiologically needed to eat. On the one hand, practiced nutrition served as a control and corrective for laboratory experimentation. On the other, dietary studies could also reveal which nutritional practices were uneconomical in regard to the relationship between food purchases and nutritive content. If poor nutrition was due to poor dietary practices, then nutrition education, not wage increases, was the solution to the problem.[49]

Bringing the Field into the Lab

By the early twentieth century, Atwater, Voit, and the physiologists, home economists, and social surveyors associated with them had generated a thicket of data detailing the dietaries of individuals and families in various income classes, countries, cities, and regions. They studied the food consumption of people in voluntary individual and communal living situations, such as boarding houses, private households, college dormitories, and factory canteens, and surveyed the dietary practices of groups as diverse as Chinese agricultural laborers in California, Swedish civil servants and Finnish farmers, the destitute poor of Naples, the lumbermen of the Maine woods, and the nurses of Japan.[50] Most physiologists, philanthropic organizations, and social policymakers accepted either the Voit or the Atwater standard or took a position between the two, depending on their country of origin.

Nonetheless, the discrepancy between the two standards highlighted the insecure nature of nutritional knowledge, and the protein standard, particularly, was questioned by both individual physiologists and dietary reformers and vegetarians.[51] In 1904, critics received strong support from the physiological chemist Russell Chittenden, Director of the Sheffield Scientific School at Yale University.

Significantly, when Chittenden questioned whether the recommended dietary standards reflected actual needs, he framed this question as a critique on methodology. As he noted, these standards had been derived by what he called the "statistical method," that is, by collecting data through surveys and averaging it to determine norms. These methods, he claimed, only recorded what people ate, not what their bodies required. They revealed the "apparent tendency" for people in different cultures to consume similar quantities of foodstuffs, despite the regionally different foods, but they actually only confirmed the status quo of customs and eating habits. Chittenden argued, in essence, that the field, with its observation-based methodology and statistical results, was not a reliable site for the generation of physiological knowledge. He writes: "Arguments predicated on custom, habit, and usage have no physiological basis that appeals strongly to the impartial observer. . . . The true food requirements of the body, under any conditions cannot be ascertained with any degree of accuracy by observations of what people are in the habit of eating; . . . customs and habits are not a safe index of true physiological needs."[52] Practiced food consumption was contingent, cultural, and malleable, not physiological and rational. Instead, Chittenden insisted, only controlled experiments that were conducted with groups of individuals over a sufficiently long period that they became "real world" conditions were capable of revealing the true physiological needs of the body and providing a basis for the knowledge of dietary norms. He noted his intention in a draft: "Dietetics to be raised from an observational to an experimental science."[53]

Chittenden's skepticism was based both on conflicting laboratory studies of nitrogen balance and on his observations of Horace Fletcher, a popular dietary reformer. Known as the "Great Masticator," Fletcher recommended chewing food until it turned into a tasteless fluid in the mouth to improve the absorption of nutrients. This, he claimed, would allow the body to subsist on a radically lower calorie and protein diet than assumed.[54] In 1902–3, Chittenden had the opportunity to study Fletcher's diet, physiology, and physical fitness over a period of several months. Although unconvinced about the efficacy of the mastication regimen, he was so intrigued by Fletcher's ability to remain in such robust health on a diet far below the norms that he tried to replicate the results in a controlled laboratory situation.

In three series of experiments, Chittenden placed relatively homogeneous groups of men—professors, athletic students, and soldiers—on low protein and calorie diets for several months and studied how they and their bodies reacted. The primary group was the soldiers, who stayed on this diet for six months. Chittenden analyzed their urine and feces, weighed them, had them do calisthenics, and took verbal protocols on their subjective well-being. He concluded from these studies that an average, active man—the equivalent of an "average worker"—required only about 50 grams of protein and less than 3,000 calories a day to maintain health and strength.[55] Less active men such as the professors could remain healthy on much less. More food, he claimed, was unnecessary and put undue strain on the body, which had to invest energy in ridding itself of this excess and potentially toxic material.

Chittenden's conclusions and especially his protein recommendations aroused both interest and condemnation.[56] Although Liebig's theory had long been discarded, the protein norms presented by Voit, Atwater, and even proposed by Rubner were only slightly lower than his had been.[57] By 1907, however, a number of international physiologists confirmed through the study of vegetarians and self-experimentation that the body could remain healthy on much lower amounts of protein, at least for the experimental period.[58] Rubner also began to question the protein standard and to look not toward the optimal protein consumption, but to minimal protein requirements, specifically those of the average worker.[59] This was a question with economic implications, since animal protein foods were expensive compared with calorie-supplying fats and carbohydrates. If protein needs were lower than the accepted standards, institutions and laborers could follow physiological economy and reduce their food costs.

Rubner took a curious path to determine minimal protein requirements, looking neither to experiment nor observation, but beginning, instead, with the macronutrient content of human milk. Reasoning that, with its 5 percent protein content, it provided full nutrition to a growing organism with high protein needs, he concluded that an average worker required only 31.4 grams dietary protein to fulfill its needs, if total calorie intake was sufficient.[60] Rubner was, however, far from recommending consumption according to physiological minima. He emphasized that norms needed to allow considerable leeway for increased needs, whether due to individual differences or changing life circumstances, and was prepared to accept Voit's norms not as an expression of the body's physiological needs, but as a reflection of observed nutritional practices, which were themselves based on conventions, appetite, and physical and psychological comfort.[61]

The dispute between Chittenden and mainstream physiologists was, as the discussion of Rubner indirectly shows, not only about protein requirements, but also about the appropriate place to look for physiological knowledge. The laboratory with its experiments and controlled conditions could generate one kind of knowledge, but even long experiments ended, and the experimenter could not consider and assess the effects of all possible environmental variables. The field, with its study of nutritional practices, was imprecise and contingent, but it allowed for generalizations about the effects of dietary practices on the health, productivity, and well-being of large populations and, by integrating humans of all ages, over the course of a lifetime.

Although some physiologists criticized Chittenden's methods, others were willing to accept his data, but only within the confines of his experiment. They questioned whether such a diet was sustainable over a longer period, whether the perceived improvements in health were due merely to suggestion or to the acknowledged benefits of a regular lifestyle, and whether the analyses had been carried out with the appropriate care and precision. Numerous studies seemed to indicate a direct and likely causal relationship between protein consumption and national productivity.[62] As Atwater's protégée and former assistant, Francis Gano Benedict, pointed out in his 1906 critique of Chittenden's experiments,

"Dietary studies all over the world show that in communities where productive power, enterprise, and civilization are at their highest, man has instinctively and independently selected liberal rather than small quantities of protein."[63] Low-protein experiments could provide useful knowledge about nitrogen metabolism, but in terms of successful application, the results of dietary practices seemed to contradict those of the laboratory.

The question of the relationship between laboratory and field knowledge and dietary norms remained unresolved. In 1916, Benedict returned to the topic of lower nutritional norms. In the intervening decade, the context of nutritional research had radically changed. The First World War, the hunger blockade against Germany, scarcity and rationing in Europe, American food exports, and voluntary food solidarity initiatives had created a situation in which limits on resource availability presented a new set of problems. Minimum requirements, not maximum potential, became scientifically and politically increasingly interesting. Nutrition researchers had long studied the physiology of undernutrition and fasting, but these were extreme conditions and, over a longer period, were not compatible with health and a productive working life. Reports from Germany, which had been plagued by food shortages and restrictions since early in the war, raised the question of whether a sustained reduced diet was possible. For nutritional physiologists, the German population had become an involuntary experimental subject for the study of the effects of a long-term low calorie and protein diet.[64]

American researchers could not travel to Germany, and with all postal communication with Germany interrupted, they had little information on German conditions. The food consumption of the civilian population could be only roughly estimated, and data on their health and metabolism under these conditions was lacking. Benedict received some internal information through Alonzo E. Taylor, a member of the US embassy in Berlin. Taylor provided his own observations on German rationing, and relayed data from Rubner, whom the German War Ministry had assigned the task of assessing the food needs of the German population and advising the government on food policy.[65] According to the information Benedict received, the German population seemed to have subsisted for an extended period on a severely restricted diet and to have adjusted itself physiologically and metabolically to this new nutritional situation.

Since a direct observation of dietary practices under the blockade was impossible, Benedict turned the methodological vector around and used the laboratory as a means to generate knowledge of the field. To test the physiological effects of this diet, he tried to replicate the conditions of the German population, or aspects of their situation, under controlled laboratory conditions. He solicited a group of students from a men's Christian college, divided them into experimental and control subjects, and gradually reduced the diet of the experimental group until they had lost 10 to 12 percent of their body weight and stabilized. He then studied digestion, metabolism at rest, metabolism during muscular work, reaction times, endurance, and so on, over a four-month period.[66] He found his subjects lost weight, felt cold, and had lowered pulse rates, skin temperature, and heat output, but were nonetheless able to conduct their daily lives as usual on a diet of 2,300 calories, and concluded that "the whole period of lowered food intake had no untoward effect upon the physical or mental activities, and the men were able to continue successfully their college duties."[67]

Benedict did not claim, as Chittenden had done, that a diet at the minimal maintenance level was desirable and beneficial to health, conceding only that it was not immediately detrimental and had application possibilities for American citizens. Reducing food consumption, he claimed, was a "patriotic duty," a means for American civilians to contribute to the war effort by making sacrifices that would benefit the suffering, hungering European allied nations, who were dependent on American food shipments.[68] As an emergency measure, a reduced diet was appropriate to the current wartime situation, in which calories had become a limited resource that had to be invested carefully and efficiently.

Chittenden's and Benedict's experiments are noteworthy in that both attempted to combine laboratory control with survey representativeness by experimenting on groups over extended periods. In some ways, the experiments owed more to the lab than the field, in that the experimental "populations" were treated not statistically, but as a group of individuals. Chittenden's thirteen soldiers had not only body weights, heights, and tables with their nitrogen balance and other data describing their physical reaction to the experimental diets. They also had names. Benedict's students had, in addition, brief personal biographies, describing their medical history and field of study, physical activity level, and well-being during the experiment. They were identified in the tables of measurements and named in the descriptive summaries. This form of data collection enabled Chittenden and Bendict to simultaneously identify general tendencies and individual idiosyncrasies, that is, to combine knowledge of the individual and individual variability with knowledge of the group, of regularities that applied to populations. By the second decade of the twentieth century, this approach to the group through the individual was, however, already in the process of change. Benedict conducted part of his respiration measurements for this study in a large respiration chamber capable of holding twelve men. Twelve individuals entered that chamber, but only one set of data emerged—the average metabolism of a group that could no longer be traced back to its individual members.

Conclusion

As this essay has shown, the search for dietary norms was anything but straightforward. Nutritional knowledge was generated at numerous sites by a wide range of actors using a variety of methods and tools. Physiologists and physicians, public health specialists and social reformers, statisticians and home economists produced and collected data in laboratories, homes, and institutions by observing real-life conditions and creating artificial ones. This diversity of places and practitioners reflects the complex network of interests that constitute the science of nutrition.

Looking at the historical development of dietary norms through the interaction of the laboratory and the field is a useful way to structure this diversity.[69] In nutritional physiology, the laboratory was the site for precise experiments by highly trained researchers on individuals under controlled conditions. Owing to their time-consuming and elaborate nature, as well as the high degree of skill and the high expense of the apparatus they required, relatively few full nutrition experiments were conducted in the period covered here. In these experiments, the individual subjects served as representative exemplars for larger groups of untestable but presumably comparable individuals. The aim was to find the laws of metabolism—regularities that applied to all normal individuals.

Nonetheless, physiologists were aware that the prerequisites for coherent experimentation differed greatly from the conditions of everyday life and actual dietary practices and that bodies, diets, and life circumstances showed more variability than could be effectively studied in the lab. This was a crucial problem, since human nutrition research offered enormous potential for applications. Since the early nineteenth century, governments and their various representatives, social reformers, and public health experts had become increasingly interested in the diets of certain social groups, owing to the demographic changes of the industrial revolution, the effects of political upheaval and conflict, and changes in perceptions of a state's responsibility for its citizens.

As much as the study of nutrition dealt with physiological processes, it was also deeply intertwined with questions of public health and social welfare, and in this regard it dealt with populations. What the lab offered on precision, the field offered in numbers. Surveys and studies of groups promised to generate large amounts of data and information about the dietary practices of populations. Sacrificing precision, surveys could better adapt to diversity and variability. Although there was some overlap of actors between laboratory studies and dietary surveys, the latter were carried out for the most part by home economists, many of whom had a similar training to the research physiologists, by social reformers and labor leaders, various public and private bodies concerned with the condition of the working classes, and public health and medical practitioners. These field actors often worked in tighter or looser collaboration with the physiologists and their laboratories.

Field researchers conducting studies of human dietary practices found themselves facing similar practical and methodological questions as social scientists. They needed to build relationships and develop structures for collecting information. Methodologically, they needed to devise means for reducing diversity to quantifiable and comparable units, and to explore relationships between the individual, the group, and the average, while continuously evaluating the potential and limits of statistical data and knowledge. Although the respective status of these sites was subject to dispute in these early decades, lab and field were complimentary. Dietary norms and standards emerged from a combination of both, mediated by cultural and scientific assumptions and historical contingencies.

Notes

1. Kenneth John Carpenter, *Protein and Energy* (Cambridge: Cambridge University Press, 1994); Frederic L. Holmes, "Carl Voit and the Quantitative Tradition in Biology," in *Transformations and Tradition in the Sciences: Essays in Honour of I. Bernard Cohen*, ed. Everett Mendelsohn (Cambridge: Cambridge University Press, 1984), 455–70; Frederic L. Holmes, "The Formation of the Munich School of Metabolism," in *The Investigative Enterprise: Experimental Physiology in Nineteenth-Century Medicine*, ed. William Coleman and Frederic L. Holmes (Berkeley: University of California Press, 1988), 179–210; Nikolaus Mani, "Die wissenschaftliche Ernährungslehre im 19. Jahrhundert," in *Ernährung und Ernährungslehre im 19. Jahrhundert*, ed. Edith Heischkelt-Artelt (Göttingen: Vandenhoeck & Ruprecht, 1976), 22–75.

2. Naomi Aronson, "Nutrition as a Social Problem: a Case Study of Entrepreneurial Strategy in Science," *Social Problems* 29 (1982): 474–87; Naomi Aronson, "Social Definitions of Entitlement: Food Needs, 1885–1920," *Media, Culture, and Society* 4 (1982): 51–61; Harvey Levenstein, *Revolution at the Table: The Transformation of the American Diet* (Berkeley: University of California Press, 2003). Following in Levenstein's footsteps, more recently Helen Zoe Veit has explored connections between diet, social values, and politics in Progressive-era America. Helen Zoe Veit, *Modern Food, Moral Food: Self-Control, Science, and the Rise of Modern America Eating in the Early Twentieth Century* (Chapel Hill: University of North Carolina Press, 2013).

3. For example: Frederick W. Clements, *A History of Human Nutrition in Australia* (Melbourne: Longman Cheshire, 1986); Jakob Tanner, *Fabrikmahlzeit: Ernährungswissenschaft, Industriearbeit und Volksernährung in der Schweiz 1890–1950* (Zürich: Chronos, 1999); James Vernon, *Hunger: A Modern History* (Cambridge, MA: Belknap Press, 2007).

4. François Magendie, "Mémoire sur les propriétes nutritives des substances qui ne conteniennent pas d'azote," *Annales de Chimie et de Physique* 3 (1816): 66–77; William Prout, "On the Ultimate Composition of Simple Alimentary Substances," *Philosophical Transactions of the Royal Society of London* 117 (1827): 355–88; Gerardus Johannes Mulder, "Zusammensetzung von Fibrin, Albumin, Leimzucker, Leuein u.s.w.," *Annalen der Pharmacie* 28 (1838): 73–82.

5. See Introduction to this volume.

6. For Liebig's theory, see Frederick Holmes, "Introduction," *Animal Chemistry, or Organic Chemistry in Its Application to Physiology and Pathology*, by Justus von Liebig, ed. William Gregory and John W. Webster (New York: Johnson Reprint Corporation, 1964), vii–cxvi.

7. This group included Emil Du Bois-Reymond and Hermann Helmholtz. Paul F. Cranefield, "The Organic Physics of 1847 and the Biophysics of Today," *Journal for the History of Medicine and Allied Sciences* 12 (1957): 407–23; Timothy Lenoir, "Social Interests and the Organic Physics of 1847," in *Instituting Science: The Cultural Production of Scientific Disciplines*, ed. Timothy Lenoir (Stanford, CA: Stanford University Press, 1997), 75–95.

8. Protein remained a crucial component of diet, since it was deemed necessary for tissue renewal, but it no longer occupied a special position as the source of muscular work. For more detail, see Carpenter, *Protein and Energy*; Mani, "Ernährungslehre."

9. Theodore Porter, *The Rise of Statistical Thinking* (Princeton, NJ: Princeton University Press, 1986); Alan Derosières, *The Politics of Large Numbers: A History of Statistical Reasoning* (Cambridge, MA: Harvard University Press, 1998).

10. Ian Hacking, *The Taming of Chance* (Cambridge: Cambridge University Press, 1990); Ian Hacking, "Biopower and the Avalanche of Printed Numbers," *Humanities in Society* 5 (1982): 279–95. For a contemporary assessment, see John Theodore Merz, *A History of European Thought in the Nineteenth Century*, vol. 2 (Gloucester, MA: Peter Smith Publisher, 1976), 548–626.

11. See the essays in Lorenz Krüger et al., eds., *The Probabilistic Revolution*, 2 vols. (Cambridge, MA: MIT Press, 1987).

12. Lorenz Jellinghaus, *Zwischen Daseinsvorsorge und Infrastruktur: Zum Funktionswandel von Verwaltungswissenschaften und Verwaltungsrecht in der zweiten Hälfte des 19. Jahrhunderts* (Frankfurt am Main: Vittorio Klostermann, 2006), chap 2.

13. See Ulrike Thoms, *Anstaltskost in Rationalisierungsprozeß: Die Ernährung in Krankenhäusern und Gefängnissen im 18. und 19. Jahrhundert* (Stuttgart: Frank Steiner Verlag, 2005); and Ulrike Thoms, "Setting Standards: The Soldier's Food in Germany, 1850–1960," chapter 4 of this volume.

14. Justus Liebig, *Die Thier-Chemie oder die organische Chemie in ihrer Anwendung auf Physiologie und Pathologie* (Braunschweig: Vieweg & Sohn, 1842), 289–95.

15. Max Pettenkofer and Carl Voit, "Untersuchungen über den Stoffverbrauch des normalen Menschen," *Zeitschrift für Biologie* 2 (1866): 459–573. See Holmes, "Carl Voit."

16. They did not specify what data provided their average, but it was considerably higher than the Queteletian average of 62.7 kilos. Alphonse Quetelet, *A Treatise on Man and the Development of His Faculties* (Edinburgh: W. and R. Chambers, 1842), 67.

17. Pettenkofer and Voit, "Untersuchungen über den Stoffverbrauch," 523.

18. Ibid., 459. The diabetes study was published a year later. See Max Pettenkofer and Carl Voit, "Ueber den Stoffverbrauch bei der Zuckerharnrohr," *Zeitschrift für Biologie* 3 (1867): 380–444.

19. Georges Canguilhem, *The Normal and the Pathological* (New York: Zone Books, 1991), esp. 151–80 (French original pub., 1966); Joachim Büttner, "Die Herausbildung des Normalwert-Konzepts im Zusammenhang mit quantitativen diagnostischen Untersuchungen in der Medizin," in *Normierung der Gesundheit: Messende Verfahren der Medizin als kulturelle Praktik um 1900*, ed. Volker Hess (Husum: Matthiesen Verlag, 1997), 17–32.

20. Hacking, *Taming of Chance*, 163–69.

21. In 1914 Francis Gano Benedict tried to clarify this uncertainty, defining "average" in relationship to the pair "normal" and "pathological." "Average" values were no longer only quantitative, but qualitative as well: "values obtained from people in presumably good health." Francis Gano Benedict et al., "The Basal, Gaseous Metabolism of Normal Men and Women," *Journal of Biological Chemistry* 18 (1914): 139–55.

22. Valerie J. Johnstone, *Diet in Workhouses and Prisons, 1835–1895* (New York: Garland, 1985); Thoms, *Anstaltskost.*

23. Carl Voit, *Ueber die Kost in öffentlichen Anstalten* (München: Oldenbourg 1876); Carl Voit et al., *Untersuchung der Kost in einigen öffentlichen Anstalten* (München: Oldenbourg 1877).

24. Voit et al., *Untersuchung der Kost,* 11.

25. Ibid., 9.

26. Hans J. Teuteberg, "Der Verzehr von Nahrungsmitteln in Deutschland pro Kopf und Jahr seit Beginn der Industrialisierung (1850–1975)," *Archiv für Sozialgeschichte* 19 (1979): 331–88, on 334.

27. Ernst Engel, "Die Productions- und Consumtionsverhältnisse des Königreichs Sachsen." Appendix 1 to Ernst Engel, "Lebenskosten belgischer Arbeiterfamilien früher und jetzt," *Bulletin de l'Institut International de Statistique* 9 (1895): 1–54, on 28, 30.

28. Voit, *Ueber die Kost,* 21. He suggested the carbon needs be covered by 56 grams of fat and 500 grams of starch.

29. Jakob Moleschott, *Die Physiologie der Nahrungsmittel,* 2nd ed. (Gießen: Ferber, 1859); Lyon Playfair, *On the Food of Man in Relation to His Useful Work* (Edinburgh: Edmondston and Douglas, 1865).

30. See Friedrich Wilhelm Beneke, *Zur Ernährungslehre des gesunden Menschen* (Cassel: Kay, 1878).

31. Hamilton C. Bowie, "Ueber den Eiweissbedarf eines mittleren Arbeiters," *Zeitschrift für Biologie* 15 (1879): 459–84, on 466. All translations by EN. Carpenter notes this as well. Carpenter, *Protein and Energy,* 89.

32. Voit, *Ueber die Kost,* 21.

33. Bowie, "Eiweissbedarf," 459.

34. Carroll D. Wright [and W. O. Atwater], "Food Consumption: Quantities, Costs, and Nutrients of Food-Materials," in *17th Annual Report of the Bureau of Statistics of Labor* (Boston: Wright and Potter, 1886), 237–326. For a description of the collaboration, see A. P. Bryant, "Some Results of Dietary Studies in the United States," *Yearbook of the United States Department of Agriculture* (1898): 439–52, on 439–40.

35. For example, M. E. Jaffa, *Nutrition Investigations among Fruitarians and Chinese at the California Agricultural Experiment Station, 1899–1901* (Washington DC: Government Printing Office, 1901); W. O. Atwater and A. Bryant, *Dietary Studies in Chicago in 1895 and 1896* (Washington DC: Government Printing Office, 1896).

36. E. R. L. Gould, *The Social Condition of Labor* (Baltimore, MA: Johns Hopkins University Press, 1893), 32. An alternative method was Engel's proposal of "person units" in the early 1880s. Since Wright was familiar with Engel's work, it is possible that the idea of assessing family members in consumption ratios was suggested to Atwater by Wright. See Ernst Engel, *Das Rechnungsbuch der Hausfrau im Wirtschaftsleben der Nation* (Berlin: L. Simion 1882).

37. Wright and Atwater, "Food Consumption," 266–67.

38. Rubner determined the potential energy in 1 gram of protein, of fat, and of carbohydrate as resp. 4.1, 9.3, and 4.1 calories. Max Rubner, "Calorimetrische Untersuchungen II," *Zeitschrift für Biologie* 21 (1885): 337–410, on 377.

39. Atwater presumably used: Josef König, *Die menschliche Nahrungs- und Genussmittel, ihre Herstellung, Zusammensetzung und Beschaffenheit, ihre Verfälschungen und deren Nachweisung: Mit einer Einleitung über die Ernährungslehre* (Berlin: Springer, 1880). He included heat value in his reanalysis of the survey data in 1891 and in his table of American foodstuffs in 1896. W. O. Atwater, "American and European Dietaries and Dietary Standards," *Fourth Annual Report of the Storrs Agricultural Experiment Station* (1891), 106–61, on 129–30; W. O. Atwater and C. D. Woods,

The Chemical Composition of American Food Materials (Washington DC: Government Printing Office, 1896).

40. Josef Forster, "Beiträge zur Ernährungslehre," *Zeitschrift für Biologie* 9 (1873): 381–10; Voit et al., *Untersuchung der Kost.* Voit summarizes the specialized studies in: Carl Voit, "Physiologie des allgemeinen Stoffwechsels und die Ernährung," in *Handbuch der Physiologie* vol. 6, book 1, ed. L. Hermann (Leipzig: F. C. W. Vogel, 1881), 518–45.

41. W. O. Atwater and C. D. Woods, *Dietary Studies in New York City in 1895 and 1896* (Washington DC: Government Printing Office, 1898), 6.

42. A family consisting of a man, a woman, and eight children of varying ages could be expressed as the equivalent of 6.8 men, and their monthly consumption as equivalent to that of one average worker for two hundred days. Wright and Atwater, "Food Consumption," 299.

43. Both contemporary and recent studies have also pointed to the generally lower food prices in the United States compared with European countries. See Gould, *Social Condition,* 28–29; Trevon D. Logan, "Nutrition and Well-Being in the Late Nineteenth Century," *Journal of Economic History* 66 (2006): 313–41.

44. Wright and Atwater, "Food Consumption," 324–25.

45. Atwater, "American and European Dietaries"; W. O. Atwater, *Methods and Results of Investigations on the Chemistry and Economy of Food* (Washington DC: Government Printing Office, 1895), 141–213.

46. Atwater, "American and European Dietaries," 149.

47. Similar sentiments are expressed in Gould, *Social Condition of Labor.*

48. A. F. Bryant, "Some Results of Dietary Studies in the United Stated," *Yearbook of the United States Department of Agriculture* (1898): 439–52, on 440–41.

49. W. O. Atwater, "Pecuniary Economy of Food: The Chemistry of Foods and Nutrition. V." *Century Magazine* 35 (1887–88): 437–46.

50. Jaffa, *Fruitarians and Chinese;* E. Hultgren and E. Landergren, *Untersuchung über die Ernährung [der wohlhabenderen Stände] bei frei gewählter Kost* (Stockholm: Samson & Wallin, 1889); Luigi Manfredi, "Ueber die Volksernährung in Neapel vom hygienischen Standpunkte," *Archiv für Hygiene* 17 (1893): 552–617; Kintaro Oshima, *A Digest of Japanese Investigations on the Nutrition of Man* (Washington DC: Government Printing Office, 1905); Sigfried Sundström, *Untersuchungen über die Ernährung der Landbevölkerung in Finnland,* Universität Helsingsfors Physiologische Institut, Thesis (doctoral), Kaiserliche Alexanders-Universität in Finnland, 1908; Charles D. Woods and E. R. Mansfield, *Studies of the Food of Maine Lumbermen* (Washington DC: Government Printing Office, 1904).

51. V. O. Siven, "Ueber das Stickstoffgleichgewicht beim erwachsenen Menschen," *Skandinavisches Archiv für Physiologie* 10 (1900): 91–148; Felix Hirschfeld, "Untersuchungen über den Eiweissbedarf des Menschen," *Pflügers Archiv* 41 (1887): 533–65.

52. Russell Henry Chittenden, *The Nutrition of Man* (New York: Frederick A. Stokes, 1907), 159, 165.

53. Russell Chittenden, "Economy in Nutrition" notes (1904), Russell Henry Chittenden Papers, MS611 box 2, folder 28, back of page 1, Manuscripts and Archives, Yale University Library, New Haven, CT.

54. Horace Fletcher, *The New Glutton or Epicure*, 2nd ed. (London: Frederick A. Stokes, 1903); Horace Fletcher, *The A.B.–Z. of Our Own Nutrition* (New York, 1906). On Fletcherism see: Margaret Barnett, "Fletcherism: The Chew-Chew Fad of the Edwardian Era," in *Nutrition in Britain: Science, Scientists and Politics in the Twentieth Century*, ed. David F. Smith (London: Routledge, 1997), 6–28.

55. Russell Henry Chittenden, *Physiological Economy in Nutrition* (New York: Frederick A. Stokes, 1904).

56. See Levenstein, *Revolution*, 90–94.

57. Max Rubner, *Lehrbuch der Hygiene*, 7th ed. (Leipzig: Deuticke, 1903), 473–77; Max Rubner, "Physiologie der Nahrung und Ernährung," in *Handbuch der Ernährungstherapie und Diätetik*, ed. E. v. Leiden, 2nd ed. (Leipzig: Thieme, 1903), 21–161, on 150–55.

58. See Corinna Treitel, "How Vegetarians, Naturopaths, Scientists, and Physicians Unmade the Protein Standard in Modern Germany," chapter 2 of this volume.

59. Max Rubner, "Die Frage des kleinsten Eiweissbedarfs des Menschen," in *Volksernährungsfragen*, ed. Max Rubner (Leipzig: Akademische Verlagsgesellschaft, 1908), 1–143.

60. Rubner, "Die Frage," 16–20. Analyses had shown that it contained 5 percent protein and 95 percent fat and carbohydrate.

61. Rubner, "Die Frage," 34–39.

62. Francesco S. Nitti, "The Food and Labour-Power of Nations," *Economic Journal* 6 (1896): 30–63.

63. Francis Gano Benedict, "The Nutritive Requirements of the Body," *American Journal of Physiology* 16 (1906): 409–37, on 430.

64. Francis Gano Benedict et al., *Human Vitality and Efficiency under Prolonged Restricted Diet* (Washington DC: Government Printing Office, 1919), 3. See also Max Rubner, "Die Nahrungswahl des Menschen," 22, Abteilung III, Repositorium 8, 138/11, Archive of the Max Planck Society, Berlin.

65. Benedict, *Human Vitality*, 3, 37–38.

66. Benedict, *Human Vitality*.

67. Francis Gano Benedict, "Physiological Effects of a Prolonged Reduction in Diet on Twenty-five Men," *Proceedings of the American Philosophical Society* 57 (1918): 479–90, on 485. Benedict plays down the negative effects of this diet in this short summary. The longer monograph presentation shows that the reduced diet had more pervasive effects on the subjects. Benedict concluded himself that the men "underwent profound metabolic changes." Benedict, *Human Vitality*, 687.

68. Benedict, "Physiological Effects," 489.

69. For a characterization of lab and field, the construction of boundaries and overlap, see the outstanding work of Robert Kohler, *Landscapes and Labscapes: Exploring the Lab-Field Border in Biology* (Chicago: University of Chicago Press, 2002).

Chapter Two

How Vegetarians, Naturopaths, Scientists, and Physicians Unmade the Protein Standard in Modern Germany

Corinna Treitel

Introduction

How is biopolitical knowledge made? Encompassing everything from pro- and antinatalist tax policies to antismoking campaigns, biopolitics refers to a wide spectrum of scientifically informed practices that aim to optimize the human resources of modern nations. In recent years, historians have devoted significant effort to understanding the role of scientists, doctors, and social planners in creating and administering biopolitical regimes. In the German context, for instance, scholars have carefully unpacked how ambitious young "genetics doctors" in the 1930s worked in concert with the state to establish research centers and implement policies for assessing and improving the nation's racial fitness.[1] Excellent as this scholarship has been, it has largely assumed something that the following essay questions: that the most important players in modern biopolitical dramas have been technocratic elites working through the state in a largely top-down manner. In this context, modern nutrition science offers many opportunities for expanding how we think about biopolitics. As a field seeking to understand and manage the physical fitness of vast human populations via diet, modern nutrition science is certainly an important example of modern biopolitics, yet one to which historians have devoted little attention. It is, moreover, a particularly instructive field because it has encompassed such a diversity of actors. As we might expect, experimentalists, clinicians, and policymakers played star roles in inventing and implementing nutrition science. More surprisingly, however, lay people with little to no scientific training also participated in this effort and, indeed, often pushed experts to change what they thought they knew about diet. As a field of biopolitical knowledge and practice, in other words, nutrition science has been made by a heterogenous group of players whose dynamics do not follow the top-down model. This essay develops that claim by focusing on a specific episode in the history of nutrition science, the unmaking of the protein standard in late nineteenth- and early twentieth-century Germany, yet also aspires to raise larger methodological questions about how scholars approach the history of biopolitics more generally.

Scholarly accounts of the protein standard typically unfold in three phases:

1. *Enthroning protein.* Building on the discovery of protein, the chemist Justus Liebig "enthroned" protein as the only true nutrient in his 1842 book *Animal Chemistry.* Only protein could make or replace tissue, which meant in turn that only protein, albeit indirectly, could produce physical work. As a concentrated source of protein, moreover, meat was the human nutrient par excellence, a view summed up in the pithy phrase "meat makes meat."
2. *Setting the protein standard.* Protein's enthronement then fueled the quest to set the so-called protein minimum, the minimum amount of daily protein needed by the average German worker to maintain health and vigor. In a series of important public lectures and studies undertaken at hospitals and other public institutions between 1876 and 1881, Carl Voit, a physiologist who had trained in Liebig's laboratory in the 1850s, set the daily amount of protein required for an average working adult eating a "nutritious" meat-based diet at 118 grams.[2]
3. *Overthrowing the protein standard.* Voit's 118-gram standard collapsed at century's turn. Two books—Russell Chittenden's 1904 *Physiological Economy of Nutrition* and Mikkel Hindhede's 1906 *Protein and Nutrition*—marked the end. Their accounts of experiments with low-protein and/or vegetarian diets convinced many researchers that Voit's standard was too high and that the Liebig school had overvalued meat. As Hindhede put it after converting to a meatless diet himself, the "rich protein diet is not only useless but probably harmful."[3]

This scheme works well as a strictly factual account of the rise and fall of the protein standard, but fails to explain the surprising role of vegetarian diets in moving the action along. How did scientists, who frequently and loudly dismissed vegetarians as fanatics and sectarians, overcome their distaste to study vegetarian diets in their labs? How did vegetarianism, a rogue epistemological player in the field of university science, change what scientists thought they knew about protein and meat? What, in short, is vegetarianism doing in the story of the protein standard?

This essay seeks answers by reconstructing the "nutritional networks" through which scientists encountered vegetarian diets. It returns to the mid-nineteenth century to argue that the sudden appearance of vegetarianism after 1900 is an illusion. In fact, vegetarians and scientists had been trading words with each other since at least the 1850s. All had a major stake in the so-called social question of what to do with the poor, but disagreed over what the nation should eat to head off revolution, instill its inhabitants with citizenly virtues, and become an industrial power. Although scientists and lay people largely talked past one another in the 1850s (section 1), continued engagement led by the late 1860s to the emergence of an incipient nutritional network of key figures in increasingly intimate contact with one another (section 2). This network then helped undermine the protein minimum by century's turn, even as the 118-gram standard and all it implied about meat remained the state's prescriptive yardstick (sections 3 and 4). As even this brief sketch suggests, my story is less one of the margins moving the center than a wakeup call to revise the way we think about the history of nutrition in particular, and about the making and unmaking of modern biopolitical programs in general.

Meat and the Social Question

Diet occupied a central place in liberal discussions of the social question in the 1850s, a discussion in which scientists, doctors, and vegetarians all participated avidly.[4] The physiologist Jacob Moleschott kicked off this debate in 1850 when he published *The Science of Food, for the People.* A radical democrat who witnessed the revolutionary consequences of the hungry forties, Moleschott made access to good food a liberal imperative, arguing that an adequate diet freed and civilized both individuals and societies. Historians have justifiably attended to Moleschott's efforts on this front, but inexplicably ignored the larger conversation about diet that he catalyzed.[5] Two figures in particular deserve mention here: the doctor and "professor" Hermann Klencke and the Swiss naturopath Theodor Hahn. Both Klencke, who was not a vegetarian, and Hahn, who was, agreed that diet grounded the social question, but took Moleschott and his academic colleagues to task for assuming that its best foundation was meat.

Born in poverty and trained as an army doctor, Klencke aspired to earn academic credentials at the university. Blocked from achieving this goal, he simply assumed several titles, including "professor," and built a national reputation as a leading medical reformer, scientific popularizer, and historical novelist in the years before 1848.[6] Given this track record, it is perhaps not surprising that Klencke decided to intervene in the dietary debate unleashed by Moleschott. In his 1855 *The Food Question in Germany,* one of the most important dietary treatises of the century, Klencke aimed "to guide practical men so far as possible to balance appropriateness and economy . . . in their food needs and production, and to obtain a real benefit for human lifestyle, agriculture, and cooking through the influence of natural science." Acknowledging that humans were usually omnivorous, Klencke also argued at length that a meatless diet could be nutritionally adequate and economically much more rational (that is, cheaper) than a meat-based one. Indeed, Klencke's political sympathies came out clearly in his scathing critique of the nutritional economy. Why was so much arable German land devoted to producing nutritionally worthless products like sugar beets, beer hops, and potatoes destined for the distillery? Why were the fields around factories used for grazing cattle that could provide meat only for the owner and his family while leaving the "crying masses" hungry? Arable land, Klencke declared, should be sown instead with pulses and legumes—"the meat and milk of the plant world"—to provide cheap and nutritious food for all.[7]

Also addressing himself to "the people," Theodor Hahn set out in his influential *The Natural Diet, the Diet of the Future* (1859) "to break new ground in the field of dietetic physiology." Taking aim at "new physiologists" such as Moleschott, Hahn declared that the best diet was the natural diet: one that was "pure, simple, unadulterated and unchanged from God's hand," lacking in meat and other stimulants (alcohol, spices, etc.), and eaten in moderation. Nor did Hahn neglect the social and political aspects of diet. To those who saw meat as essential to the progress of civilization, Hahn replied, "If we banned meat from the European table and fed instead ten or twenty million proletarians (destitute because of the meaty diet of the rich and educated), we would have field hands, factory workers, and urban laborers feasting on bread and fruit rather than being consumed with communist desires!"[8]

As all of this suggests, by the late 1850s meat and the social question had become part of a liberal discourse being conducted "for the people" by figures both in and out of academic circles. University-based scientists like Moleschott assumed that boosting meat consumption held an important key to the social question, whereas lay commentators concerned with moral or economic categories of "natural" or "rational" questioned that very assumption. Would a meat or meatless diet best optimize the human resources of the nation? In 1860, this question had yet to be settled as players only dimly aware of one another began to stake out competing positions.

Setting the Protein Standard in Context

In the 1860s to 1870s, as Voit and his collaborators moved toward the 118-gram standard, scientists and lay people continued to debate the question of what to eat in an ever more intimate fashion. But if the reference point of the 1850s had been the hungry forties and the unresolved political questions of 1848, the new context of discussion in the 1860s was unification, industrialization, and what these meant for Germany's emergence as a great European power. What should Germans eat? The answer hinged, at least in part, on who Germans wanted to become.

Whereas Moleschott, a physiologist, had catalyzed the discussion in the 1850s, a vegetarian, Eduard Baltzer, kicked off the next round of this debate in 1867 when he published the first two volumes of his *The Natural Lifestyle*.[9] The leader of a radical Protestant sect known as the *Lichtfreunde* (Friends of Light), Baltzer became a prominent republican in the Prussian revolution of 1848, then faced state persecution in the 1850s. In the 1860s, he reemerged as a crusader for interfaith dialogue, German democracy, and a vegetarian diet, to which he converted after reading Hahn's *The Natural Diet.* Vegetarianism, he argued, promoted health, happiness, and mental acuity, saved time, energy, and money, and helped prevent war and bloodshed. Most important, he insisted, the vegetarian diet held the solution to the social question. Transposing the language of revolutionary republicanism from politics to diet, Baltzer extolled the virtues of vegetarianism with the following words:

> Through [the vegetarian diet] we learn to own and use the invaluable possession of greater personal independence, especially in economic and civic (*bürgerlich*) relations, [an independence] that is the foundation of all humane living and the only liberation. The more artificial our needs are, especially in food, the more they will be distorted by human greed. . . . The vegetarian return to simplicity relieves us from striving after pure moneymaking and no one throws away his life's work on professions that are trivial or even harmful to the public good.[10]

Devoting hundreds of pages to a thorough critique of the nation's consumption habits, Baltzer concluded that by simplifying human needs, the vegetarian diet would produce citizens who could govern themselves politically as well. For Baltzer, in short, a vegetarian diet was the nutritional foundation of a future German republic.

Much more intellectually sophisticated than Hahn and with impeccably left liberal credentials to boot, Baltzer drew the ire of three of Germany's leading crusaders for science and liberalism: Rudolf Virchow, Otto Funke, and Carl Ernst Bock.[11] In a public lecture delivered before a Berlin workers' association in 1867, for instance, Virchow flagged a meat-containing diet as central to the social question:

> The getting and preparing of food grounds all human activity to such a great extent that not only the individual but society and the state are also determined by them . . . it would be a great mistake if one were to forget that in the tangled relations between modern society and the state the food question is always the first and most important one . . . that in [the food question] is rooted the feared social question. Bread and meat, sugar and salt, beer and wine, tobacco and coffee, these are the mighty resources on which the welfare and prosperity of the greatest states rest, and often through their availability or scarcity quiet and order, peace and harmony are maintained or disrupted.

Of particular public concern, Virchow noted, was the question of whether "meat, apparently the most natural substitute for our own flesh, is really nothing more than the carrier of putrefaction and death in our body?" A direct reference to the writings of Hahn and Baltzer, this comment also set the frame for his discussion of dietary politics. Dismissing the meatless diet "as one of the worst and most unnatural errors of the human race," Virchow used evidence from anatomy, anthropology, and history to argue that vegetarian claims about the "naturalness" of their diet were both unscientific and harmful to the public good. Pointing out that "the highest achievements of the human race come from nations that eat and have eaten a mixed diet," Virchow led his listeners to the inescapable conclusion that Germany would have to become a nation of meat eaters to become a great power.[12]

Both Baltzer and Hahn responded quickly to this physiological critique. In his *Letters to Virchow about His Essay* (1868), Baltzer thanked Virchow for becoming the first scientist to engage respectfully with the vegetarian position, but criticized him for ignoring his own evidence that many peoples in the world had thrived for generations on a meatless diet. The real problem, Baltzer noted, was that scientists and vegetarians alike suffered from a dearth of facts. In a call that would become common in this conversation between meat-avoiding lay people and meat-extolling scientists, Baltzer invited Virchow and his colleagues to test vegetarian diets in the laboratory so as to erect once and for all a "stringently scientific diet."[13]

Not to be outdone, Hahn and Klencke also stepped into the fray. Lambasting Virchow and other liberal professors as "princes of science," Hahn faulted all of them for assuming what needed to be investigated. Was a mixed diet featuring meat really the best diet? The quantitative evidence was nowhere to be found. Nor did he buy the claim, widely reprinted in the scientific literature, that a meatless diet produced weak and slavish peoples. The meat-eating Germans certainly loved war, he pointed out tartly, but who in 1869 could accuse them of loving freedom?[14]

For his part, Klencke took a position that would eventually become the consensus view by century's turn. Invited by a popular journal to provide an evaluation of this debate, Klencke strived to maintain strict neutrality on the question of whether meat belonged in the human diet. Instead, he investigated the merits and demerits of both positions. The hostility shown by university-trained scientists, he speculated, reflected their conservative reluctance to cede power to lay people as well as their slavish adherence to bourgeois mores. Meat had become part of the modern "luxury kitchen," eaten less for reasons of nourishment than taste and fashion. Germans seemed blind to the fact that in times of socioeconomic stress humans became "forced vegetarians" with no harm to their vigor or longevity. Claims about the "naturalness" of the vegetarian diet might be spurious, he conceded, but vegetarians had shown that their lifestyle had undeniable benefits. Did Germans eat too much meat to the detriment of themselves and the nation? And what made the vegetarian diet so healthful? Klencke urged scientists to put these questions to the test.[15]

By the time the furor over Baltzer's books died down in the early 1870s, scientists, vegetarians, and lay commentators had not agreed on meat's dietary value, but they had begun an exchange that would continue into the twentieth century. A common class background in the educated bourgeoisie, a common politically liberal outlook, and a common stake in the nutritional aspects of the social question facilitated their conversation. So, too, did the emergence of a national press and national venues in which they could air their disagreements before a German public. This emerging "nutritional network" did not settle the question of what Germans should eat, but it did make clear that a great diversity of players had a stake in this struggle for the stomach of the nation.

Challenging the Protein Standard

The experiential knowledge of lay reformers and the experimental knowledge of laboratory scientists evolved together. Lay reformers had always shaped their claims about the benefits of natural diets in relation to natural science, most obviously by co-opting the chemical language of proteins, fats, and carbohydrates that emerged in the 1830s and then by adding the physical language of calories in the 1880s. They had also repeatedly called scientists out for making unfounded claims about the role of meat and protein in human nutrition. Co-optation and calling out, however, also worked in the opposite direction. Physiologists took careful note of what vegetarians claimed to be achieving with their odd diet. They puzzled over how to explain, or explain away, the health and vigor of lay reformers while also criticizing them for being unscientific in their outlook. From the 1880s until at least the First World War, reformers and researchers engaged in a lively, if not always gracious, exchange of ideas and practices that resulted in a fundamental shift in the way that experts thought about meat and protein and their role in human diet. And because experts also had the ear of the state, changes in what physiologists thought they knew had immediate relevance to *Volksernährung* (public nutrition), a vast new arena of biopolitical action.

This dynamic of co-opting and calling out emerges with particular clarity in the story of the protein standard, set in the 1870s by the physiologist Carl Voit and then overturned in the early twentieth century by a heterogeneous group of scientists and laymen. As the following two sections detail, German experts set the terms of debate, but other actors—especially German vegetarians and Japanese physicians studying German medicine—drove the conversation to its outcome. The story of the protein standard, indeed, suggests that modern biopolitical knowledge is made and unmade not just in a top-down diffusionist manner, but also in a bottom-up or perhaps more simply "sideways" fashion as different groups confront a common problem together—in this case, "what should we eat?"

Carl Voit unwittingly initiated the debate over protein in the 1870s when he recommended that an average German worker eat no less than 118 grams of protein each day. A professor at the University of Munich, Voit had made a name for himself as a world expert on metabolism and nutrition. His reputation was based in no small part on his technical success in developing and using an apparatus that could measure precisely what a research subject took in and put out, whether oxygen, water, and food, or carbonic dioxide, urine, feces, and sweat. By carefully controlling and comparing intake with output, Voit and his collaborators set the fledgling science of nutrition on a solid laboratory footing.[16]

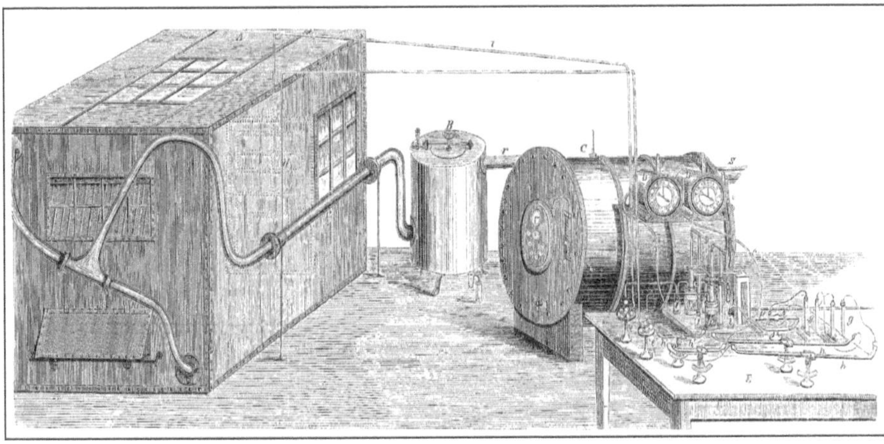

Figure 2.1. Pettenkofer-Voit Respiration Apparatus. In Elie de Cyon, *Atlas zur Methodik der Physiologischen Experimente und Vivisectionen* (Giessen, Germany: Carl Ricker, 1876), 30. Max Planck Institute for the History of Science, http://vlp.mpiwg-berlin.mpg.de/technology/data?id=tec209 (accessed October 28, 2011).

His status as an experimentalist established, Voit expanded in the 1870s to research with more direct social applications. A study of what healthy German workers ate every day became the basis for Voit's prescription about what the average German worker *should* eat. This amounted to 118 grams of protein, 500 grams of carbohydrates, and 56 grams of fat every day, with half of the protein coming from animal sources, preferably meat. Presented in 1875 at a medical congress in Munich, these standards were of immediate interest to Voit's audience, which consisted mostly of doctors and civil servants charged with running prisons, hospitals, public kitchens, and other sites of mass feeding.[17] The 118-gram protein standard received particular attention because protein was considered the human nutrient par excellence, essential for building muscle and enabling the body's physical labor. Because meat was widely held to be one of the most concentrated and easily digestible sources of dietary protein available, moreover, Voit's 118-gram standard became virtually inseparable from support for a meaty diet. Meat makes muscle, the thinking went, and Voit's 118-gram standard with its implicit privileging of meat quickly became the yardstick for evaluating diets across the industrializing world.[18] In Germany, the official *Gesundheitsbüchlein* (Health booklet) disseminated the standard widely and its color-coded chart of "nutritive values" became ubiquitous in popular nutritional culture.[19]

But just as Voit's 118-gram standard was climbing to prominence, so too were natural diets beginning to pique the interest of natural scientists. The physiologist Traugott Cramer, for instance, read the vegetarian treatises of Sylvester Graham, the doctor Anna Kingsford, the naturopath F. W. Dock, and the botanist Leonhard Baltzer (son of Eduard Baltzer) with increasing dismay. Concerned that the unfounded claims being made by lay advocates might prompt an ignorant public to alter its diet for the worse, Cramer invited a sixty-four-year-old vegetarian male into his laboratory for a three-day study in 1882.[20] Although forced to admit that the diet nourished his subject adequately and cheaply, Cramer nonetheless concluded that a vegetarian diet remained "an eminently impractical method for feeding the masses, since one can produce for the same price a much greater quantity of mixed and thus more digestible food."[21] Cramer may have hoped to end debate there, but a younger generation of physiologists refused to let the matter rest. Gustav Bunge, a *Privatdozent* (junior lecturer) at the University of Basel, took the lead in 1885 in a public lecture simply titled "Vegetarianism."[22] "Laughing is indeed easier than thinking," he admonished his academic audience, but "neither a scientific rejection of nor scientific justification for [the vegetarian] doctrine has yet been attempted." Based on his reading of the major vegetarian works, Bunge admitted, the anatomical, historical, and ethical reasons offered to justify the diet were scientifically worthless. Still, the scientist within him could not ignore the obvious. Vegetarians are healthy and vigorous, Bunge pointed out, and we do not know why. His own hypothesis was that vegetarians owed their health less to avoiding meat than to refraining from alcohol, but whatever the reason, Bunge concluded, it was high time for scientists to study the undeniable benefits of vegetarian diets in their labs.[23]

The first vegetarian to walk through the door opened by Bunge was August Aderholdt, a close collaborator of Eduard Baltzer. Doubtful about the 118-gram standard and what it implied about meat, Aderholdt contacted Voit in 1889 about working with a local vegetarian volunteer. Without bothering to read any publications by lay reformers, Voit proclaimed that "only an experimental study is able to decide the matter," thereby co-opting vegetarianism as a purely physiological matter, and accepted the offer. He proceeded to conduct two experiments: one on the volunteer Leopold Grün, a twenty-eight-year-old paper hanger who ate his normal diet of cold vegetables, whole grain bread, raw fruit, and oil, and the other on an employee who was normally a meat eater but ate Grün's diet for the study.[24] Whereas Grün comfortably maintained nitrogen balance and continued his physically demanding job with only 54 grams of protein each day, the normally carnivorous employee found the large volume of Grün's diet unpleasant to digest and indeed showed an overall protein loss.[25] Could workers maintain health and vigor on such a diet? Voit admitted that under strict laboratory conditions the answer for Grün must be yes, but he doubted that these results were generalizable or even sustainable by Grün over the long term. The issue, Voit speculated, was protein rather than meat. Japanese, Italian, and Bavarian peasants all performed hard physical labor on what was effectively a vegetarian diet, he reasoned, but its generous use of dairy made it a high-protein one. The exclusively plant-based diet of urban vegetarians such as Grün, in contrast, contained dangerously little protein and required eating in large volume, which led to frequent and uncomfortable bowel movements. Practically speaking, he concluded, a vegetarian diet of this kind was eminently unsuitable for the general population.[26] When the results were published in Voit's own journal, the *Zeitschrift für Biologie*, adherents of the natural lifestyle were predictably incensed. To Voit's admission that Grün seemed healthy and fit, for instance, the editors of *Die neue Heilkunst* (a naturopathic-vegetarian journal associated with Louis Kuhne) commented sarcastically: "Yeah, yeah, science is making progress. If this continues, it will next determine that circles are round, triangles three-sided, and rectangles four-sided, never mind that blue is blue and red red."[27]

Voit's experiments with Grün may not have yielded the conclusion that Aderholdt and other reformers wanted, but three more studies published in 1889 cast further doubt on the 118-gram standard. That all three studies brought a distinctively Japanese perspective to German debates over protein, moreover, signaled a new demographic dimension to the German life sciences. Japan entered the debate as a result of professional exchange between modernizing Japanese reformers and their German advisers. Young Japanese doctors had begun flocking to Germany in the 1860s to study Western medicine, physiology, and chemistry as part of a push by the Meiji state to build Japan into the world's first non-European great power.[28] At the same time, German scientists took up academic positions in Japan, mostly at the newly founded University of Tokyo.[29] With the fresh eyes of those encountering radically different dietary norms, both sets of researchers began to question the very same assumptions about meat and protein that German vegetarians had already begun to raise. At stake were questions of great national import: Did the Japanese diet contain enough protein? Should meat and bread displace rice and fish on the table of the Japanese soldier? Should the Japanese masses, who ate much rice but little to no fish, change too? Should Japan, in short, "Europeanize" its diet? Germans and Japanese alike went to the laboratory to find out.

Written by Oscar Kellner and Y. Mori and published in the same issue of the *Zeitschrift für Biologie* as Voit's article about Grün, the first study endorsed an orientalized version of Voit's standard for Japan. The common Western view that the Japanese diet was "almost vegetarian" and by implication insufficient had galvanized the two researchers into action. Both worked at the University of Tokyo. Kellner, a professor of animal nutrition, had been there since 1881, and Mori, his twenty-three-year-old lab assistant and research subject, was a local.[30] Mori tried three diets for six days each:

1. A vegetarian diet of rice, miso, tofu, soy sauce, and vegetables typically eaten by poorer Japanese workers inland, containing 71 grams of protein.
2. The same diet supplemented with a little fish, typically eaten by workers with more money or access to waterways, containing 109 grams of protein.
3. A German-style diet with beef and dairy, containing 123 grams of protein.

Based on Mori's inability to maintain nitrogen balance in the first experiment, the researchers concluded that the vegetarian Japanese diet was inadequate. However, based on the results of the second and third experiments, they concluded that the mixed diets, in both Japanese and German form, were. Having opened the door to Western diets rich in beef and dairy, however, the authors quickly closed it on the basis of cost concerns and instead recommended the mixed Japanese diet that included fish as most appropriate for mass feeding. By raising concerns about the adequacy of the forced vegetarianism of most Japanese while also endorsing an "orientalized" version of Voit's standard for these same Japanese masses, Kellner and Mori had remade Western prescriptions for East Asian bodies.[31]

The Japanese physician Toichiri Nakahama, however, refused to let the matter rest. Son of the famed Manjiro Nakahama, one of the first Japanese to make contact with the United States, Nakahama had been sent by his government in the 1880s to study at the University of Leipzig. Bothered by the discrepancy between scientific claims about defects in the Japanese diet and the simple observation that Japanese workers were healthy and fit, Nakahama used his post at the Physiological Institute in Leipzig to put the matter to experimental scrutiny.[32] Using himself and twelve German laborers, Nakahama found that with both low meat and fully vegetarian diets averaging 85 grams of protein each day, everyone maintained full mental and physical vigor. Since Japanese workers typically ate a comparable amount of protein, Nakahama concluded that Japanese diets in both vegetarian and mixed forms were perfectly nutritious. In an 1889 article published in the *Archiv für Hygiene*, moreover, he asserted boldly that Japan had no need to embrace "Western" foods. This was not the orientalized endorsement that Kellner and Mori had given Voit's standard, but neither was it yet an explicit challenge to the Western yardstick. To be sure, Nakahama implied that Voit's standard might be too high, but declined to pursue the matter further.[33]

A third Japanese researcher, Muneo Kumagawa, had no such qualms about openly challenging Voit's standard. Sent by his government in the 1880s to study at Rudolf Virchow's Pathology Institute in Berlin, Kumagawa took himself as a research subject. Over several weeks, he ate a series of "European" (mixed, with beef and pork), "Japanese" (mixed, with fish), and "Japanese vegetarian" diets and concluded, like Nakahama, that the last diet was perfectly nutritious and that Japanese workers had no need to change their ways. In the article published later that year in *Virchows Archiv*, moreover, Kumagawa used his research to turn the tables on Voit. With only 54.7 grams of daily protein intake and a net nitrogen gain, he pointed out, his own body had shown that Voit's 118-gram standard was much too high.[34] If Kellner and Mori had adapted a Western yardstick for Japanese use, Kumagawa broke the yardstick and threw the pieces back at his German hosts.

Taken together, these four studies from 1889 signaled a shift in nutritional research. For one thing, they raised sensitive questions about existing standards. Voit may have declined to see the obvious—that 118 grams of protein might be too high, that meat might not be crucial—but other researchers were intrigued. As the physician Felix Hirschfeld put it that year, the Japanese researchers had posed a "great riddle." According to Voit's standard, the vegetarian Japanese diet was inadequate, yet those living on it, the majority of the Japanese population, were healthy and fit. How was this possible? His own hunch was that Voit had drastically overshot the true protein minimum. It was not the Japanese diet, he speculated, but nutritional knowledge about the human diet that was at fault.[35] The four studies of 1889 also marked the entry of a new type of diet to the science of nutritional physiology. Virtually ignored before 1889, vegetarian diets now became the object of frequent study and publication in Germany's main biomedical journals. The *Zeitschrift für Biologie*, founded and edited by Carl Voit, carried Voit's study of Grün as well as the article by Kellner and Mori. Nakahama published in the *Archiv für Hygiene*, founded and edited by Max Pettenkofer, Germany's leading hygienist as well as Voit's collaborator. And Kumagawa published in *Virchows Archiv*, founded and edited by Rudolf Virchow, Germany's top pathologist and a well-known liberal politician to boot. A more illustrious set of journals or editors could hardly be imagined. These journals had set the agenda for German research in the life sciences, and these scientists were advising the German state on everything from sanitation and forensic science to laboratory medicine and mass feeding. Finally, these four studies ushered in new types of people to the German research enterprise, whether as subjects (Japanese workers, German vegetarians) or as investigators (Japanese), yet incorporated them in different ways.[36] German researchers such as Voit and Kellner may have deigned to study vegetarian diets in their labs, but they never became research subjects themselves; German vegetarians, for their part, entered the laboratory as research subjects, but never became investigators. The Japanese, in contrast, did both. They were, of course, not simply doing science but also using science to defend Japanese foodways, either by showing that they confirmed Voit's standards in an oriental setting (Mori) or by casting doubts on the universality of Voit's standards altogether (Nakahama, Kumagawa). But the pattern was larger than Japan, for in the years ahead an uncrossable line between German vegetarians and German researchers persisted, while non-German researchers proved willing to become vegetarians in order to prove with their bodies that the 118-gram standard was flawed. By 1889, in short, new diets and new people in the laboratories of German nutritional physiology had raised enduring questions about Voit's yardstick.

Toppling the Protein Standard

The research that finally broke the consensus among German physiologists about the 118-gram standard came, once again, from a diverse group of outsiders: German vegetarians, German researchers working in satellite institutions, and non-Germans. The process began in 1899, when V. O. Sivén, a Finnish researcher working at a physiological laboratory in Stockholm, conducted a series of experiments on himself. Intrigued by Kumagawa's findings, Sivén tried a low-meat, low-protein diet and found that for at least a short time he could sustain himself well with just 28.3 grams of daily protein. Two years later, he reached the same conclusion with a series of vegetarian diets containing even less protein.[37] In Germany, academics working far from the leading institutes of nutritional research in Munich, Leipzig, and Berlin bowed to pressure from the vegetarians. In Hamburg, for instance, a local vegetarian named Paul Ortmann showed up at a popular medical lecture given by Theodor Rumpf, a professor of medicine at the university. After listening politely while Rumpf extolled the benefits of meat and protein, Ortmann rose to offer his own body, healthy and vigorous yet nourished with no meat and little protein, as counterevidence meriting laboratory investigation. Intrigued, Rumpf teamed up with the medical chemist Otto Schumm to study the matter further and was amazed to find that Ortmann maintained health and vigor and even gained nitrogen on less than 74 grams of plant protein per day.[38] In Berlin, meanwhile, the physician Albert Albu concocted a new kind of study that followed vegetarians in real life. Long interested in the lively local vegetarian scene, Albu jumped at the chance in 1901 to work with a female vegetarian who was auditing courses at the University of Berlin.[39] Although he held a position as a *Privatdozent* at the Physiological Institute, Albu eschewed the laboratory, relying instead on his scientifically literate vegetarian to collect real-life data about her own intake and output. The results showed that this woman got by on just 34 grams of protein per day. Rumpf, Schumm, and Albu all concluded that a low-protein vegetarian diet could cover the needs of a working body adequately, yet concurred, as Albu put it, that for now the diet should remain "only a child of necessity." Bland and monotonous, it had to be eaten in uncomfortably large volume and often produced gas, making it unsuitable for mass feeding. Expressing a disdain widely shared among experts, moreover, Albu closed with the comment that "we must . . . deny vegetarians credit for having drawn general conclusions about human nutrition from their experiences, which have been poor, personal, immature, and incorrectly understood."[40]

Even this cautious endorsement of the vegetarian diet encountered skepticism from an entire generation of physicians who had been schooled in Voit's standard. This became clear in 1901, when Albu, still a *Privatdozent*, presented a paper entitled "An Assessment of the Vegetarian Diet" at a meeting of the Berlin Medical Society presided over by none other than Rudolf Virchow. Albu's bald assertion that Voit's standard might be as much as 30 percent too high provoked a lively debate.[41] Ernst Grawitz, a professor of medicine at the University of Berlin, worried that Albu had given the vegetarian "fanatics" a tool for propagating their cause and asserted that cases like Albu's female vegetarian notwithstanding, the normal body required more protein, especially from meat. The only two physicians who came to Albu's defense were also outsiders: Erwin Baelz, a retired professor of medicine who had been at the University of Tokyo since 1876, and Karl Bornstein, who was just emerging as a pioneer of German social hygiene. Baelz was a particularly interesting case because although he belonged to an older generation, he had vast experience of the non-German world. In a full-length paper supporting Albu's claims, indeed, Baelz blasted European scientists for their irrational prejudice against vegetarians. Too rooted in their own cultural frame to see the facts clearly, he scolded, Voit and his followers had simply taken their own diet as the world standard.[42] These studies and comments by Sivén, Rumpf, Schumm, Albu, Baelz, and Bornstein hardly gave a ringing endorsement to German vegetarians, but nonetheless co-opted vegetarian diets to pursue a scientific agenda that overlapped considerably with that of lay reformers.

The studies that finally confirmed the nutritional value and everyday practicality of low-protein vegetarian diets, the very opposite of Voit's prescription for a high-protein, meat-based diet, came in a burst from 1903 onward. In the United States, the American lay reformer Horace Fletcher convinced Russell Chittenden, a German-trained professor of physiology at Yale, to study his meatless diet. Dismissing Fletcher's vegetarianism as unscientific, Chittenden nonetheless suspected that Fletcher's health and vigor stemmed from his low-protein diet and put this hypothesis to the test in a series of very elaborate experiments with almost meatless diets in which he himself participated. His conclusion that 60 grams of daily protein, from either plant or animal sources, could sustain "physiological economy in nutrition" was a direct strike against Voit's standard.[43] In Denmark, the physician Mikkel Hindhede came to the same conclusion by experimenting on himself and his family. Both distanced themselves from the outlandish claims of lay reformers, whom they knew either personally or through their writings, so as to more effectively co-opt and rebrand lay discoveries as their own. And in Berlin, in two studies published in 1903 and 1905, Wilhelm Caspari became the first German physiologist to assert without caveats that one could exist healthfully and practically on less than 30 grams of protein per day, all of it from plant sources. Caspari may have been a physiologist, but he was merely a *Privatdozent* and did his research not at the Physiological Institute associated with the University of Berlin but at the second-tier Institute for Animal Physiology associated with a newly established Königliche landwirtschaftliche Hochschule (Royal Agricultural College).[44] Caspari's research was symptomatic of the convergence that had finally been achieved between lay reformers and scientific experts. Not only were his research subjects prominent members and even leaders of the German vegetarian movement, but he allowed them to appear in his published articles as themselves, that is, as robust subjects with both voices and bodies.[45] This was particularly evident in his 1905 article, published in *Pflügers Archiv,* where he gave his research subject, an army officer in his fifties, a full twelve pages in which to explain his diet, provide a medical autobiography, and air his critique of contemporary health practices. Scientists and physicians, the vegetarian wrote, should study the techniques and successes of naturopaths and other lay reformers rather than arrogantly dismiss them without cause. "Vegetarianism opens a new and valuable bright spot in the physiology and therapy of the future," he wrote, "and is thus a source of new pathbreaking truths that deserve to be studied thoroughly. This is something that

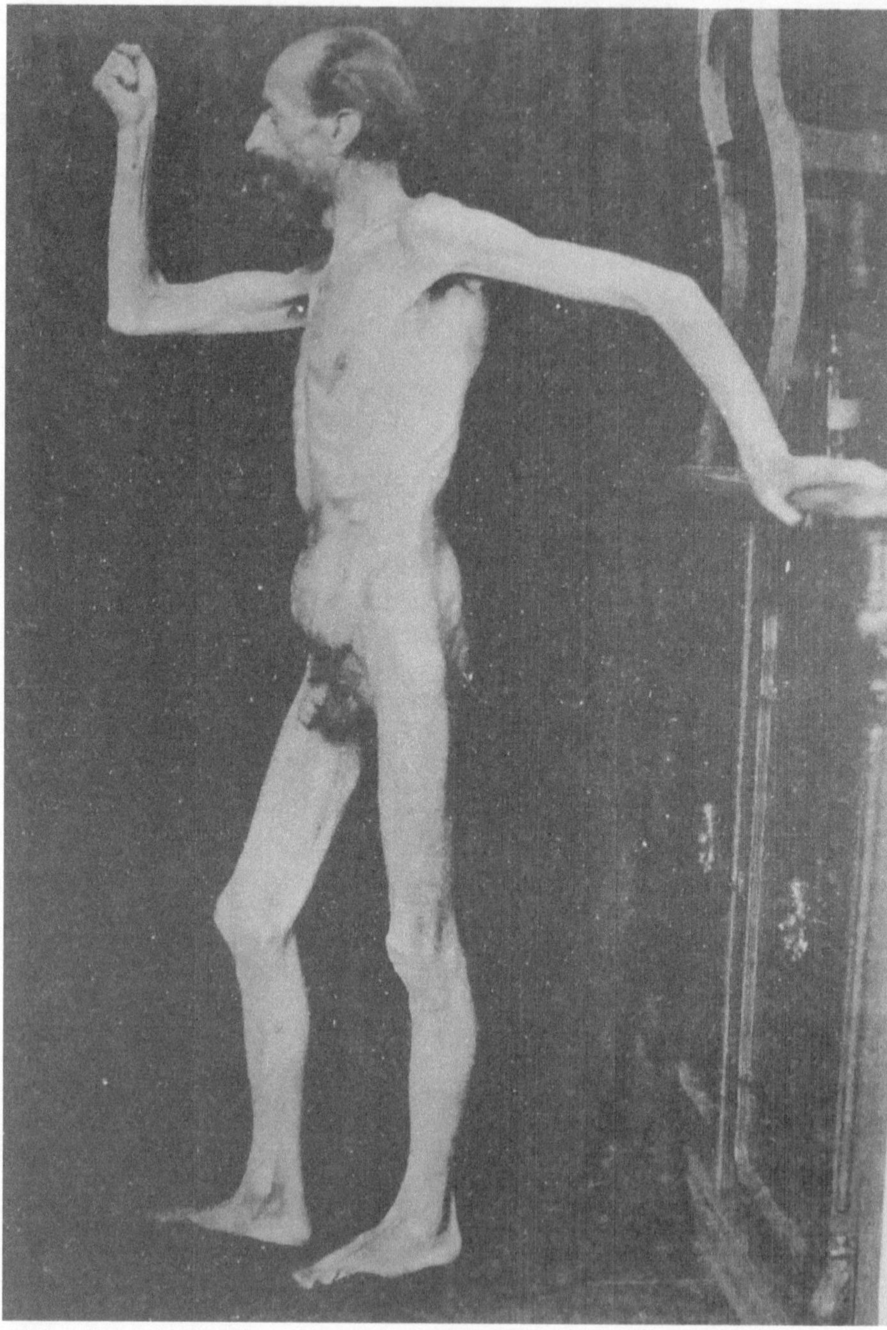

Figure 2.2. "Herr Hauptmann H at the End of the Trial." Note the full beard, a mark of health and masculinity. Dr. W. Caspari, "Physiologische Studien über Vegetarismus," *Pflügers Archiv für die gesammte Physiologie des Menschen und der Thiere* 109 (1905): Tafel 9.

one learns best through unbroken self-observation of one's own body, namely, through regularly observing and investigating one's own urine and feces." Nude photos of the officer taken at the end of the nearly three-month-long study, moreover, showed a very thin man whose full beard and well-developed muscles testified to his physical fitness.

Caspari confirmed the vegetarian's robust masculinity, indeed, when he reported that the officer had spent his days working out in the gym, writing essays, doing mathematical exercises, and translating from Latin, French, and English before finally emerging at the end of the study to wrestle several of Germany's leading physiologists, including Nathan Zuntz, to the ground.[46] Zuntz, indeed, provided a fitting end to the story of the protein standard in his 1909 *Textbook of Human Physiology*. After reviewing the literature on human protein needs, Zuntz bypassed Voit's standard to recommend that adults not go below an intake of 80 grams of protein a day. Then he added a surprising follow-up that would have warmed the hearts of Hahn, Klencke, Baltzer, and countless others who were now long dead. "If one chooses well," he wrote, "this amount of protein can be met very well with vegetables alone."[47]

Conclusion

The unmaking of the protein standard reveals a dynamic of co-optation and critique in the making of modern biopolitical knowledge. Indeed, the wide variety of players seems to have fostered this dynamic. Voit, Rubner, König, and other prominent professors of physiology developed the epistemological, technological, and institutional foundations of modern nutrition science and controlled the prescriptions and tools of dissemination that codified the 118-gram standard. Yet from the 1880s onward, other epistemological players—lay reformers, physicians, junior lecturers, and non-Germans—penetrated the terrain of nutritional physiology both by force and by invitation. These new players challenged the 118-gram standard from a wide variety of perspectives and for a wide variety of reasons, yet all shared a commitment to bringing experience and experiment into line with each other. The experience of Japanese workers with low-protein diets prompted Japanese physicians to conduct important experiments in the 1880s that brought Voit's standard into question. Similarly, the experience of vegetarians with low-protein diets prompted researchers both in and out of Germany to conduct experiments in the early twentieth century that further undermined the protein standard and all it implied about meat. And finally, although lay reformers and experts certainly both deserve credit for unmaking the protein standard, they were never really collaborators. Scientists repeatedly co-opted the experience of lay reformers by declaring the laboratory as the only legitimate site for the production of knowledge. Yet lay reformers also co-opted the laboratory in order to force their own experiences into the sightline of German experts. In this back and forth of critique and co-optation, biopolitical knowledge—understood both as what is produced in a laboratory as well as what is revealed by one's own bodily experience—emerged as the result of exchange between different players pursuing different agendas in response to a single question of massive biopolitical import: What should we eat?

All of this has a bearing on how we think about biopolitics in general. Historians, I think, are still too inclined to invoke a simple Foucauldian model that frames biopolitical programs as sinister top-down affairs foisted off by experts on the unsuspecting masses. On this front, the unmaking of the protein standard provides a cautionary tale. Lay people also create, follow, and persuade others to follow biopolitical programs, and their views and practices can and do alter expert opinion. This episode shows that new ideas and practices can "trickle sideways" from lay circles into expert opinion and official policy.[48] And this, in turn, suggests that we need to look well beyond doctors and scientists to write the history of modern biopolitics properly.

Notes

1. This topic has garnered a vast scholarly literature. See, for instance, Robert Proctor, *Racial Hygiene: Medicine under the Nazis* (Cambridge, MA: Harvard University Press, 1989); Hans-Walter Schmuhl, *The Kaiser Wilhelm Institute for Anthropology, Human Heredity, and Eugenics 1927–1945* (Dordrecht: Springer, 2008); and Sheila Faith Weiss, *The Nazi Symbiosis: Human Genetics and Politics in the Third Reich* (Chicago: University of Chicago Press, 2010). For an important rethinking of the German case, see Edward Ross Dickinson, "Biopolitics, Fascism, Democracy: Some Reflections on Our Discourse about 'Modernity,'" *Central European History* 37 (2004): 1–48.

2. In the 1890s, Wilbur Atwater, who had worked with Voit and Max Rubner in Munich, raised this standard for American workers to 125 grams. Kenneth J. Carpenter, *Protein and Energy: A Study of Changing Ideas in Nutrition* (Cambridge: Cambridge University Press, 1994), 105.

3. Mikkel Hindhede, *Eine Reform unserer Ernährung: Lebe gesund! Lebe kräftig! Lebe billig!* (Leipzig: K. F. Koehler, 1908), 177. Unless otherwise noted, all translations from the German are my own. For historical accounts of the protein standard, see Carpenter, *Protein and Energy*, chaps. 3–6; Sabine Merta, *Wege und Irrwege zum modernen Schlankheitskunst: Diätkost und Körperkultur als Suche nach neuen Lebenstilformen 1880–1930* (Wiesbaden: Franz Steiner Verlag, 2003), 153–62 and 190–96; and Ulrike Thoms, *Anstaltskost im Rationalisierungsprozeß: Die Ernährung in Krankenhäusern und Gefängnissen im 18. und 19. Jahrhundert* (Stuttgart: Franz Steiner, 2005), 345–48, 356.

4. For liberalism and science in this period, see Andreas Daum, *Wissenschaftspopularisierung im 19. Jahrhundert: Bürgerliche Kultur, naturwissenschaftliche Bildung und die deutsche Öffentlichkeit 1848–1914* (Munich: R. Oldenbourg, 2002).

5. Harmke Kamminga, "Nutrition for the People, or the Fate of Jacob Moleschott's Contest for a Humanist Science," in *The Science and Culture of Nutrition, 1840s–1940s*, ed. Harmke Kamminga and Andrew Cunningham (Amsterdam: Rodopi, 1995), 15–47. Jacob Moleschott, *Lehre der Nahrungsmittel, für das Volk* (Erlangen: Ferdinand Enke, 1850).

6. See Hermann Klencke, *Das deutsche Gespenst* (Leipzig: Wienbrack, 1846) and *An Seine Majestät den König von Preußen: Eine öffentliche Stimme des christlichen und*

wissenschaftlichen Bewußtseins über Lebensrecht und Volksfreiheit im Staate (Leipzig: Christ. Ernst Kollmann, 1849).

7. Hermann Klencke, *Die Nahrungsmittelfrage in Deutschland oder: Welches sind die Naturanforderungen menschlicher Ernährung, wie müssen sie durch die deutsche Küche erfüllt und wie dann dem Unbemittelten eine billige und kräftige Nahrung geboten werden? Vom Standpunkte der praktischen Naturwissenschaft beantwortet* (Leipzig: Eduard Kummer, 1855), iii, 109, 112–13.

8. Theodor Hahn, *Die naturgemässe Diät, die Diät der Zukunft: Nach Erfahrung und Wissenschaft aller Zeiten und Völker* (Cöthen: Paul Schettler, 1859), x, 12, 274–75, 278–322.

9. Eduard Baltzer, *Die natürliche Lebensweise*, 4 vols. (Nordhausen: Förstemann, 1867–72). Vol. 1, *Der Weg zu Gesundheit und sozialem Heil*, and vol. 2, *Die Reform der Volkswirtschaft vom Standpunkte der natürlichen Lebensweise*, appeared in 1867. Vol. 3, *Briefe an Virchow über dessen Schrift: "Nahrungs- und Genussmittel"* (1868), is discussed below; vol. 4, *Vegetarismus in der Bibel*, appeared in 1872. The series went through multiple editions.

10. Eduard Baltzer, *Flugblatt 2 Die naturgemässe Lebensweise* (approx. 1878), 3 (unpaginated), Frecot Collection 72 00134, Stanford University Library Archive, Stanford, CA.

11. Carl Ernst Bock was a professor of physiology at Leipzig, a vocal liberal, and a nationally known scientific popularizer. Otto Funke was a professor of physiology at the University of Freiburg. Both launched attacks on Baltzer and Hahn in the bourgeois periodical *Die Gartenlaube*. Carl Ernst Bock, "Zur Nahrungssorge," *Gartenlaube* 12 (1868): 185–87; Otto Funke, "Die Diätetik der Vegetarianer," *Die Gartenlaube* (1870): 454–57 and 470.

12. Rudolf Virchow, "Ueber Nahrungs- und Genussmittel," *Sammlung gemeinverständlicher wissenschaftlicher Vorträge*, ed. Rudolf Virchow and F. von Holtzendorff (Berlin: C. G. Lüderitzsche Verlagsbuchhandlung, 1867), 5–6, 7–8, 30, 33, and 35.

13. Eduard Baltzer, *Briefe an Virchow über dessen Schrift: "Nahrungs- und Genussmittel"* (Nordhausen: Ferdinand Förstemann, 1868), 2, 25–26, 32–37, 62–68, 74.

14. Theodor Hahn, *Die Ritter vom Fleische: Offene Brief über die Ernährungsfrage an Prof Dr med. Virchow, Voit, Liebig, Bock, Moleschott, Stengel, Seegen, Medizinalrath Dr med C. A. W. Richter, Hofrath Dr med Steinbacher, Dr Bersch und Ule, an den Staatsanzeiger von Württemberg, Daheim, Berner Sonntagspost, Wiener konstitutionelle Vorstadt-Zeitung und an den Stuttgarter Beobachter zugleich ein Beitrag zur Lösung der sozialen Frage* (Berlin: Theobald Grieben, 1869), 15, 48–50, 70–77, 87.

15. Hermann Klencke, *Fleisch- oder Pflanzenkost? Eine populäre Antwort der Wissenschaft auf die Streitfrage: Soll der Mensch natur- und gesundheitsgemäß auch Fleisch genießen, oder sich nur von Vegetablien ernähren?* (Leipzig: Carl Minde, 1869), iv, 12, 15, 21, 50–53. The book began as a commissioned essay for the journal Über Land und Meer.

16. For the rise of laboratory medicine at midcentury, see *The Laboratory Revolution in Medicine*, ed. Andrew Cunningham and Perry Williams (Cambridge: Cambridge University Press, 1992). For Voit and his impact, see Frederic Holmes, "The Formation of the Munich School of Metabolism," *The Investigative Enterprise: Experimental Physiology in Nineteenth-Century Medicine*, ed William Coleman and Frederic L. Holmes (Berkeley: University of California Press, 1988), 179–210.

17. Carl Voit, "Ueber die Kost in öffentlichen Anstalten," *Zeitschrift für Biologie* 12 (1876): 1–59. Voit also returned to these numbers in Carl Voit, *Untersuchung der Kost in einigen öffentlichen Anstalten* (Munich: R. Oldenbourg, 1877), 20; and Carl Voit, "Physiologie des allgemeinen Stoffwechsels und der Ernährung," in *Handbuch der Physiologie*, vol. 6, ed. L. Hermann (Leipzig: Verlag F. C. W. Vogel, 1881), 518–28. The average worker was a male of 70 kilograms engaged in moderate physical labor as, for example, a peacetime soldier or a carpenter. Workers eating a mostly plant-based diet, Voit also claimed, would have to eat even more than the standard 118 grams of protein because vegetable protein was so much less digestible than animal protein.

18. Thoms, *Anstaltskost*, 345–48 and 356. Many physiologists recommended as much as 165 grams of daily protein, depending on the type of work being performed. See Graham Lusk, *The Elements of the Science of Nutrition* (Philadelphia: W. B. Saunders, 1921), 335–36. For an example of the international uses of Voit's standards, see Francesco S. Nitti, "The Food and Labour-Power of Nations," *Economic Journal* 6 (March 1896): 34–36. Nitti served as economics minister in Italy during the First World War and then became the prime minister in 1919.

19. Kaiserliches Gesundheitsamt, *Gesundheitsbüchlein* (Berlin: Julius Springer, 1899), 57 and 60. The tables were based on Joseph König, *Chemie der menschlichen Nahrungs- und Genussmittel* (Berlin: Julius Springer, 1879), which went through five more editions at the same press under the modified title *Die menschlichen Nahrungs- und Genussmittel* by 1920. König was an extremely prominent food chemist who also served at the *Reichsgesundheitsamt*. For König's work on setting standards for food markets, see Uwe Spiekermann, "Redefining Food: The Standardization of Products and Production in Europe and the United States 1880–1914," *History and Technology* 27 (March 2011): 15–16.

20. His research subject had been a vegetarian for eleven years, which means that he converted in the era when Eduard Baltzer's *Natural Lifestyle* series was making a splash.

21. Traugott Cramer, "Die Ernährungsweise der sog: Vegetarier, vom physiologischen Standpunkte aus betrachtet," *Zeitschrift für physiologische Chemie* 6 (1882): 346–85, on 384. For an early hygienist's critique of vegetarianism, see Max Gruber, "Ueber die Kostreform der Vegetarier," *Deutsches Wochenblatt für Gesundheitspflege und Rettungswesen* 1 (1884): 165–68, 177–79, and 189–93. Gruber later became a prominent eugenicist who worked with many of the social hygienists discussed later in this chapter.

22. Bunge had been interested in vegetarian diets since the 1870s when he was doing studies on the role of salt in human metabolism. Relying perhaps in part on data that his father had gathered in his travels with Humboldt, Bunge linked his chemical studies to an anthropological observation that largely meat-eating races avoided salt, whereas largely plant-eating races craved it. See C. M. McKay, "Gustav B. von Bunge," *Journal of Nutrition* 49 (1953): 6.

23. Gustav von Bunge, *Der Vegetarianismus: Ein Vortrag* (Berlin: August Hirschwald, 1885), 4, 16–17, 39–41. Bunge continued to express skepticism over Voit's standard in the following years. See, for example, Gustav von Bunge, *Lehrbuch der physiologischen und pathologischen Chemie*, 4th ed. (Leipzig: F. C. W. Vogel, 1898), 78–79. The first edition was 1887.

24. There is also a helpful summary of the dozens of studies on the protein minimum by R. O. Neumann, "Experimentelle Beiträge zur Lehre von dem täglichen Nahrungsbedarf des Menschen," *Archiv für Hygiene* 45 (1902): 1–87.

25. Voit focused on nitrogen because the only nitrogen-containing nutrient is protein. A nitrogen loss meant that a research subject lost more protein from his body through work than he assimilated into his body from food. Continued nitrogen loss led to starvation. Nitrogen balance meant that the research subject assimilated as much protein from food as he excreted in urea. This was a desirable state for the maintenance of health and physical fitness. A nitrogen gain, finally, meant that the research subject had assimilated more protein from food than he had excreted. Researchers disagreed on the benefits and drawbacks of nitrogen gain. For an overview, see Lusk, *Elements of the Science of Nutrition*, 26–27 and 47–52. As Karl Rothschuh put it more metaphorically, the respiration apparatus allowed Voit to study "the metabolic turnover in the organism . . . in the same fashion as one would be able to surmise indirectly the work of a factory by examining the entering raw materials, end products and emerging waste." Karl E. Rothschuh, *History of Physiology* (Huntington, NY: Robert E. Krieger Publishing, 1973), 293.

26. Carl Voit, "Ueber die Kost eines Vegetariers," *Zeitschrift für Biologie* 25 (1889): 232–36, 255–88. He did not cite any vegetarian works.

27. "Briefkasten," *Die neue Heilkunst* 1, no. 4 (March 21, 1889): 39.

28. Pierre-Yves Donzé, "Studies Abroad by Japanese Doctors: A Prosopographic Analysis of the Nameless Practitioners, 1862–1912," *Social History of Medicine* 23 (August 2010): 244–60. Between 1862 and 1912, 763 young doctors went abroad to American and European universities. Almost 86 percent of those holding public scholarships went to Germany, most of them going to the University of Berlin. Most of these scholarship holders, moreover, arrived in Germany with some grounding in Western medicine, received from German professors teaching at the Faculty of Medicine in Tokyo. Among these was Erwin Baelz, who appears later in this section.

29. Robert S. Schwantes, "Foreign Employees in the Development of Japan," in *The Modernizers: Overseas Students, Foreign Employees, and Meiji Japan*, ed. Ardath W. Burks (Boulder, CO: Westview, 1985), 207–17.

30. "Kellner, Oscar," WBIS (World Biographical Information System) Online, document number D645-484-9.

31. O. Kellner and Y. Mori, "Untersuchungen über die Ernährung der Japaner," *Zeitschrift für Biologie* 25 (1889): 102, 113–15, 118–20. They reasoned that 109 gr. was close enough to 118 gr. when the smaller stature and lighter weight of Japanese workers was taken into account. Voit referred to this study, as well as the study by Nakahama discussed below. Voit, "Ueber die Kost eines Vegetariers," 246 and 254. For how this debate affected Japanese dietary recommendations, see Katarzyna J. Cwiertka, "Popularizing a Military Diet in Wartime and Postwar Japan," *Asian Anthropology* 1 (2002): 1–30.

32. Manjiro Nakahama (1826–98, also known as John Mung) was also an adviser to the Japanese government. "Nakahama, Toichiro," WBIS Online, document number V46695.

33. T[oichiri] Nakahama, "Ueber den Eiweissbedarf des Erwachsenen mit Berücksichtigung der Beköstigung in Japan," *Archiv für Hygiene* 5 (1889): 78, 81,

100–101. The workers were miners, drillers, plumbers, and other kinds of physical laborers.

34. Muneo Kumagawa, "Vergleichende Untersuchungen über die Ernährung mit gemischter und rein vegetabilischer Kost mit Berücksichtigung des Eiweissbedarfs," *Virchows Archiv* 116 (1889): 370–72. Mori and Nakahama also did experiments on themselves. Although writing from Japan, Kumagawa had done these experiments at the Pathological Institute in Berlin, run by Rudolf Virchow.

35. Felix Hirschfeld, "Betrachtungen über die Voit'sche Lehre von dem Eiweissbedarf des Menschen," *Archiv für die gesamte Physiologie des Menschen und der Thiere* 44 (1889): 432 and 462. Hirschfeld had already cast doubt on the 118-gram standard, in Felix Hirschfeld, "Untersuchungen über den Eiweissbedarf des Menschen," *Archiv für die gesamte Physiologie des Menschen und der Thiere* 41 (1887): 533–65. He was a *Privatdozent* at the University of Berlin.

36. Germany was the first but not only place that this happened. See, for instance, Myer E. Jaffa, *Nutrition Investigations among Fruitarians and Chinese at the California Agricultural Experiment Station, 1899–1901* (Washington, DC: Government Printing Office, 1901); and Myer E. Jaffa, *Nuts and Their Uses as Food* (Washington, DC: Government Printing Offices, 1908), which studied the low-protein diet of Asian laborers in California.

37. V. O. Sivén, "Ueber das Sticksotffgleichgewicht beim erwachsenen Menschen," *Skandinavisches Archiv für Physiologie* 10 (1899): 106–27 and 142–48. V. O. Sivén, "Zur Kenntniss des Stoffwechsels beim erwachsenen Menschen, mit besonderer Berücksichtigung des Eiweissbedarfs," *Skandinavisches Archiv für Physiologie* 11 (1901): 308–32.

38. Th[eodor] Rumpf and O. Schumm, "Ueber den Stoffwechsel eines Vegetariers," *Zeitschrift für Biologie* 39 (1899).

39. In 1890, Albu had been involved as an "opponent" with the thesis defense of Carl Peters, a medical student at the University of Berlin. See Carl Peters, "Ueber die Berechtigung einer ausschliesslichen Pflanzennahrung für den Menschen (Vegetarismus)" (PhD diss., Friedrich-Wilhelms-Universität Berlin, 1890).

40. Albert Albu, "Der Stoffwechsel bei vegetarischer Kost," *Zeitschrift für klinische Medizin* 43 (1901): 77 and 82–83.

41. Albert Albu, "Zur Bewerthung der vegetarischen Diät," *Verhandlungen der Berliner medicinischen Gesellschaft* 32 (1902): 140–55; Anon., "Discussion zu dem Vortrage des Hrn. Albu," *Verhandlungen der Berliner medicinischen Gesellschaft* 32 (1902): 84–86. Albu also invoked the papers of Hirschfeld, Kumagawa, and Sivén here.

42. Baelz, "Ueber vegetarische Massenernährung und über das Leistungsgleichgewicht," *Verhandlungen der Berliner medicinischen Gesellschaft* 32, part 2 (1902): 181–82. "Discussion zu dem Vortrage des Hrn. Albu," 65–66 and 72.

43. Russell H. Chittenden, *Physiological Economy in Nutrition: An Experimental Study* (New York: Frederick A Stokes, 1904), 475. Robert Suchier, a physician interested in meatless diets, translated an extract of this book into German as Ökonomie in der Ernährung (Munich: Gmelin, 1910).

44. The institute at which Caspari worked was run by the physiologist Nathan Zuntz, a pioneer of sports hygiene and later the rector of the college. Caspari and Zuntz, close friends, were both Jews (though Zuntz had himself baptized in order to become a professor in the 1880s) and their careers were hampered by academic

anti-Semitism. See Hanns-Christian Gunga, *Nathan Zuntz: His Life and Work in the Fields of High Altitude Physiology and Aviation Medicine* (Amsterdam: Elsevier, 2009), 76–77.

45. Wilhelm Caspari and Karl Glaessner, "Ein Stoffwechselversuch an Vegetariern," *Zeitschrift für diätetische und physikalische Therapie* 7 (1903): 475–85. Wilhelm Caspari, "Physiologische Studien über Vegetarismus," *Pflügers Archiv für die gesammte Physiologie des Menschen und der Thiere* 109 (1905): 473–595. See also Albert Albu and Wilhelm Caspari, "Bericht über die Untersuchungen an den Dauergehern beim Distanzmarsch Dresden-Berlin, am 18./19. Mai 1902," *Deutsche medizinische Wochenschrift* 29 (1903): 252–54, discussed in the second section of this chapter. Caspari and Glaessner studied a married vegetarian couple: the engineer J. K., a vegetarian since 1883 and a leader in the national movement, and his wife, a vegetarian since 1899. Caspari and Glaessner, "Ein Stoffwechselversuch an Vegetariern," 477–79. Note that Albu briefly studied the engineer J. K. too. See Albu, "Der Stoffwechsel bei vegetarischer Kost," 83–84. For a photo of this muscular man in the nude, see Caspari, "Physiologische Studien über Vegetarismus," Tafel X.

46. The research subject was the army officer L. H. and his illness narrative followed a common pattern. Born in 1853, L. H. suffered poor health as a child, then as a young soldier came down with a host of ailments, including gonorrhea (treated with mercury) and nose polyps (treated with cocaine). L. H. became so sick that he lost his beard and hair. In 1892 he converted to vegetarianism and his health improved immediately. After becoming a fruitarian and embracing naturopathy, he found that his health improved even further. Caspari, "Physiologische Studien über Vegetarismus," 487–99, 567–68, and Tafel IX.

47. Nathan Zuntz and Adolf Loewy, *Lehrbuch der Physiologie des Menschen* (Leipzig: F. C. W. Vogel, 1909), 688. Note that Zuntz had already reached similar conclusions at least as early as 1905. See N. Zuntz, "Neuere Erfahrungen und Gesichtspunkte über den Eiweissbedarf des Menschen," *Fortschritte der Medizin* 22 (1905): 565–74.

48. For a parallel example, see Lynn Nyhart, *Modern Nature: The Rise of the Biological Perspective in Germany* (Chicago: University of Chicago Press, 2009).

Chapter Three

Of Carnivores and Conquerors

French Nutritional Debates in the Age of Empire, 1890–1914

Deborah Neill

Could meat eating change your personality? In the early nineteenth century, some French commentators argued that it could, and that meat eating could even define the collective character of a people. Julien-Joseph Virey, a pharmacist and anthropologist, proclaimed in 1813 that consuming meat had made the Romans "vigorous, energetic and bellicose," and that the retention of Roman meat-eating habits by northern Europeans, particularly the Germans and the English, had given them the same characteristics. In the modern states of Greece and Rome, in contrast, Virey argued, the people had embraced a more vegetable-heavy diet and consequently had lost some of their "force and vigor." Meat, Virey suggested, made for an aggressive, passionate, and forceful population, a population that could embark on the conquest of others.[1] This message was popular throughout much of the nineteenth century, and in the 1890s most scientists still agreed that meat should hold a central place in the French diet. Yet there were also signs that experts were starting to revisit the meat question. For example, in 1893 the military doctors Louis Henri Polin and Henri Joseph Labit, in their text *L'hygiène alimentaire,* while stating that "meat-eating peoples are robust and strong," also conceded that it was possible to live without meat. As they noted, "it is incontestable and demonstrated by experience: being deprived of meat is more easily supported perhaps than being deprived of vegetables."[2] Jean Rouget and Charles Dopter, two researchers from the Val-de-Grâce military hospital, went even further in their book, also called *Hygiène alimentaire*, which was published in 1906. For them, the ideal dietary preference found a balance between meat and vegetables. But then they added: if a vegetarian supplemented his or her diet with butter, milk, eggs, cheese, and other fats, then this diet "was eminently rational."[3] In other words, vegetarianism was not only a viable but perhaps in some cases a logical choice as well for French men and women in the modern age.

Why did questions arise about the role of meat in the French diet in the late nineteenth and early twentieth centuries? In the tropical colonies, as I have argued elsewhere, a belief in the need for reduced meat diets arose from fears that warm climates and the stresses of colonial life had a negative impact on French digestive systems.[4] But although they were far more hesitant, some scientists in metropolitan France also argued that meat's primacy in the diet was worth interrogating. In what follows I explore this development from four related angles. First, I examine the broad context in which nutrition studies in France developed at the turn of the century, particularly the new opportunities available to researchers with an interest in diet. Second, I explore the related anxieties about depopulation and degeneration and how this helped to shape the study of diet. Third, I turn to the contributions of alimentary hygienists, therapeutic specialists, and chemists. And finally, I examine how French scientists were influenced by studies about the diets of people across the world, particularly those who practiced vegetarianism. In highlighting the relationship between broader trends in society and changing ideas among professional experts on diet and nutrition, I also argue that even as meat's centrality and purpose was subject to greater scientific scrutiny, what remained consistent was how deeply embedded social and cultural assumptions informed protein recommendations and shaped scientific findings.

The Context: New Opportunities, New Ideas

In France, dietary choices vary significantly by region, but certain foods and traditions have over time come to be known as distinctly "French." Rooted in the culinary habits of the aristocracy, the "national" diet of France privileges meats in rich sauces, uses significant amounts of milk, cream, butter, and cheese, and relies heavily on bread, root vegetables, green beans, mushrooms, and fresh seasonal fruit. In the nineteenth century, as more products became available for mass consumption, those who could afford it indulged in fine wines, champagne, coffee, tea, and chocolate.[5] But for many French people, diets were primarily informed by cost, regional availability, and the urban-rural divide. Meat consumption—from red meats to pork, chicken, horse, and mutton—amply demonstrates these divides: although meat eating was steadily increasing in France, from an average annual consumption per head of 24 kilograms in 1856 to 35 kilograms in 1877, urban dwellers, with their consumption of 66 kilograms per head in 1877, ate far more meat than their rural counterparts, whose consumption was a mere 24 kilograms per head.[6] Despite the variations, however, the country as a whole experienced an increase in meat consumption, and in urban centers, meat was usually the main component of the meal.

For much of the nineteenth century, the scientific assumption was that meat should be the center of the French diet. The study of nutrition in France had rapidly developed in the eighteenth century in what the historian Kenneth Carpenter has called "a new beginning for nutritional science."[7] Antoine Lavoisier's pioneering research on respiration was cut short by his execution during the Reign of Terror, but scientists such as François Magendie and Jean Baptiste Boussingault took up his work on nitrogen, chiefly found in protein, and they, together with other scientists, argued that "foods that do not contain nitrogen cannot continue to support life."[8] Foodstuffs were therefore valued for their protein content, more generally measured as albumin or nitrogen, and since meat is high in protein, it was highly prized. By the mid-nineteenth century, Justus von Liebig was arguing that protein "was the only true nutrient, providing both the machinery of the body and the fuel for its work."[9] An increasing knowledge about the digestive process and the chemical breakdown of specific foods led Liebig and other scientists to refer to the body as an ideal "machine" that could reach its full potential by finding the right fuel. This position made way for a variety of studies of different dietary regimens to determine how to maximize energy efficiency for the completion of necessary human tasks.[10] A central belief, that protein provided muscle, led to the view that physical and mental strength resulted primarily from a diet heavy in meat.

In fin de siècle France, interest in dietary questions was facilitated by political and social developments that offered new opportunities for researchers. The growth of France's empire in Africa and Asia provided scientists with information about other cultures' dietary habits and brought new foodstuffs into the country. A strong economy, which brought industrial and technological progress, made transportation easier; thanks to technologies such as refrigerated steamships, the movement of food around the empire could be expanded and expedited. Food preservation technologies were also important. For example, in 1896, over five thousand workers in France were working in 254 canning factories, producing about 120 million cans a year.[11] Better communication systems and significant advances in education promised tangible benefits to all French men and women, and scientists were called on to broaden their reach and instruct new audiences about the value of their work. They found support in new institutions, like the Pasteur Institute (opened 1888), which was dedicated to uncovering the microbiological agents that caused disease, and the Musée Social, a national society founded in 1894 by the wealthy politician Aldebert de Chambrun, which sought to improve the housing, daily lives, and health of French workers, and in doing so, affect lasting social change.[12] And the development of dedicated societies, journals, and conferences brought not just French scientists together but also connected them to a wider community of international experts eager to build a network of people interested in diet and nutrition. Conferences dedicated to food questions developed between the 1880s and 1914, first as a result of discussions at the International Conference on Hygiene and Demography and the Congrès de laiterie, both of which took place in Brussels in 1903. These meetings furthered the resolve of delegates who vowed to address "alimentary falsifications and frauds," and in 1908 and 1909 delegates met to do just that at the International Congress on Pure Foods and Alimentary Substances.[13] Smaller gatherings also furthered the field. The French established a League for School Hygiene in 1903, and international conferences on this subject were held in 1904 in Nuremberg, and in 1906 in both London and Paris.[14] Research on infant dietary needs was enriched by discussions at the First International Congress of Gouttes de Lait, held in Paris in 1905. A second, held in London in 1906, focused on infant mortality.[15]

French scientists were inspired to form dedicated societies in part because of these international discussions. The Brussels conferences of 1903 spurred the formation of the Société scientifique d'hygiène alimentaire et d'alimentation rationnelle de l'homme (Scientific Society for Alimentary Hygiene and the Rational Feeding of Man), which had the chemist Armand Gautier as its president and published a bulletin in which members could present their dietary research.[16] In 1906 this group helped to launch the Congrés international d'hygiène alimentaire et de l'alimentation rationnelle de l'homme (International Congress on Alimentary Hygiene and the Rational Feeding of Man) in Paris, with a second conference held in Brussels in 1910.[17] Both congresses emphasized the importance of scientists as reformers and celebrated the ways in which science would make practical improvements to people's lives.[18] Gautier revealed the increasingly ambitious goals of dietary reformers in his opening speech at the 1906 meeting: he hoped that experts could formulate dietary recommendations and set standards for the wide variety of groups in modern society, including workers, the elderly, women, children, and the infirm; he expressed his belief that technology and the laboratory could help with diversifying and protecting the food supply; he believed that dietary studies would reveal which foods were capable of "augmenting physical energy, moral courage, and cerebral activity" for modern populations; and he hoped that collectively the experts would answer the question of whether meat could be substituted for other foods without sacrificing strength and power.[19] In his opening speech at the 1910 congress, the Belgian Minister of the Interior Paul Berryer reiterated some of these ideas and argued that some of the greatest challenges facing modern nations would be solved by scientists: physiologists, who studied the workings of the human body in the hopes of improving health and function; bacteriologists, who understood pathogens in food; chemists, who could trace falsifications and adulterations; engineers, who could provide scientific advice on potable water; and jurists and officials, who could enact appropriate protective legislation.[20]

A burgeoning economy, a vast empire, new technologies, and the ambitions of reform-minded political and scientific elites provided a framework in which there were new opportunities to ask questions about the relationship of diet to the requirements of modern life. But if promising technological, political, and international developments facilitated a rising attention to diet, French reformers were also motivated to address dietary questions because of their considerable anxiety that France was falling behind its neighbors as a leading global power.

National Anxieties

French anxieties about depopulation and degeneration greatly increased after Prussia's victory in the war of 1870–71, which led to the loss of Alsace-Lorraine and the rise of a newly united Germany potentially threatening France on the eastern border. Many politicians and social commentators worried about France's ability to compete militarily because of the declining birth rate. Between 1872 and 1911, Germany's population grew by 58 percent, Great Britain's by 43 percent, whereas France's climbed by a mere 10 percent.[21] For those who feared that France was falling behind its rivals, the declining birth rate seemed to indicate a reluctance or an inability of the French populace to bear healthy children, and they lamented that vice, prostitution, and ill health were the primary causes.[22] As the historian Joshua Cole notes, among politicians after 1870 there were "nearly unanimous" fears about depopulation and "politicians and publicists endlessly discussed measures to increase the birthrate in the decades leading up to World War I."[23] What were some of the proposed solutions? Reformers embraced a series of policies designed to improve the "quality and quantity" of the French population.[24] These included combatting infectious diseases through research and public hygiene programs, promoting family-friendly policies and pronatalism, and creating or revitalizing healthy private and public spaces for the working classes who were perceived to be at the most risk for illness and degeneration.[25] Doctors and scientists with an interest in dietary reform—and the meat question in particular—found a ready place among groups intent on a program of national regeneration.

Historians have discussed the degeneration and social hygiene debates in considerable depth, particularly the fears of middle-class activists about vice, sexually transmitted diseases, tuberculosis, and alcoholism.[26] Although they acknowledge the importance of diet in these debates, scholars have spent less time detailing contemporary views on the relationship between a poor diet and degeneration.[27] In fact, many nineteenth-century social reformers believed that improving the diet of the French populace—particularly the working classes—could go some way to not only preserving the health of the current generation but also of their potential children, since many assumed that acquired characteristics could be passed down to future generations.[28] The stage was set by the psychiatrist Bénédict-Augustin Morel, who argued in his 1857 treaty on degeneration that among other things, alcohol and poor dietary choices were to blame for population decline.[29] Halting degeneration required activist scientists to intervene; as Rafael Huertas has argued, Morel "drew the practical conclusion that doctors must lead any attempt to improve society."[30] His ideas were taken up by the widely read German social critic Max Nordau, who echoed Morel's views that urban life, vice, stimulants, and alcohol contributed to degeneracy.

Large working populations in unsanitary living conditions, Nordau insisted, had access to temptations unknown to their ancestors, and they were exposed to "stale, contaminated, adulterated food" that contributed to their ill-health and inability to produce healthy children. He also argued that the pace of life outstripped the body's ability to adjust, and that "our stomachs cannot keep pace with the brain and nervous system."[31] In Nordau's references to the impurities entering not just body but also the mind, we see how fears about food quality and choices intersected with larger degeneration concerns.

The links between degeneration and diet were more thoroughly elaborated in the popular book *L'alimentation et la cuisine naturelles dans le monde* (Diet and Natural Cuisine in the World) written by the physician and natural therapeutics advocate Dr. A. Monteuuis. Published in 1907 and reissued in 1910, this book also argued that scientists were ideally placed to participate in "the work of social regeneration." Monteuuis didn't just attack stimulants and alcohol; he also targeted meat, arguing that too much of it "ruins the health of the individual as it does the vigor of the race" and "constitutes a veritable social peril."[32] He linked poor dietary choices to disease and he traced generational patterns: from the second generation a bourgeois family is generally arthritic, whereas the third generation suffers from obesity, diabetes, neuropathy, and other ills, and without active attempts to counter it, either through country living or an alliance with a peasant, the family is destined to fade away completely by the fifth or sixth generation. Monteuuis's book found a wide audience and received the approval of experts. In a review of the book in the prestigious colonial medical journal *Annales d'hygiène et de médecine coloniales*, the author praised its "agreeable and precise style," its laudable advocacy of a balanced diet, and its accessible mix of advice and recipes aimed at a broad readership.[33]

As William Schneider has shown, among the physicians committed to a more public reform role there were a number who joined the French eugenics movement. Their hope was to "improve the hereditary quality of the population" through the promotion of health, medicine, and social hygiene.[34] Dietary reformers in the eugenics movement included the biologist Frédéric Houssay, who served as the first vice president of the society. He carried out experiments that included feeding an all-meat diet to chickens; among his conclusions was the view that dietary variations could cause changes in organ functions and that "a poorly balanced diet with poorly regulated organic intake can be a determinant of defects and degeneration."[35] Other dietary reformers included two of the society's presidents, Eugène Apert and Adolph Pinard; both men were infant-care specialists who had an interest in wet-nurse regulation and breast-feeding to address the problem of infant mortality.[36] And Louis Landouzy, a neurologist and tuberculosis researcher, served as part of the French consultative committee at the First International Eugenics Congress in London in 1912.[37]

Landouzy was concerned with how poverty and ill-health weakened the population's ability to fight off tuberculosis and he addressed the question of diet and meat directly in a work he published with the physicians Henri and Marcel Labbé in 1905.[38] This study analyzed dietary choices of working-class patients at a Paris clinic to determine if unhealthy eating habits led to a rise in tuberculosis.[39] The authors, reflecting middle-class assumptions about the ignorance of the working poor, concluded that workers' higher tuberculosis rates resulted in part from weak nutritional knowledge. They also lacked access, the authors argued, to healthy and inexpensive foodstuffs. The authors noted particularly the cost of meat: good quality meat was costly, whereas cheaper products were potentially unsafe and of questionable nutritive value. They therefore came to a notable conclusion: workers should reduce meat, particularly red meat, in favor of other nitrogen-rich foods. They provided tables on foodstuffs best equipped to provide albumin, and though smoked herring came first, it was followed by cheeses and dried peas. Ham came in fifth, and beef eleventh, trailing almonds, haricots, and lentils. Meat was "far from being advantageous as a reservoir of strength," the authors argued, and "the place of meat in our menus is less important than that taken by many other foods that the uninformed public feels obliged to ascribe a lesser nutritive value."[40] For these physicians, meat could be replaced with other healthy, nitrogen-rich foods, and as a practical way to improve workers diets, a reduced-meat diet was recommended to save money and protect against poor-quality meat products.

Landouzy and the Labbés' study, with its mix of clinical research and practical advice, demonstrates how dietary reformers sought to disseminate their recommendations. In the final part of their study, the authors strongly advocated for better public education because "if again today we reiterate that food hygiene should be the object of everyone's concerns, it is because everywhere it is as neglected as possible." To this end, they saw value in partnerships between researchers and popularizers of dietary reform who could reach new audiences, particularly women.[41] They praised the founder of the Paris-based École de meres (School for Mothers), Augusta Moll-Weiss, for her ongoing campaign to educate working-class mothers about dietary choices, including her papers commissioned by the Musée Social.[42] She, in turn, was influenced by their work, and in her publications she also questioned the value of meat, particularly for young children. Indeed, her 1909 book on children's diets recommended milk, butter, cheese, fruit, fish, cereals, and some select vegetables. "We will leave aside meat until age six," she declared, since children chewed poorly and might have digestion difficulties, and the freshest meat, required by children, was expensive.[43]

Improving the population became a rallying cry for many physicians, politicians, social commentators, and activists in fin de siècle France. The working classes were the major focus of reforming concern, and some experts saw the high rates of alcoholism and tuberculosis among workers as resulting from their ignorance and poverty. Their response was to advocate for better education, exchange best research with their colleagues at home and abroad, disseminate their ideas, and make practical suggestions about how to eat lighter, budget-friendly, nutritious meals with substitutions for the expensive meats so out of reach to the working poor. But it was not only cost and availability that caused a change in meat recommendations; questions about the need for meat were also informed by other developments within the scientific community. The nineteenth century saw advances in a variety of scientific disciplines that, as Julia Csergo notes, "profoundly altered the approach to food and the nutritional model," which helped to establish "the foundations of our modern diet."[44] Scientists from the burgeoning fields of alimentary hygiene, therapeutics, and chemistry came to question and modify some prevailing assumptions about the central role of meat in the French diet.

Alimentary Hygiene and Therapeutics

Saving the French population from degenerative influences led some eugenicists, popular writers, and infectious disease specialists to approve of meat-reduced diets if nitrogen could be obtained from other budget-friendly alternatives. Their fears about meat-heavy diets, however, were not based on a belief that meat was not healthy or important; rather, the issues were primarily about excess and cost. The issue of food contamination was also a major concern: Max Nordau's observations about the dangers of spoiled and adulterated foods, although not central to his own argument, reflected popular views that the food supply in France was not as safe as it could be. This concern increased in the wake of the trichinosis scare that swept France in the 1880s.[45] Salt pork imported from the United States was blamed for this outbreak, and the spread of the problem in Germany highlighted the fragility of the inspection system. The debates about banning imports or introducing other control measures gave doctors—who did not all agree on measures to be taken to stop the problem—new forums to debate their ideas and seek out a greater public role as dietary reformers, even when their views were not adopted.[46] It also led to an interrogation of the safety of meat in particular.

Scientists seeking to publish research on food safety issues found a friendly forum in the journal *Revue d'hygiène et de police sanitaire*, founded in 1879. This important publication, edited by the Val-de-Grâce hygiene professor Edmond Vallin, actively sought specialized studies concerning water purity, ventilation, housing standards, and food safety.[47] A subsection of the public hygiene advocates, comprised primarily of scientists from the fields of chemistry, therapeutics, physiology, and medicine, began to embrace the concept of "alimentary hygiene" and their goal was to guarantee the safety of the food supply through the advocacy of protective legislation, the prevention of fraud, working on improved transportation and storage, and the monitoring of abattoirs. An increased attention to spoilage and fraud in the food supply then served as an entry point into larger discussions about dietary standards.

Many of the dietary texts that emerged between 1890 and 1914 were primarily about food safety issues. Polin and Labit, both members of the Société de medicine publique et d'hygiène professionelle (Society of Public Medicine and Professional Hygiene), were both food safety experts and in 1890 coauthored a volume expressly about food poisoning, particularly from undercooked and contaminated meat. In 1892 they cowrote a second food safety volume, then in 1893 published *L'hygiène alimentaire.*[48] Although the authors were still deeply concerned with food safety, this book was more ambitious and far-reaching, describing the process of digestion, the composition and value of a wide variety of foodstuffs and of various dietary regimes (values were based, here and elsewhere, on the five priority categories of albumin, minerals, water, fats, and carbohydrates). The authors were advocates for red meat, particularly for male laborers, but they also argued that meat-centered diets might not be suitable for other professions, age groups, and women. Indeed, they speculated that in some cases, diets too rich in meat might be bad for you, quoting the studies of Dr. Huchard, who attributed to this diet a rise in arteriosclerosis, the retention of ptomaïnes, food-borne disease-causing agents, and perhaps even the growth of cancers.[49]

Dopter and Rouget's 1906 text was also primarily a food-safety manual. Both men were professors at France's preeminent military hospital Val-de-Grâce, and Dopter became a leading member at the Pasteur Institute and served as a government adviser on public hygiene.[50] The bulk of the book he wrote with Rouget discussed falsifications and adulterations, the dangers of poorly conserved or prepared food, and illnesses originating with contaminated food. But echoing Polin and Labit, the authors also assessed specific foods and offered advice about ideal regimens, arguing that "the rational and scientific alimentation of man is the source of power and of health" and therefore needed to be widely known among the population. They noted approvingly that the Society of Alimentary Hygiene had proposed to include dietary instruction in the public and private education systems.[51] These diets needed to account for differing needs, including "age, sex, size, weight, rest, work, profession, climate, season, state of health, convalescence, sickness, etc."[52] In discussing these categories, the authors came to question the role of protein in the French diet—what was acceptable for a laborer was not necessarily required for other groups.

Therapeutic specialists also entered into the meat debate, primarily as a result of their interest in food as medicine. Many physicians had long supported a meat-centered diet for preventive and curative reasons. A good example is the 1861 book by Jean Baptiste Fonssagrives, a professor at the Naval School of Medicine at Brest and later professor of hygiene at Montpellier. His 688-page text, appearing in two more editions, in 1867 and then 1881, touts the health value of milk and meat, arguing that meat in particular "constitutes, strictly speaking, the base of nourishment of the sick and the convalescent." Fonssagrives argued that since the properties found in meat naturally corresponded to the organic tissues in need of repair, that they were ideally "suitable for restoring the energetic forces without imposing a very laborious digestive process on the stomach."[53] In contrast to his strong advocacy of milk and meat, Fonssagrives treated fruits and vegetables with caution. He noted that fruits should be used judiciously and not as a replacement for "foodstuffs more substantial and more restorative." He was not averse to vegetables but argued that root vegetables such as carrots, beets, and celery, important to healthy people, played a "very secondary role" in the convalescent diet.[54]

In the 1880s, these views were challenged by Georges Octave Dujardin-Beaumetz, the editor of the *Bulletin de thérapeutique* (Bulletin of Therapeutics) and an adviser on the Sanitary Council of the Seine (a hygiene body in Paris).[55] His influential 1887 text, *L'hygiène alimentaire*, was republished in 1889 as *L'hygiène alimentaire: aliments, alimentation, régime alimentaire dans les maladies* (Alimentary Hygiene: Food, Diet, and Dietary Regimens in Disease).[56] Although he was not a vegetarian, Dujardin-Beaumetz argued that for certain intestinal and kidney problems, meat was actually problematic—indeed, he outlined a host of diseases in which a vegetarian diet was not only more acceptable but also advisable. His ideas were supported by his student Jean Laumonier, who wrote *Hygiène de l'alimentation dans l'état de santé et de maladie* (Alimentary Hygiene in Health and Disease) first published in 1894 and reissued three times.[57] Although Laumonier cautioned against a meat-free diet, arguing that albumin requirements were such that vegetarians would be obliged to consume prohibitive quantities of vegetables to meet their nutrition needs, he also argued that vegetables "were in reality complete foods" and provided excellent sustenance for people with a variety of medical problems.[58] Rouget and Dopter, for their part, were influenced by Dujardin-Beaumetz and his disciples, praising the value of reduced-meat diets for people with conditions ranging from arthritis, rheumatism, and gout to arteriosclerosis. Yet they also repeated the caution against an excess of vegetable consumption for healthy eaters, noting that "vegetable albumin is not as assimilable or as restorative as that of animals."[59] The research, therefore, led to increased attention on the value of reducing meat intake, but the findings seemed to support meat-reduced diets primarily for people with specific afflictions. Physicians stopped short of recommending vegetarianism as an appropriate diet for the healthy population, since physicians continued to believe that meat provided the necessary strength for hard physical and mental work.

Chemists, whose laboratory-based research into specific foodstuffs was vital to their colleagues, were also enthusiastic about the possibilities of setting new standards for the French population. Some were advocates of technology, hoping that the laboratory would revolutionize food production. Marcellin Berthelot, famous for his work on thermochemistry, was an advocate of synthetic foods and hoped to use the laboratory to "obtain foodstuffs that are more palatable, more fragrant, that lead to faster and easier digestion and assimilation than we have achieved with natural foodstuffs."[60] Berthelot inspired industrial developers and chemists to turn their attention toward food for profit or social-reform motives. He particularly inspired Armand Gautier, who became the leading proponent of dietary reform in France.[61] Gautier's zeal for the subject was also inspired by Wilbur O. Atwater, the American calorie counter whom he had met in Paris in 1903.[62] Atwater asked Gautier to use nutritional science for a "crusade for the benefit and defense of the poor."[63] Gautier's master work was a seven-hundred-page dietary text, *L'alimentation et les régimes chez l'homme sain ou malade*, first published in 1904, republished in 1908, and translated into English in 1906 as *Diet and Dietetics*.[64] The book was divided into three parts—"principles and methods," "foodstuffs," and "regimens"—and outlined the core principles of nutrition, the role of individual foodstuffs in digestion and bodily functions, and ideal diets established by type of work, climate, race, gender, age, and illness. This text reflected the numerous strands of the emerging nutrition movement and offered a synthesis of new research. Gautier situated himself within the broader concerns of degeneration, noting that he would first "consider how healthy and wealthy people are nourished, in order to determine how long use may have introduced abuses into the general habits—abuse of which physical degeneration and the weakening of intellectual abilities are the signs."[65] He praised new technologies and emphasized the importance of food safety. He agreed with the therapeutic specialists that a vegetable-leaning diet might counter tendencies of an arthritic or gouty nature.[66] But like his colleagues, he reiterated that reduced-meat diets, appropriate perhaps for women, children, and the elderly, were not for working men.[67] He also echoed his colleagues' view that the volume of vegetables required to achieve the required amount of nitrogen would require sometimes immense volumes of vegetable foods. He added, "the herbivorous animal is constructed so as to digest vegetables, but man, we have seen, digests them only very incompletely and laboriously."[68] Like the other dietary reformers, Gautier saw the value of questioning the emphasis on meat, but he hesitated to fully embrace a meat-free dietary regimen, qualifying his conclusions on the grounds that workers needed meat because it was easily digested and provided necessary strength and vigor.

Gautier's views were consistent with those of other scientists, and their collective research seemed to indicate that although nitrogen could be obtained from vegetables, meat remained the best foodstuff for building muscular strength and endurance. These findings, however, were not just informed by laboratory discoveries. In fact, the persistent view that meat and strength were intimately connected was also deeply embedded in broad cultural assumptions about national character, race, and power. Nowhere is this more evident than in the discussions about vegetarianism.

Vegetarianism and National Character

The influence of vegetarian societies, as well as studies of groups across the world who ate little or no meat, led to soul-searching about the effect of particular dietary regimes on national culture at a time when many French men and women were confident about France's superiority and yet insecure about how the nation was to maintain its power. Accordingly, dietary views remained beholden to aspects of the old narrative about meat's overarching importance to "character." Indeed, comparisons of the meat-based French diet with vegetarian alternatives, though demonstrating the possibility that a population could readily live on plants alone, reveal an ongoing belief that meat-eating peoples had more physical and intellectual strength than those who relied primarily on vegetables.[69]

Great Britain and Germany were the two nations that dietary reformers most frequently compared with France, and Britain's meat-eating population was particularly envied. Gautier, Rouget and Dopter and other experts made repeated references to the meat-eating habits of the British that had allowed them to prosper. Rouget and Dopter praised Britain's "veritable fleet of refrigerated ships" and lamented France's woefully inadequate supply of both refrigerated ships and depots; moreover, French reluctance to welcome foreign imports "deprived the worker population of a foodstuff of primary necessity."[70] Gautier also noted France's inadequacy in importing meat as compared with Great Britain's access to meat products from the United States, New Zealand, Australia, and elsewhere. But he then subdivided Europeans into north and south, arguing that northerners need more meat: "an Englishman or Dutchman becomes weakened by being deprived of meat fare more quickly than a Spaniard, Southern Frenchman, or Italian," he stated.[71]

Although some scientists suggested that British meat eating was to be admired, this view was countered by vegetarian arguments that meat eating had little to do with physical strength but rather was an unhealthy and unwise choice for modern peoples. Although never large, the French Vegetarian Society grew from thirty initial members in 1899 to eight hundred in 1906, and its adherents forged ties to foreign counterparts including the Belgian Vegetarian Society, collaborating on a journal, *Réforme alimentaire*.[72] Moreover, its membership actively sought to influence the population through the dissemination of magazines, tracts, pamphlets, and public lectures, so the society was more publicly present than the small official membership lists suggest. In France, the most influential vegetarian was a physician, Ernest Bonnejoy, who favored health rationales over moral arguments and maintained that vegetarianism was a valuable lifestyle in the quest to reverse decline and degeneration in the French population. As Ceri Crossley argues, he sought to "present vegetarianism as the sensible, rational way forward for the nation at large."[73] His views resonated with some influential physicians; about 10 percent of the French Vegetarian Society's membership were doctors, and even nonvegetarian doctors such as Marcel Labbé were sometimes collaborators on subjects such as alcoholism and worker dietary reform.[74] Bonnejoy even had Dujardin-Beaumetz write the preface to his 1891 book *Le végetarianisme et le régime végétarien rationnel* (Vegetarianism and the Rational Vegetarian Regimen). Having an established therapeutics specialist write the preface was a coup, even if Dujardin-Beaumetz was not an advocate of vegetarianism for people with no preexisting medical conditions.[75]

Scientists took the research of vegetarians seriously, in part because their goals and those of "rational" vegetarians like Bonnejoy were not that different. Both groups sought to stamp out adulteration, provide defences against disease, and suggest effective dietary standards for a changing population. The question became one of what kinds of animal products, if any, were acceptable and "rational." For meat advocates, the scientific problem remained one of muscular strength, but their arguments included cultural assumptions. Gautier, for example, although advocating for a mixed diet, also accepted that a "mitigated" vegetarianism (that included dairy products) was "very rational and acceptable," and that mitigated vegetarian diets "tend to make us peaceful and not aggressive, violent, or nervous beings." But he also made sweeping assumptions: "at this time the people of the white race who are the most active and enterprising are those who eat the most meat."[76] Likewise, Polin and Labit, who conceded that a vegetarian diet including eggs, cheese, and milk could be sustainable, dismissed an entirely plant-based diet. They referenced Trappist monks who did not eat meat and yet maintained their health. But, they cautioned, the physical stamina of vegetarians, unless they supplemented with dairy products, was perhaps not at the level of meat eaters. Healthy workers required meat because it provided the most strength and vitality. They noted that carnivores were conquerors; populations in Asia, who relied primarily on rice, "are obliged to ingest great quantities and yet still remain soft, lazy, and lacking in vigor."[77] They also cited the work of the antivegetarian physician Jules Arnould, whose *Nouveaux éléments d'hygiène* stated that "the people with vegetarian regimes are made to be conquered" and that abstaining from meat produced weak people with little by way of intellectual or material accomplishments."[78]

The consensus, however, was not absolute among the physicians engaged in the debate. The electrotherapy expert J. A. Rivière, who gave a speech on "rational diets" at the 1906 Congress on Alimentary Hygiene, took the opposite view and argued that the toughness of foreign peoples demonstrated how a vegetable diet created "muscular vigor." He noted that "we know of the enormous work accomplished by the Abyssinian, Indian, Egyptian proletariat, etc . . . who yet exclusively consume rice, beans, lentils, corn, figs, and dates, to the exclusion of meat, eggs, and even milk."[79] Meat preparations were "exciting" to the digestive tract and had "serious disadvantages," including producing "false hungers" that the senses found difficult to resist. It was not the same with vegetables, which "make an extended stay" in the gastrointestinal tract. Because of these findings, Rivière stated, special attention on limiting fats and albumin should be part of an overall reduction in rations.[80]

The persistent assumption that there was a relationship between meat eating and national character is particularly evident in discussions about Japan, a country whose decisive victory over Russia in the war of 1904–5 shocked many people in Europe.[81] Japanese prowess was praised in a 1905 article in the vegetarian journal *Réforme alimentaire;* the author noted that several other medical journals had praised these "vegetarians and drinkers of water" as "people whose physical strength and endurance astonish the world."[82] Rouget and Dopter also explored the Japanese case but took a different tack: they cited a study that described how Japanese doctors, schooled in Germany physiology, had become quite concerned about raising the level of albumin in their rice-heavy diet and were advocating an increase in meat. Perhaps, Rouget and Dopter speculated, this increased meat eating might have led to "modifications in the character and temperament of the Japanese," and that "may be the starting point of the current conflict." This, they noted, fit Cesare Lombroso's theories on criminality, since he had stated that meat eating was "a common cause of an addiction to crime in both humans and animals."[83] Although Rouget and Dopter conceded that such deductions were "without doubt a bit excessive," they did argue that "we cannot ignore the fact that diet has an undeniable influence on the activity of individuals and, as a result, of their lives and their customs." They added, "the study of vegetarianism has supported this view." In their view, meat eating could lead to aggression, whereas vegetarian diets could contribute to calm personalities and alert minds.[84]

Here marks an important change. Although accepting the long-standing view that meat provided significant vigor and strength to a people, Rouget and Dopter presented the Japanese shift as a cautionary tale about the perils of too much meat and the value of vegetables as a counter to aggressive behavior. For these scientists, too much meat was as bad as too much vegetarianism in shaping the character of a "race." They pursued this theme by analyzing "extreme" diets, including the meat-only regimens of "Eskimos," trappers in the Americas, northern explorers, and the Lapps, and the vegetarian diets of religious groups in India and Egypt, ethical societies in Europe, and poor peasant communities in far-flung regions of the world.[85] They concluded that the ideal diet was a balanced one, but this was not only for physiological reasons: it was also because balance improved character, both for individuals and for nations.

The dietary model emerging among alimentary hygienists, therapeutic specialists, chemists, and other scientists favored balance, but this position was formulated not just because of scientific findings regarding the relative nutritive qualities of meats and vegetables; rather it was predicated on cultural assumptions about power. This was a world where Europeans controlled much of the earth's resources and land, and part of the question of diet remained, as it had for early nineteenth-century nutrition writers, the question of the conquerors and the conquered. This hierarchical thinking contributed to the compromise position that suggested modern French men and women could safely reduce their meat consumption, which might even mitigate some of their ruder personality traits, but too little meat could create fatal weaknesses, as it had for colonial peoples. Gautier summarized it most frankly:

> Does the desirable balance not lie between the aggressive personality of a race or man who is essentially a meat eater, who plunges straight ahead, pursuing his interests above all else, with nothing, not reason, nor pity, stopping his actions or giving rise to hesitations, and the passive energy of the Hindu, eater of rice, who idly accepts his sad fate and protects all life, even that of a bug? The diet of one opens the door to violence and the abuse of force, the other to peacemaking but also to passivity. *In medio stat virtus* [virtue is found in the middle].[86]

Gautier's views demonstrate how the assessment of dietary regimes was affected by political and cultural assumptions in a highly competitive and increasingly interconnected world.

Conclusion

A hundred years after Virey's assertion that meat eaters were powerful conquerors, the idea still persisted that French people required meat to maintain their position at the top of global hierarchies. And yet, there had been a shift; more and more, dietary experts were questioning the primacy of meat and arguing for a better balance that would lead to greater health for a modern French population. In a 1913 speech to a Paris medical society, the physician Alfred Gottschalk worried about the "abuse of animal foods" and warned that "we fall into excesses in this regard very easily." He then stated: "I plainly declare that I am in agreement with the vegetarians when they argue that their regime is absolutely compatible with all of the manifestations of life, with all of the dispensing of energy."[87] By 1917 dietary textbooks were treating the belief in meat's overriding centrality as a "prejudice" left over from a less informed age. The president of the *Société de thérapeutique*, Godefroy Bardet, wrote: "It is important to combat the prejudice of alcohol's necessity for the working people just as we must combat the prejudice that meat is needed by the middle classes. These are two occasional foodstuffs that in certain circumstances can present some advantages, but their inconveniences significantly surpass their utility."[88] And Doctor Armand Hemmerdinger's meal guide and nutrition manual was equally frank: "meat is not nearly as necessary as it is believed to be," he stated.[89] Neither man advocated vegetarianism—Hemmerdinger's suggested weekly menus included significant amounts of meat products—but both saw meat as on a far more equal level with other nutrient-rich foodstuffs than their predecessors.

The slowly changing ideas about the relative value of meat demonstrates a complex relationship between national anxieties, scientific research, and cultural biases in French society. Expert information was influenced by a wide range of new scientific knowledge deriving from therapeutics, microbiology, chemistry, and other specialties. But it was also influenced by ideas about France's position as a leading power in a hierarchical world. The French compared their diets with the other great empires in their midst, and the rise of Japan as a major force in the East gave them pause as they sought to analyze how diet influenced the vitality and culture of a nation or "race." Anxious to keep their place in a global hierarchy that saw European peoples at the top and indigenous peoples at the bottom, the discourses on French and foreign eating habits reflected both justifications of French superiority and some anxiety about the dangers of a bad diet. "Modern" methods and techniques, rooted in the dictates of laboratory-based scientific rigor, sought to dispel the myths of meat in the diet and create a more rational, modern regimen suitable for forward-thinking French men and women. But the persistence of cultural stereotyping and its reshaping within the context of justifying and preserving France's global position marked nutrition studies between the 1880s and 1914.

Notes

1. Julien Joseph Virey, *Du régime alimentaire des anciens, et des résultats de la différence de leur nourriture avec celle des modernes* (Paris: D. Colas, 1813), 49. Virey was chief pharmacist at the French military hospital, Val-de-Grâce, and the founder of the field of chronobiology. For more on his work, see Alain E. Reinberg, Hadas Lewy, and Michael Smolensky, "The Birth of Chronobiology: Julien-Joseph Virey 1814," *Chronobiology International* 18, no. 2 (2001): 173–86.

2. Louis Henri August Marie Polin and Henri Joseph Jules Pierre Labit, *L'hygiène alimentaire* (Paris: Rueff, 1893), 43, 69.

3. Charles Dopter and Jean Rouget, *Hygiène alimentaire* (Paris: Baillière et fils, 1906), 142. This book is volume 4 of the series *Traité d'hygiène*, edited by P. Brouardel and E. Mosny. It is also one of two volumes they wrote together: the second was *Hygiène militaire* published in 1907. See L. Launoy, "Eloge de Charles Dopter (1873–1950)," *Bulletin de la Société de pathologie exotique* 44 (1951): 13–14.

4. See Deborah Neill, "Finding the 'Ideal Diet': Nutrition, Culture, and Dietary Practices in France and French Equatorial Africa, c. 1890s to 1920s," *Food and Foodways* 17, no. 1 (2009): 1–28.

5. Ibid., 5. On regional variations, see Julia Csergo, "The Emergence of Regional Cuisines," in *Food: A Culinary History*, ed. Jean-Louis Flandrin and Massimo Montanari (New York: Penguin, 2000), 500–515. On rural diets, see Anne Lhuissier, "Frugality as a Way of Life: French Rural Workers and Food during the Second Half of the Nineteenth Century," *Food and Foodways* 20, no. 1 (2012): 31–52.

6. Alessandro Stanziani, "Food Safety and Expertise: The Trichinosis Epidemic in France, 1878–1891," *Food and Foodways* 10, no. 4 (2002): 213–14. Urban centers are measured for towns of ten thousand or more. The author also notes that pork represented a third of the meat sold in 1877. The urban-rural divide was consistent over time. In 1908, according to Armand Gautier, the average consumption rate per head of animal foods was 38 kilograms for the country, but in Paris consumption was significantly higher at 94 kilograms per head. See Gautier, *L'alimentation et les régimes chez l'homme sain ou malade* (Paris: Masson, [1903, 1904] 1908), 162.

7. Kenneth J. Carpenter, "A Short History of Nutritional Science, Part 1 (1785–1885)," *Journal of Nutrition* 133 (2003): 638–39; Jean-Paul Aron, "Biologie et alimentation au XVIIIe siècle et au début du XIXe siècle," *Annales* 5 (October 1961): 971–77. Two excellent overviews of this period are Kenneth J. Carpenter, *Protein and Energy: A Study of Changing Ideas in Nutrition* (Cambridge: Cambridge University Press, 1994); Frederic Lawrence Holmes, *Claude Bernard and Animal Chemistry: The Emergence of a Scientist* (Cambridge, MA: Harvard University Press, 1974).

8. Carpenter, "A Short History of Nutritional Science," 640.

9. Ibid., 639–40, 641. For more on the scientific justification of meat as an ideal food in the early and mid-nineteenth century, see Alan D. Krinsky, "Let Them Eat Horse Meat! Science, Philanthropy, the State, and the Search for Complete Nutrition in Nineteenth Century France" (PhD diss., University of Wisconsin-Madison, 2001). On Liebig's life and work, and particularly his influence on the British, see William H. Brock, *Justus von Liebig: The Chemical Gatekeeper* (Cambridge: Cambridge University Press, 1997).

10. See Anson Rabinbach, *The Human Motor: Energy, Fatigue and the Origins of Modernity* (Berkeley: University of California Press, 1992).

11. Statistics are quoted in Dopter and Rouget, *Hygiène alimentaire,* 52. On canned food, see Alberto Capatti, "The Taste for Canned and Preserved Food," in Flandrin and Montanari, *Food,* 492–99; Martin Bruegel, "How the French Learned to Eat Canned Food, 1809–1930s," in *Food Nations: Selling Taste in Consumer Societies,* eds. Warren Belasco and Philip Scranton (London: Routledge, 2002), 113–30. On French refrigeration and shipping, see Alberto Capatti, *Le gout du nouveau: Origins de la modernité alimentaire* (Paris: Albin Michel, 1989), 115–17.

12. Members of the Musée Social, comprising politicians, philanthropists, urban planners, engineers, scientists, and other social reformers, sought to ameliorate the conditions of the working classes, develop a "science of society," and disseminate data in an effort to defuse social conflicts and influence the formation of social policies. See Janet Horne, *A Social Laboratory for Modern France: The Musée Social and the Rise of the Welfare State* (Durham, NC: Duke University Press, 2002), 82–83. Among the dietary studies conducted for the Musée, see, for example, Dr. Cazalis, "Enquête sur l'alimentation a bon marché en Suisse et en Allemagne," *Le Musée social: Mémoires et documents* (1907): 145–77.

13. Léon Fredericq, "Discours," in *IIe Congrès International d'hygiène alimentaire et de l'alimentation rationnelle de l'homme, Bruxelles 4–8 Octobre 1910* (Brussels: M. Weissenbruch, 1910), lxxix; Loudon M. Douglas, "International Congress on Pure Foods and Alimentary Substances," *Nature* 82, no. 2088 (November 4, 1909): 25–26. Patrick Zylberman has argued that officials modeled some of France's food adulteration legislation in 1905 on suggestions made at international gatherings of the 1880s. See Patrick Zylberman, "Making Food Safety an Issue: Internationalized Food Politics and French Public Health from the 1870s to the Present," *Medical History* 48, no. 1 (2004): 18.

14. Josep Barona, "Nutrition and Health: The International Context during the Interwar Crisis," *Social History of Medicine* 2, no. 1 (2008): 89.

15. Lawrence Weaver, "'Growing Babies': Defining the Milk Requirements of Infants, 1890–1910,'" *Social History of Medicine* 23, no. 2 (2009): 323.

16. The Société still exists and continues to function as a central repository of information and studies on nutrition in France. See Jean-Louis Multon and Max Feinberg, *La Société scientifique d'hygiène alimentaire: Cent ans d'histoire au service de l'alimentation (1904–2004)* (Paris: Société scientifique d'hygiène alimentaire, 2005). Also see the website of the Société: www.ssha.asso.fr (accessed February 6, 2013). Key supporters of the original society included the physiology and therapeutics expert Paul Brouardel, the chair of the National Advisory Council on Public Hygiene, who cowrote (with Ernest Mosny) the multivolume *Traité d'hygiène* and with Joseph Girode compiled a ten-volume *Traité de medicine et de thérapeutique* (1895–1902). Also on the list of founding members was Arsène d'Arsonval, the physiologist E. J. Marey, Albert Berthelot, and the physiologist and chemist Albert Dastre. See Fredericq, "Discours."

17. For the 1906 meeting, see "Ier Congrès International d'hygiène alimentaire," *Revue de la Société scientifique d'hygiène alimentaire et de l'alimentation rationnelle de l'homme* 3, nos. 2–6 (1906). For 1910, see *IIe Congrès International d'hygiène alimentaire et de l'alimentation rationnelle de l'homme, Bruxelles 4–8 Octobre 1910* (Brussels: M. Weissenbruch, 1910).

18. The 1906 conference saw a wide range of papers, including papers on soldier and worker diets, diets for tuberculosis patients and adolescents, digestive processes, the effects of individual foodstuffs on digestion, and several papers analyzing wine. See "Table des Matières," in *Revue de la Société scientifique d'hygiène alimentaire et de l'alimentation rationnelle de l'homme* 3, no. 2 (1906): 1463–66. For more on the goals they sought to accomplish, see Claudius Nourry, Secretary-General, speech at the "séance de cloture," idem, xxv.

19. Gautier, "Les problèmes généraux de l'alimentation humaine," *Revue de la société scientifique d'hygiène alimentaire et de l'alimentation rationnelle de l'homme* 3, no. 2 (1906): xi–xiv.

20. Paul Berryer, "Séance générale d'ouverture," in *IIe Congrès International d'hygiène alimentaire et de l'alimentation rationnelle de l'homme, Bruxelles 4–8 Octobre 1910*, lxxvii–lxxviii. French participation at the 1910 congress included three delegates from the Ministry of Agriculture, two from the Ministry of War (one was Jean Rouget), two from the Ministry of the Interior (Drs. Bonjean and Bordas), and seven from the Ministry of Public Instruction, a list that included Gautier as well as Landouzy and the Pasteur Institute biochemist Gabriel Bertrand. Britain was not among the twenty-two countries on the list, which is surprising since it had been an active participant at the Congress on Pure Foods. For a complete list of delegates, see "Liste des Délégués," *IIe Congrès International*, xxxii–xxxvi. At the 1910 congress, presentations on vegetarianism included H. Labbé, "Végétariens et végétaliens," and V. Hoton, "Le régime végétarian, est-il suffisant pour le travail manuel?" On climate, see W. Caspari, "Die Ernährung des Menschen in verschiedenen Klimaten" and Dr. Dryepondt's bizarre "L'alimentation du blanc au Congo." All are listed in "Rapports et Communications," *IIe Congrès International*, iii–x.

21. Robert Nye, *Crime, Madness and Politics in Modern France: The Medical Concept of National Decline* (Princeton, NJ: Princeton University Press, 1984), 134.

22. The extensive literature on French fears about depopulation and degeneration includes: Nye, *Crime, Madness and Politics*; Joshua Cole, *The Power of Large Numbers: Population, Politics, and Gender in Nineteenth-Century France* (Ithaca, NY: Cornell University Press, 2000); William Schneider, *Quality and Quantity: The Quest for Biological Regeneration in Twentieth-Century France* (Cambridge: Cambridge University Press, 1990); William Schneider, "Towards the Improvement of the Human Race: The History of Eugenics in France," *Journal of Modern History* 54 (June 1982): 268–91; S. Gilman and J. Edward Chamberlin, eds., *Degeneration: The Dark Side of Progress* (New York: Columbia University Press, 1985); Rachel Fuchs, "France in a Comparative Perspective," in *Gender and the Politics of Social Reform in France, 1870–1914*, ed. E. Accampo, R. Fuchs, and M. L. Stewart (Baltimore, MD: Johns Hopkins University Press, 1995); Sean M. Quinlan, "The Racial Imagery of Degeneration and Depopulation: Georges Vacher de Lapouge and 'Anthroposociology' in Fin-de-Siècle France," *History of European Ideas* 24, no. 6 (1998): 393–413; Daniel Pick, *Faces of Degeneration: A European Disorder, c. 1848–1918* (Cambridge: Cambridge University Press, 1989); Eugen Weber, *France, Fin de Siècle* (Cambridge, MA: Belknap Press, 1986), and the essays from the forum on gender, population, and the state in *French Historical Studies* 19, no. 3 (1996): 633–754.

23. Cole, *Power of Large Numbers*, 4.

24. Schneider's *Quality and Quantity* discusses in detail the eugenics movement and the optimistic goals of physicians in this project of national regeneration.

25. For more on public hygiene and the physicians, legislators, researchers, and reformers who promoted it in this period, see Murard and Zylberman, *L'hygiène dans la République La santé publique en France, ou l'utopie contrariée, 1870–1918* (Paris: Librairie Arthème Fayard, 1996).

26. On alcohol, see Patricia Prestwich, *Drink and the Politics of Social Reform: Antialcoholism in France since 1870* (Palo Alto, CA: SPOSS, 1988).

27. Nye, for example, explores the problem of alcohol as well as the role of sport in reviving the nation, but does not emphasize other preventive measures like healthy diets. Some scholars have tackled the nutrition question through the study of vegetarians: for example, Ceri Crossley's *Consumable Metaphors: Attitudes towards Animals and Vegetarianism in Nineteenth-Century France* (Oxford: Peter Lang, 2005) has useful material on the rise of science, health, and vegetarian debates within the context of anxiety about French national decline (see 239–87).

28. These beliefs were built on theories outlined by the famed botanist Jean-Baptiste Lamarck (1744–1829). More on Lamarck can be found in L. J. Jordanova, *Lamarck* (Oxford: Oxford University Press, 1984). For information on neo-Lamarckian ideas in the French eugenics movement, see Schneider, "Towards the Improvement of the Human Race," 268–91; Schneider, *Quality and Quantity.*

29. B. A. Morel, *Traité des dégénérescences physiques, intellectuelles et morales de l'espèce humaine et des causes qui produisent ces variétés maladives* (Paris: Masson, 1857).

30. Rafael Huertas, "Madness and Degeneration, I: From 'Fallen Angel' to Mentally Ill," *History of Psychiatry* 3, no. 12 (1992): 391–411, 402.

31. Max Nordau, *Degeneration* (London: William Heinemann, [1892] 1895), 35. Nordau notes that although degeneration was occurring in many countries, in France it had reached massive proportions because of the "awful catastrophe" of 1870 when the loss against Germany led to "a veritable epidemic of mental diseases" known as "siege-madness" (see 42–43).

32. A. Monteuuis, *L'alimentation et la cuisine naturelles dans le monde* (Nice: Visconti, [1907] 1910), 25–29.

33. Book review of Monteuuis, "De l'alimentation et de la cuisine naturelles dans le monde (Paris, 1907)," in *Annales d'hygiène et de médecine coloniales* no. 10 (1907): 482–83.

34. Schneider, *Quality and Quantity*, 8.

35. Schneider, "Towards the Improvement of the Human Race," 271.

36. In the 1860s and 1870s, concerns about infant mortality led to campaigns to promote breast-feeding by mothers and protective legislation regulating the wet-nurse industry. See Joshua Cole, "A Sudden and Terrible Revelation: Motherhood and Infant Mortality in France, 1858–1874," *Journal of Family History* 21, no. 4 (1996): 419–45. William H. Schneider, "Puericulture, and the Style of French Eugenics," *History and Philosophy of the Life Sciences* 8, no. 2 (1986): 269–70.

37. On the list of delegates at the eugenics congress, see *Problems in Eugenics: Papers Communicated at the First International Eugenics Congress, London, July 24–30, 1912* (London: Eugenics Education Society, 1912), xxi–xiii; and the detailed list in Schneider, *Quality and Quantity*, 84–87.

38. Landouzy was not alone in this fear; as Barona notes, for many scientists, "poor nutrition was claimed to be the main factor for impaired organic resistance as a previous stage to infection" (see "Nutrition and Health," 89). But although the question of diet's relationship to tuberculosis was raised frequently in the alimentary hygiene guides and in the major journals, it has not been a major focus of tuberculosis historians. David Barnes's otherwise thorough account, *The Making of a Social Disease: Tuberculosis in Nineteenth-Century France* (Berkeley: University of California Press, 1995), does not focus on dietary concerns, and although Jack Ellis notes that dietary reform became "a recurring theme" among physician-legislators, he primarily focuses his remarks on diet to food safety issues in the campaign against tuberculosis. See Jack D. Ellis, *The Physician-Legislators of France* (Cambridge: University of Cambridge Press, 1990), 76, 196–200.

39. Louis Landouzy, Henri Labbé, and Marcel Labbé, *Enquête sur l'alimentation d'une centaine d'ouvriers et d'employés parisiens* (Paris: Masson, 1905). The authors first presented their research at the International Tuberculosis Conference of 1905. See F. H. Renaut, "Review of Drs. Louis Landouzy, Henri Labbé, and Marcel Labbé, *Enquête sur l'alimentation d'une certaine d'ouvriers et employés parisiens*" (Paris: Masson, 1905), in "Bibliographie," *Revue d'hygiène et de police sanitaire* 28 (1906): 897–98.

40. Landouzy, Labbé, and Labbé, *Enquête sur l'alimentation*, 56.

41. Ibid., 69, 71. The authors argued that mothers were the "safeguards of moral health and national health [*physique du pays*]."

42. For example, see Moll-Weiss, "L'enseignement ménager en Allemagne," in *Musée social, mémoires et documents* (1905): 345–80, 353.

43. Augusta Moll-Weiss, *L'Alimentation de L'enfant de 2 à 6 ans dans la famille et à l'école maternelle* (Paris: G. Steinheil, 1909), 23. For more on Moll-Weiss, see Sandrine Roll, "'Ni bas-bleu, ni pot-au-feu' la conception de la femme selon Augusta Moll-Weiss (France, tournant des XIXe–XXe siècles)," *Genre et Histoire* 5 (Automne 2009): 1–15.

44. Julia Csergo, "Entre faim légitime et frénésie de la table au XIXème siècle: la constitution de la science alimentaire au siècle de la gastronomie," http://www.lemangeur-ocha.com/wp-content/uploads/2012/04/faim_legitime_frenesie_table_int6.pdf (accessed February 16, 2013).

45. Trichinosis is an infection with the roundworm *Trichinella spiralis* and is spread primarily through undercooked meat. For more, see Alessandro Stanziani, "Food Safety and Expertise: The Trichinosis Epidemic in France, 1878–1891," *Food and Foodways* 12 (2002): 215–16.

46. The debates ultimately led to the passing of the French Food Adulteration Act in 1905. For more on trichinosis and food safety, see Zylberman, "Making Food Safety an Issue," 1–28. For more on the economic drivers behind food safety legislation, see Stanziani, *Histoire de la qualité alimentaire XIXe–XXe siècle* (Paris: Seuil, 2005).

47. Edmond Vallin, "De l'étude et de l'exercice professionel de l'hygiène," *La Revue d'hygiène et de police sanitaire* 1, no. 1 (1879): 1–8. For more on Vallin and his deeply held beliefs about the social value of improving public hygiene, see Murard and Zylberman, *L'hygiène dans la République*, 58–60.

48. Louis Henri August Marie Polin and Henri Joseph Jules Pierre Labit, *Étude sur les empoisonnements alimentaires (microbes et ptomaïnes)* (Paris: Octave Dion, 1890); Polin and Labit, *Examen des aliments suspects* (Paris: Gauthier-Villars, 1892); Polin and Labit, *L'hygiène alimentaire.*

49. Polin and Labit, *L'hygiène alimentaire,* 44.

50. In 1918 Dopter became Medical Inspector General of the French Army. See Launoy, "Eloge de Charles Dopter," 8–15.

51. Dopter and Rouget, *Hygiène alimentaire,* 143.

52. Ibid., 139.

53. J. B. Fonssagrives, *Hygiène alimentaire des malades, des convalescents et des valétudinaires: ou, du régime envisagé comme moyen thérapeutique* (Paris: Baillière, 1881), 93.

54. Ibid., 173, 202, 239.

55. Biographical details on Dujardin-Beaumetz (1833–95) are taken from the obituary page of *The British Medical Journal* 1 (March 16, 1895): 621.

56. Georges Octave Dujardin-Beaumetz, *L'hygiène alimentaire: Aliments, alimentation, régime alimentaire dans les maladies* (Paris: Octave Dion, [1887] 1889).

57. Jean Laumonier, *Hygiène de l'alimentation dans l'état de santé et de maladie* (Paris: Félix Alcan, 1894). Subsequent editions were published in 1898, 1904, and 1911. Laumonier also wrote other texts for professional and lay audiences, including *L'hygiène de la cuisine* (Paris: Félix Alcan, 1896).

58. Laumonier, *Hygiène de l'alimentation,* 32–33.

59. Dopter and Rouget, *Hygiène alimentaire* 142.

60. Marcellin Berthelot, *Science et libre pensée* (Paris: Calmann-Lévy 1905), 190.

61. Gautier mentions Berthelot's ideas in his speech, "Les problèmes généraux de l'alimentation humaine," xi–xvii.

62. See Elizabeth Neswald, "Nutritional Knowledge between the Lab and the Field: The Search for Dietary Norms in the Late Nineteenth and Early Twentieth Centuries," chapter 1 of this volume.

63. Gautier, "Les problèmes généraux de l'alimentation humaine," xvi.

64. Gautier, *L'alimentation et les régimes chez l'homme sain ou malade*; Gautier, *Diet and Dietetics* (London: Archibald Constable & Co. Ltd, 1906). Earlier works included *Chimie appliquée à la physiologie, à la pathologie et à l'hygiène* (Paris, 1894).

65. Gautier, *L'alimentation et les régimes chez l'homme sain ou malade,* 11.

66. Ibid., 566.

67. Like other alimentary hygienists, Gautier broke his analysis down by age and gender. Most of the experts in this period believed that women had peculiar physiological and emotional needs and required different rules to govern their diets.

68. Gautier, *L'alimentation et les régimes chez l'homme sain ou malade,* 555, 556. For more on Gautier's ideas, see Neill, "Finding the Ideal Diet," 5–8.

69. British scientists faced similar cultural barriers when they promoted wholemeal bread over white bread. As Ina Zweiniger-Bargielowska argues, consumers preferred white bread in part because they saw it as a symbol of British superiority. See Ina Zweiniger-Bargielowska, "'Not a Complete Food for Man': The Controversy about White versus Wholemeal Bread in Interwar Britain," chapter 6 of this volume.

70. Dopter and Rouget, *Hygiène alimentaire,* 61. Comparisons with Britain and fears about the dangers of reduced meat consumption were also prevalent in other countries.

For example, an 1894 essay in *La riforma sociale* by Francesco Nitti argued that Italian laborers consumed half as much meat as French workers and one-quarter as much as British workers. "This deficit of protein will not kill them," Nitti noted, "but the population or group in question will slowly waste away or simply not develop." Quoted in Carol Helstosky, *Garlic and Oil: Food and Politics in Italy* (Oxford: Berg, 2004), 22.

71. Gautier, *Diet and Dietetics*, 377.

72. Crossley, *Consumable Metaphors*, 241–42, 242n15. On British vegetarianism, see James Gregory, *Of Victorians and Vegetarians: The Vegetarian Movement in Nineteenth-Century Britain* (London: I. B. Tauris, 2007); on the American case, see Adam D. Shprintzen, *The Vegetarian Crusade: The Rise of an American Reform Movement, 1817–1921* (Chapel Hill: University of North Carolina Press, 2013).

73. Crossley, *Consumable Metaphors*, 247. Arnaud Baubérot agrees that the movement was concerned with the hygienic and medical reasons for avoiding meat; in the writings of vegetarian advocates one finds little concern with the social and economic conditions related to the production of meat. See "Un projet de réforme hygiènique des modes de vie: Naturistes et végétariens à la Belle Époque," *French Politics, Culture and Society* 26, no. 3 (2008): 7. Baubérot explores the relationship of the vegetarian movement to "naturalist" medicine that was highly critical of modern life in France and advocated a variety of hygienic practices to combat it.

74. Crossley, *Consumable Metaphors*, 242; Bauberot, "Un project de réforme," 10.

75. Crossley notes that Dujardin-Beaumetz was "a real catch" for vegetarians because even though he did not advocate a vegetarian diet, he gave some vegetarian arguments "scientific credibility." See Crossley, *Consumable Metaphors*, 248–49. Vegetarians played an important role in challenging prevailing protein orthodoxies in Germany as well, as Corinna Treitel argues in "How Vegetarians, Naturopaths, Scientists, and Physicians Unmade the Protein Standard in Modern Germany," in chapter 2 of this volume.

76. Gautier, *L'alimentation et les régimes chez l'homme sain ou malade*, 17, 557–60, 161. On vegetarians embracing Gautier, see Crossley, *Consumable Metaphors*, 249–51. For more on Gautier's specific views on vegetarianism, see Neill, "Finding the Ideal Diet," 8.

77. Polin and Labit, *L'hygiène alimentaire*, 69–71, 79.

78. Ibid., 43–44.

79. J. A. Rivière, "Considérations sur le régime alimentaire rationnel," *Revue de la Société scientifique d'hygiène alimentaire et de l'alimentation rationnelle de l'homme* 3, no. 2 (1906): 1089, 1093.

80. Ibid., 1093.

81. It was not only in France that Japanese diets attracted interest. Treitel notes the importance of studies on the Japanese among groups mounting challenges to Carl Voit's protein standard in Germany. See Treitel, "How Vegetarians, Naturopaths, Scientists, and Physicians Unmade the Protein Standard in Modern Germany," chapter 2 of this volume.

82. Anonymous, "Japonais tous végetariens et buveurs d'eau," *Réforme Alimentaire* 9 (1905): 12. The journals the author quotes are *Revue française de médecine et de chirurgie*, the *Medical Record*, and the *Edinburgh Medical Journal*, all from 1904.

83. Dopter and Rouget, *Hygiène alimentaire*, 141. The study they cite on Japanese dietary choices is by Lapique (no full citation is provided). Lombroso, a physician

and psychiatrist, argued that measuring heads and evaluating facial features and body types could reveal whether a human had innate tendencies toward criminality. His views were very popular in late nineteenth-century Europe, particularly for some eugenicists and those who feared social degeneration. For more, see Pick, *Faces of Degeneration*.

84. Dopter and Rouget, *Hygiène alimentaire*, 141–42.

85. Ibid., 140–41.

86. Gautier, *L'alimentation et les régimes chez l'homme sain ou malade*, 558.

87. Alfred Gottschalk, "Le régime végétarien et les régimes de sobriété: Communication faite à la société médicale du IXe arrondissement de Paris, le 8 mai 1913," *Réforme Alimentaire* 7 (1914): 43–44.

88. Dr. G. Bardet, *La ration normale: Moyens pratiques de l'établir: Guide pratique d'hygiène alimentaire* (Paris: Octave Dion et Fils, 1917), 80.

89. Armand Hemmerdinger, *Leçons pratiques d'alimentation raisonnée* (Paris: Masson et Cie., 1918), 32–33.

Chapter Four

Setting Standards

The Soldier's Food in Germany, 1850–1960

ULRIKE THOMS

In his classical work on military tactics, *The General Principles of War*, Friedrich the Great (1712–86) stated that anyone wanting to build an army must start with the belly.[1] Procuring sufficient food was crucial in warfare, since food supply influenced both the soldiers' performance and their morale.[2] Nevertheless, provisions were basic. Friedrich's soldiers were supplied with just two pounds of bread per day,[3] and food procurement and preparation were largely left to the individual soldier. Military food consumption thus followed traditional, regional, and social differences. Whereas officers ate in restaurants, with their families, or with householders, the common soldiers prepared their foods in cooperative cooking communities called *Menagen*. They purchased food collectively and hired a cook or cooked in turn. As a result, the peacetime food of regular soldiers was similar to that of the civilian population. It was shaped by custom and varied according to rank.

During wartime, food was requisitioned from the civilian population, which was obligated to accommodate soldiers and reimbursed for its expenses. The army organized food provision only when larger forces were assembled and where opportunities for self-catering or quartering seemed uncertain.[4] This began to change only during the eighteenth century, after the establishment of standing armies and permanent barracks. Two decrees, announced in 1827 and 1831, emerged from these changes and opened the possibility that some food would be centrally supplied during campaigns. However, the state did not provide complete and healthy food in peacetime.[5] When the army supplied only bread, soldiers continued to purchase the rest of their food from marketers in or near garrisons, and marketers accompanied the army on military campaigns. More fundamental change had to wait until 1858 when the food provision regulation (*Verpflegungsreglement*) was enacted.[6]

This essay follows developments in the soldier's rations between 1850 and 1960, focusing not on organizational changes but on scientific and medical discourses on dietary standards, which began in the middle of the nineteenth century. Two developments shaped these discourses. They were, first, deeply influenced by the Crimean War (1853–56). Military tactics had changed from static to mobile warfare, and the experiences of the war showed that the military was unable to supply adequate food to its more mobile troops.[7] There was simply no time to set up traditional systems of provisioning. Second, the army became increasingly interesting to physiologists, statisticians, and anthropologists, who saw it as a kind of laboratory for investigating food questions and for testing hypotheses and new products.

During the preparatory phases of the 1863 International Statistical Congress, Rudolf Virchow (1821–1902) argued that medical examinations of potential recruits presented opportunities for collecting statistics on the physiques of young men. This would enable physicians to draw conclusions about the physical condition and health of the population. Virchow was not alone in his interest in the health of military recruits. Some of his contemporaries feared that, if these recruitment survey reports represented broader developments, they were an alarming sign of physical deterioration in the population.[8] Poor nutrition and infectious diseases among working- and lower-class boys produced frail bodies that did not conform to the general male body ideal of the strong and healthy warrior.

Medical researchers and anthropologists were interested in army food for another reason. The army offered opportunities for experimentation and for the collection of consistent and long-term data. In soldiers they had a group of healthy, active males of roughly the same age who lived under comparable and controllable conditions. Moreover, soldiers were accustomed to strict hierarchies and were required by law to acquiesce to medical treatment. In addition, the common soldiers came from the working class, whose performance, health, and nutrition was already a subject of concern. For these reasons, the army was seen as an ideal field for nutritional experimentation, especially since statisticians, physicians, scientists, and administrators expected that better food would improve performance.

A detailed investigation of the development of soldiers' rations and of soldiers' reactions to attempts to alter their diets are beyond the scope of this essay. Instead the focus here is on the construction of various kinds food standards: the social standards of officers and recruits, and physiological, toxicological, hygienic, and technological standards. As will be seen, military food standards were used as a reference point for civilian practices. Attempts to write a history of German military food standards are difficult owing to the country's political history. Although the administrative practices of the German armies converged after the foundation of the North German Confederation (Norddeutscher

Bund) in 1867 and the German Reich in 1871, considerable regional variations remained. Therefore this essay concentrates on the food of the Prussian Army, although even the Prussian dietary schemes also varied across the different regions within Prussia.

Rational Nutrition: Physiological Standards and the Army

For many centuries, the soldier's ration was based exclusively on bread. Around the mid-nineteenth century, proponents of the model of "rational nutrition," according to which food intake should satisfy bodily needs in the most financially economical way, began to turn their attention to army food.[9] Once chemists like Antoine Lavoisier (1743–94) and physiologists such as François Magendie (1783–1855) had shown that protein was necessary to sustain life and to maintain performance, the search for the protein minimum and inexpensive protein sources began. Foods were ranked according to the relation between price and protein content. This search clearly linked science and political and social welfare, and researchers such as Jakob Moleschott (1822–94) were proponents of leftist ideas of social and political reform. The moderate political perspective of Justus von Liebig (1803–73) relied on an analogy between the state and the human body. Just as muscles, nerves, and tissues formed parts of the animal body and played roles in metabolism, every individual participated in the state in an appropriate proportion to the capacities of his body and mind.[10] The task of the state was to maintain and restore the life of the state's body.[11] This included the obligation not to ask for more than individuals were able to contribute. If the state increased its demands, it was obliged to increase its investment, that is, to provide more food to the people. For Liebig food was not only a question of physiology but also the core element of culture. It was equivalent to the economy of power and connected to the wise use of resources, whereas waste in agriculture, industry, and science was, in his eyes, barbarism, or a deficit of culture.[12]

Although the relevant figures are hidden in an appendix to Liebig's *Thier-Chemie*, the data on which he based his assumptions included calculations of the food intake of 855 soldiers.[13] For one month he weighed the food served to these soldiers by the cooking communities and estimated the foods they had purchased at the small shops in the garrison. Based on analyses of the foodstuffs and the soldier's excretions (urine, faeces), he calculated the average nutrient intake of the soldiers. Liebig's work had far-reaching consequences and solidified the protein paradigm, which would dominate research for decades.[14] According to Liebig, the soldiers received 112 grams of beef, about 30 grams of pork, 157 grams of vegetables or 556 grams of potatoes or 13 grams of dried beans, 13 grams of dried lentils, 12 grams of dried peas, and 2 grams of fat per day.[15]

Numbers such as these gained importance from the emerging power of science. Military physicians expected that "the study of the laws of nature and the utilization of their immeasurable powers in the field of military hygiene will furnish the soldier with an abundance of endurance, power, and courage and make him capable of achieving his lofty goals."[16] Although doubts remained about the specific diets proposed by physiologists,[17] the attitude behind them spread. Simultaneously, the army took on increasing responsibility for the daily needs of its members, including food provision.

The Crimean War, the first war widely covered in the news media, was crucial. Many reports described the disastrous living conditions of soldiers, and it was clear that their needs had been neglected.[18] This influenced the assessment of the soldier's diet in Prussia. In 1858 new rules replaced those of 1831. They kept the differentiation between campaign and peacetime. As before, the new regulations provided for only 630 grams of rye bread daily in peace, but the soldier was now entitled to extra pay, the food rate (*Verpflegungssatz*). This was calculated on the basis of a virtual ration, which fixed certain physiological food needs as "normal." It was revised every three months to conform with price changes. In peacetime it included 130 grams of meat, either 80 grams of rice or 102 grams of barley or 204 grams of pulses, 0.75 litres of potatoes, and 7 grams of salt. During campaigns the ration was increased to 220 grams of meat, 102 grams of rice, 131 grams of groats, and 270 grams of pulses per day to cover the higher physical needs. Moreover, the salt ration was increased and even coffee was included, an acknowledgment of the effect of physical stimulants.[19]

This Prussian decree was extended to all states of the North German Confederation and to all German member states in 1867. Although it set quantities, it left enough flexibility to allow adaptation to regional dietary customs and special situations.[20] Nevertheless, social standards still played a role. Only the diet of the lower ranks was rationed, whereas officers were free to purchase whatever food they desired. Moreover, the regulations of 1858 were relative. If a regular soldier was provided with food and board by civilians during campaigns or on marches, he was not entitled to more or better food than his hosts. Although the state was responsible for his provision, his claims could not exceed what was customary for civilians in the region.[21]

Nevertheless, the situation had changed significantly, insofar as the state acknowledged its responsibility for the soldiers' well-being and increasingly took scientific knowledge into account. One major problem remained. Although medicine and physiology now held the authority to judge on physical needs, the medical service had almost no influence on the administrative branch, which was responsible for practical food provision. This caused many problems, since the improvements suggested by physiologists also raised costs, whereas the army administration wanted to keep the food simple and inexpensive. For psychological and disciplinary reasons, they also took the soldier's food preferences into account.

Physiologists argued that spending more on food was an investment that would pay for itself through increased performance and health.[22] The soldier could be taken as an *homme moyenne* (average man), as defined by Adolphe Quetelet,[23] and the most economical way of meeting his needs could be calculated. Although the military administration still hesitated to adopt this approach, military medicine did not. Like the many handbooks on general and social hygiene,[24] those on military hygiene contained large sections on the food of the soldier as one major factor of health.[25]

These handbooks show that until the mid-1860s, food provisioning was seen primarily as an administrative task. But from then on, the new results of physiology were integrated into the military doctor's knowledge. The scientific findings helped in two ways. First, they underlined the importance of physiology and were an important argument for the professionalization of military medicine.[26] Second, they demonstrated that the case for army food reform was not unreasonable, but, instead, was justified by science.

These developments took place against the background of a broader discussion on degeneration, as more and more recruits seemed to be unfit for military service.[27] In the 1850s the medical doctor Wilhelm Hildesheim stressed the correlation of this finding with the nutritional situation of the people. He stated: "The fact that physical examination shows that most conscripts are unfit for military service implies a discrepancy between the diet and the dietary needs of the people in general. It would be desirable to find out the reasons through thorough examination of the diet, in order to counteract increasing decline in the generations to come."[28] One important point here is that tuberculosis, which was often diagnosed in poorly nourished people such as prisoners, was often found in young conscripts as well. This not only provided a significant argument in support of the state's obligation to satisfy all of the soldiers' physiological needs. It also made better food seem a rewarding investment. Hildesheim, for example, spoke directly of the importance of strong bodies for the national economy.[29]

Giving the young soldiers sufficient nourishment would enable them to serve their fatherland in war and in peace, after which they would return home to a productive working life.[30] This same argument drove changes in prison diets in Prussia in 1872. In order to reduce mortality and to improve the physical condition after release, prisoners were entitled to a regular portion of meat every other day, and even to real coffee and spices, which were deemed to have a stimulating effect on digestion.[31]

The physiologist Carl Voit addressed the Bavarian Ministry of War several times in order to improve the food rations of soldiers. His first initiative was a memorandum he wrote in 1860.[32] In 1877 he and his student circle published a comprehensive collection of articles on institutional feeding, after he had given a lecture at the Association for Public Health (Verein für öffentliche Gesundheitspflege) in Munich.[33] Voit emphasized, "The state has a great interest in making soldier's bodies strong, not weak, because it wants to have strong men available when a war starts."[34] At the same time Voit bitterly complained that whereas in every other field of military life new science and technology were readily applied to reduce waste, this was not so in the case of food. Farmers had quickly realized the advantages of modern food science, he claimed.[35] Mistakes in livestock feeding led to financial losses, but no one cared whether a prisoner fell ill owing to insufficient food or whether a soldier was forced to supplement his *Menagen* provisions from elsewhere. Repeatedly, Voit pointed out the importance of nutrition science for the administration of public institutions. In his eyes it could help improve the health of inmates so that they would able to work and earn their living. He campaigned for the full provisioning of soldiers, arguing that it would reduce costs through high-volume purchases and allow for savings in less nutritious or superfluous foods, such as the enormous bread portions that soldiers did not eat completely. The improved diet would not necessarily be more expensive. Nevertheless, Voit's argument was not purely philanthropic. He spoke of the soldiers as "war material." Just as the commander needed gunpowder, he also needed his soldiers and had to care for their proper nutrition.[36] For Voit, professional motives were even more important, since one could learn much from studies of soldiers and get new ideas for further scientific work. Other authors followed this general line.[37]

Finally, their words were heard. In January 1878 a new guideline for the medical service was issued in Prussia. It set the ratio of different nutrients in the army's diet, and military physicians were given the responsibility of examining and controlling the nutrient content of the menus on a regular basis. Consequently, the *Menagen* commissions were no longer completely free to follow the preferences of the soldiers. They had to fulfil general minimum nutritive requirements and to follow the expertise of the physicians who controlled them.[38] Two years later, the Bavarian king called a special commission in Munich to study army food and propose changes. Extensive investigations were made using the very methods Voit and his students had developed in their studies of institutional feeding in 1877. The special commission came to the same conclusion as Voit: soldiers needed above all more animal protein.[39]

The Protein Standard

The importance of albuminous substances for proper nutrition was long known.[40] Liebig regarded protein metabolism as the primary metabolism and used nitrogen excretion to measure it. Scientific discussions of military provisioning focused on the daily amount of meat that the soldiers should receive, but the real reasons for the emphasis on meat in the soldier's diet were a mixture of physiology and psychology. Meat was the traditional food for warriors and men, whereas women, children, servants, and marginalized groups such as prisoners followed a largely meatless diet.[41] Some of this can be attributed to social differentiation. Meat was expensive and therefore unaffordable for the lower classes and especially for workers. Therefore it was a prestige food and the food of those in power. Meat was also associated with aggression, with cruelty, and thus with struggle and fighting. Rationalizing the diet meant looking for ways to increase protein intake without increasing cost and finding ways to balance higher expenses for meat with lower expenses for other foods.

Apart from these factors, meat had additional advantages for mass provisioning. Not only did its pleasant taste enliven an otherwise bland diet, but it was also practical, as a handbook from 1858 pointed out. In contrast to other foods, it could be easily transported in the form of livestock. Moreover, cattle could be procured anywhere and meat could be easily and quickly prepared even under the basic conditions of field kitchens.[42]

From around 1850 onward, efforts to reform the soldier's diet aimed at increasing its protein content. To that end, newly developed products such as meat extract and pulse flour were integrated into the diet, while more animal protein came from the introduction of cheese and sea fish.[43] Nineteenth-century nutritional physiologists heavily criticized the high fiber content of the diet of the lower classes, from which most soldiers were recruited, and recommended more meat in their diet. For example, in 1858 Johannes Ranke described the bloated bodies of soldiers who had been nourished primarily with bread. Because of its low cost, coarse rye bread seemed appropriate in times of peace, but in times of war, performance made high meat rations necessary.[44] Suggestions for appropriate rations resembled those that Voit had fixed for the worker with moderate physical labor, but the soldier's field ration was adjusted to higher performance levels. Although Voit rejected Liebig's idea of protein as the source of muscle power, he demanded a field diet that contained 500 grams of raw meat per day. This enormous amount was justified by the claim that meat was an easily digestible, concentrated food, whereas large amounts of vegetables and especially of coarse rye bread were seen as a heavy burden for the fighting body, since they slowed down the process of digestion.[45]

Although physiological thought and writing focused almost exclusively on the question of protein,[46] this was criticized and was the subject of intensive debate over several decades. Doubts such as those formulated by the physicians Hans Lichtenfelt and Felix Hirschfeld since the late 1880s increased among the members of the physiological and medical community. Much of this can be traced to the impact of life reform and vegetarianism.[47] Consequently, the belief that man could do with lower meat rations gained ground. On the basis of his scientific expertise and credibility, Max Rubner pleaded for a reduction of the high meat rations.[48] Nevertheless, as can be seen from table 4.1, the daily meat ration during the First World War was still fixed at the high standard of 375 grams of raw, salted, or frozen meat. After the First World War, life reform and vegetarianism gained ground. But although the National Socialists favored these ideas, meat was still considered indispensable for physiological and, even more, for psychological reasons. The main argument was the food habits of the soldiers. Pointing to personal and practical experience, the administrators refused changes because they thought that reducing the meat ration would affect the troops' morale.[49] Moreover, scientists again stressed the importance of protein for physical performance. This view received support from a systematic examination of the diets of sportsmen during the 1936 Olympic Games, which showed that successful participants ate large amounts of meat.[50] Consequently, large amounts of meat were still deemed essential.

Table 4.1. Meat rations in the soldier's diet (grams per head per day)

	In the garrison	During war
1858, Verpflegungsreglement	97	117
1867, Verpflegungsreglement		770
1870, Bavaria and Prussia		500
1876, Voit's norm for the soldier	250	500
1898, Friedensverpflegungsvorschrift	180	250
1914–18		375
1939	200	200

Sources: Voit, "Anforderungen," 29; Kirchner, *Lehrbuch der Millitärhygiene,* 17, Bickel, "Eiweiss," 25, 29.

The Army and Control Technologies

Overall, the intensity of the meat discussion declined at the beginning of the twentieth century, although control of the soldier's diet was extended. As mentioned, army physicians were required to control the nutrient content of the diet from 1878. Nevertheless, this control covered only the midday meal and bread ration, because it was left to the individual troop units to decide whether or not to establish full provisioning. Many efforts were made to install a system of full provisioning that would completely control the food budget and quality. Self-catering was regarded as more expensive and, since soldiers often spent money that was intended for food on other things such as alcohol, centralized provisioning allowed better control of the quality of the diet and of the daily food intake.[51] Army kitchens and full provisioning were important means to discipline appetites and bodies and make the latter fit for high-performance tasks. Although the process of establishing kitchens and full provisioning cannot be precisely traced through the nineteenth century, at the beginning of the twentieth, new instructions for provision in peace and war were issued (in 1900 and 1902). They were followed by instructions for the administration of troop kitchens and for the regular inspection of the food and calculations of its nutrient content.[52] Ironically, once this standardization had taken place, guidelines were introduced that allowed considerable variability. In 1913 there were six different meal schedules with greater or lesser amounts of meat and vegetables.[53] Increasing variety and quality had become more important than fixating on meat and on uniform amounts of calories and nutrients.

The experiences of the First World War drove this development forward, especially since the troops bitterly complained about monotonous meals. Consequently, more variety was introduced through an increased number of vegetables and other nonmeat products and more varied recipes. The firm establishment of nutritional knowledge and of a basic dietary norm allowed foods to substitute one another as long as the overall nutrient requirements were fulfilled, and physicians assessed the diet for physiological adequacy.[54] This allowed the army administration leeway to adapt to local market conditions and dietary customs.

Whereas physicians remained responsible for ensuring the diet was sufficient and healthy, controlling food quality was the task of pharmacists, who formed part of the army control boards.[55] Practical food chemistry and food control in Germany were closely connected to the work of pharmacists. Beginning in 1879, pharmacists could earn a degree in food chemistry with an additional year of university study. The working field of the army pharmacists was extensive. They analyzed food and water and conducted toxicological examinations. Meat, however, was inspected by army veterinarians. Both food chemists and veterinarians published numerous reports on their findings in journals for military medicine and developed quality standards that were then included in provision regulations (*Beschaffungsvorschriften*).[56]

Included in the supply contracts with marketers and producers were quality standards that defined the quality of the articles to be delivered according to existing knowledge and market customs.[57] Institutions that fed large groups, such as hospitals and prisons, adopted the army's provision regulations. One example is the Berlin Charité Hospital. Many of the directors of these institutions had formerly worked in the military and were familiar with the regulations.[58] In institutions that produced some of their own food, such as sausages, as did the Moabit Hospital in Berlin, military practices served as a model.[59] The army had a reputation for handling food-supply questions economically, and army standards were viewed as well-grounded in practice.[60]

The famous wholemeal bread of the German Army (*Kommissbrot*) is a good example of a highly standardized military food. Even today the word *Kommiss* is used as a synonym for the army, which can be explained by the central position of this bread in army food, especially during the first half of the nineteenth century. It became a symbol of military service.[61] In addition, its quality became a reference point for the bread in prisons and other public institutions.[62] Given its importance, its quality was closely regulated. Until 1872 only 5 percent of the flour was sieved out as bran, but under the influence of the nutritional sciences and the rising standard of living, this percentage was increased to 15 percent.[63] Around 1900, the physician Wenzeslaus Plagge and the chemist Georg Lebbin from the Academy for Military Medicine in Berlin researched the question of army bread. They reviewed the extensive literature, collected calculations on the digestibility of army bread, and performed eighty-five experiments between 1891 and 1896 on which kind of bread would have the highest nutritional value.[64] Their conclusions confirmed what soldiers had reported repeatedly: the coarse army bread was hard to digest, especially since it was often of poor quality.

Setting New Standards: Army Food and Food Technology

Plagge and Lebbin's book on army bread demonstrates that the army tried to improve the food through technology and encouraged scientists to search for technological solutions to food problems. The consequences of the Crimean War can hardly be overstated. In the aftermath, all European states increased their efforts to improve the soldier's food and especially emergency food, the so-called iron rations needed when supply trains could not reach army units. Canned and preserved foods were introduced as foods that were ready to eat, low in volume and weight, nutritious, and cost efficient.

The Franco-Prussian War (1870–71) served as a catalyst for the introduction of foods such as preserved meat, dried soup powders, and bouillon cubes.[65] Experiments with foods that formed a complete meal had been made since the early nineteenth century when meat zwieback and meat extracts were introduced.[66] Their success was limited because of problems with large-scale production and high prices, and also because soldiers were still responsible for their own provisioning. But as the army took on more responsibility for the food of the troops, and with the outbreak of the Franco-Prussian War in 1870, these products were finally integrated into the rations, first into the field ration. Discussion about the value of the new products resumed after the end of the war.[67] These products meant more than mere foods. They were signs of modernity, since they promised to solve the problems of provisioning by technological and scientific means. This can be easily seen in the detailed descriptions of their manufacture in medical journals. Many efforts were made to create an industrial product that united the assumed physiological need for high protein content with the economic limitations. There was a firm belief in the possibilities of physiology and technology. One day it would possible to create an economical food that would satisfy all physiological and practical needs.

Not only industrial entrepreneurs but also chemists and chemically interested physicians such as Carl A. Meinert were active in this field. In 1880, Meinert published an extensive study of army food in which he tried to determine the nutritive value of a meat powder produced by Franz Hofmann.[68] Such products were fashionable. They were heavily marketed through popular channels and to the medical and scientific public.[69] They were received with great interest, as they seemed to be the realization of the long-existing idea of a perfect food for soldiers.[70]

Meat powders never gained an important economic position, since they were expensive and did not taste very good. The case was different for many soup products, which used meat extracts and legume powders as ingredients. The idea of concentrating the strength of meat in bone and meat extracts and soup cubes had been researched by chemists such as Magendie, Sigismund Friedrich Hermbstaedt, and Liebig. Liebig's product, in particular, was a market success,[71] as was the so-called pea sausage of the Berlin cook Heinrich Grüneberg (1819–72), who presented his ingenious invention in 1870. Grüneberg's product was prepared from a mixture of dried pea powder, fat, spices, and dried bacon. It was cooked into a pasty mixture and filled into sausage casings, which were then dried and packed. A soldier needed only to dissolve the mass in boiling water to have a complete meal. The Prussian Army was enthusiastic and bought the production secret for the immense sum of 37,000 Thaler. During the Franco-Prussian War, 1,900 people were employed in the daily production of sixty to seventy thousand pea sausages per day, and by the end of the war forty million sausages had left the factory. The factory was then handed over to the private entrepreneur Louis Lejeune and continued in production until the 1940s because pea sausage became integrated into the daily diets of civilians. Other firms, such as that of Friedrich Scheller (1822–1900) from Thüringen, produced similar products,[72] sometimes to improve product quality or to introduce new variations. Scheller experimented with other preparations and created pressed dried soup concentrates, which he offered in four variations to the Prussian Army: rice, brown flour, milled wheat, and pea soup. For fifteen years he sold large amounts of these, which were also exported to the United States. Scheller's products lost ground only after the large companies Knorr and Maggi began to make similar products, among them a pea sausage, and marketed them with large advertising campaigns.[73]

The food quality standards of the army were high, and not all new products made their way into the army kitchens. Dried vegetables, for example, were rejected because of their poor taste, and other items proved too expensive.[74] But they were ideal for the "iron ration," as they were lightweight, took up little space, and were easy to pack and to store. As for canned meat, the army was neither satisfied with the quality of existing products nor did it trust the producers. It therefore built two army canneries, the first in Mainz in 1876, following an idea from the commander of the army in France, Edwin von Manteuffel. Its production was larger than one might expect. It included a mill, bakery, vegetable processing section, butchery with kitchen, and a room for the preparation of coffee. In the second factory, opened in Spandau in 1892, three thousand oxen were slaughtered daily and canned as beef.[75] In contemporary publications, industrial products of this kind seemed to be the solution to all the provisioning, hygienic, and physiological problems of army food.

In the early decades of the twentieth century the focus changed after the emergence of the "vitamin" concept, and vegetables, brown bread, and fruit acquired new importance. Dietary schemes were reformed in general. At the same time, it became clear that further progress depended not so much on theoretical knowledge, counting calories, and measuring nutrients, but on practical skills and food technology. It is important to note that until the 1930s, army cooks were almost always untrained, whereas under National Socialism training for cooks was established. This not only helped ensure more culinary variety, but also that the cooks knew how to preserve vitamins and to create a balanced diet by calculating the nutrient content.[76]

These changes were driven by Wilhelm Ziegelmayer from the Military Administration. Ziegelmayer was a chemistry graduate and teacher who worked in nutrition science and education in the 1920s before entering the Army High Command in 1937. His book, *Food Resources for the Nutrition of the General Population*, followed the official National Socialist food policy in that he strongly argued that Germany should be self-sufficient in food and encouraged the use of forgotten, traditional foods as well as new ones. Based on Ziegelmayer's efforts, the army issued a new diet scheme in 1939, released an army cookbook, and established a department for food experimentation at the Army Administration School in Munich. Ziegelmayer was convinced that the nutrition question would prove the modernity of the German Army. He believed that science would win the war.[77] In contrast to nineteenth-century military provisioning, now only physical needs determined the food ration. Any social distinction in the diets provided to officers and soldiers was abolished, and Hitler himself was often portrayed sharing a meal with soldiers in the field kitchen at the front, putting himself on the level of the simple soldier.[78] Thus, the shared meal was used to produce a community, and it is not by accident that the term *Gemeinschaftsverpflegung* (community provisioning) was created during these years to designate mass catering.[79]

In addition, at the reopened Military Medical Academy in Berlin, where physiological and chemical research on army food was conducted, a specialized teaching group (Lehrgruppe) on scientific research in physiology was established. It had a strong focus on nutrition. In 1940 a special army food working group (Arbeitsgemeinschaft Ernährung der Wehrmacht) was formed, where officers from all army divisions, scientists, and people from industry met to solve problems of food provision. Tellingly, it was founded as a working group on vitamin questions, which were very fashionable at the time. Like the public, administrative organizations were obsessed with vitamins and how to provide them.[80]

This obsession led to state-financed and nationwide vitamin initiatives, during which workers, school children, and soldiers received daily vitamin drops in order to increase their performance and resistance to infections.[81] The meat and the protein problem was therefore completely replaced in public discourse by the question of how to consume a sufficient amount of vitamins. Vitamins were regarded as "silver bullets," although deficiency diseases were rare.[82] Instead, researchers collaborated with Hoffmann La Roche, the main producer of vitamin C, to construct so-called hypovitaminosis, a latent deficiency, which was said to cause numerous, albeit not dramatic, symptoms. According to this theory, people with vitamin deficiencies would feel miserable, sleep badly, tire quickly, and be short-tempered. Articles reported on experiments that had shown that sportsmen showed increased vigor and capacity once an existing deficit had been remedied.[83] This resulted in demands for vitamin-rich foods and the prophylactic use of vitamin preparations, which were integrated into field rations in the form of vitamin drops.

Many scientists and physicians followed the vitamin line, some of them for the sake of their professional positions. Industry eagerly jumped on this bandwagon in order to promote and sell vitamins and supplemented products.[84] Much was done to increase the vitamin content of the diet, for example by integrating raw foods and fruit on a regular basis. Administrators and physiologists also spoke out strongly for a reduction in the size of meat portions, which were deemed too large from the physiological and too expensive from the administrative point of view. Instead, soy products and meat surrogates were introduced and promoted as major achievements of modern nutritional research and technological development.[85] More salad and vegetables were to be served, and better seasoning of meals was to be used to improve taste, which had previously been supplied by meat. After Wilhelm Ziegelmayer had taken over the initiative, the army presented itself as the leader of food innovations. In 1940 the army proudly announced at the Leipzig fair that it had developed 140 new foods since 1936.[86] From about 17,000 patents of the Nazi period, 9,540 dealt with food technology, of which roughly one-third concerned production and two-thirds processing.[87] Many were simply improvements or continuations of innovations that had been introduced earlier, for example, vegetable drying. Even the introduction of frozen meat and fish, which was strongly promoted by the army and especially by Rudolf Heiss, the specialist in this field, dates back to the First World War. What had changed was that the administration was now much more generous with expenditure, and the reduced meat portions allowed more freedom in other items. Even more important is the fact that the quick integration of modern food technology was an important element of the self-presentation of the Wehrmacht as a modern army that relied on the results of scientific research and engineering. This is obvious not only in Ziegelmayer's publications, but also in the journal of the army administration, which in 1939 published a report on Hitler's tour along the Westwall. It proudly stated that all efforts had made by the provisions office (*Verwaltungsamt*) to solve the problems of army provision. New foods were displayed to the Führer and used for a test meal.[88] Moreover, the new field cookbook was displayed. It was noted that Hitler was very satisfied and was especially interested in crispbread. Many articles were published in the public press to reassure relatives at home that the army cared for its soldiers and provided them with sufficient and healthy food.[89]

During these years the view of army food as model food was promoted and purposefully exploited in National Socialist food propaganda. The former concentration on the *homme moyenne* was replaced by a focus on the Nazi concept of the *Volkskörper* (racial body). Army food was now regarded as having a decisive educational influence on the dietary habits of soldiers and their families, since they would carry the new and epidemiologically useful habits home with them.[90] Under Nazi rule various forms of *Gemeinschaftsverpflegung* were extended, for example, via the Hitler youth camps and the factory canteens, in order to extend control of the food budget and to steer consumption.[91]

The nutritional physiologists of the German armed forces, however, were skeptical about many of the claims made for vitamins and opposed the common public opinion that vitamin C increased physical performance. Instead they pointed to the danger of undersupply with protein as early as 1940 and countered the vitamin enthusiasts by underlining the importance of calories and protein, arguing that the real danger was not vitamin deficiency but undernourishment and starvation.[92] Studies on work efficiency conducted by army physiologists had shown that a high level of performance depended on high-value animal protein. This became more important under poor living conditions and with the demanding duties of a soldier. A dissertation on the problem pointed at the fact that fertility increased with higher consumption of animal protein and implied that the poor physical condition and low reproduction rate of Italians was due to their consumption of only 60 to 70 grams of protein per day.[93] Finally, as previously mentioned, studies of the diet of Olympic athletes seemed to encourage higher meat consumption.[94]

For propaganda reasons, the army concealed the food supply problems that arose from fast movement of the troops. Military strategists refused to reveal any information to the public and stated explicitly, "The topic hunger is not to occur in the reports."[95] The existence of hunger was well-known at home through soldiers' letters.[96] Nevertheless, none of the six hundred doctors in encircled Stalingrad dared to speak of hunger in their reports. Until June 1942, army physicians and military commanders were officially puzzled about the accumulation of edema cases. Standards and reality crashed in a cruel and irreconcilable manner.

Conclusion

This essay has analyzed how the army integrated nutritional knowledge from 1850 onward. The army served as a site for the production of nutritional knowledge, as it formed a seemingly ideal place for nutritional investigations. The importance of the health and fitness of soldiers was also a perfect argument for researchers to underline the value of their investigations, opening up new professional opportunities. Almost from the beginning of nutritional sciences, scientific knowledge of food was integrated into the bureaucratic procedures of the German Army. It had an important position in the context of health policy, since the improvement of diets was deemed an important tool in the fight against the physical degeneration of the population, demonstrated by the poor health of new recruits. The discourse on army food resembled the discourse on workers' food and was similarly shaped by the state's need for healthy and strong bodies. This development peaked during National Socialism when the soldier's body became an emblem of the healthy *Volkskörper* to come, and significant efforts were made to improve the soldier's diet after the experiences of the First World War. Even before 1939, several innovations had been made to improve the soldier's diet under field conditions. During the Second World War these efforts were exploited for propaganda purposes to display the army as modern and up-to-date in science and technology. At the same time, the army was seen as a means to familiarize recruits with a healthy diet. It was hoped that they would take their new customs home and follow them for the rest of their lives. What remained was the idea of the soldier as a warrior whose power was related to some long-standing, almost magical ideas about the importance of meat for virility and the will and ability to fight. Even though nutritionists realized that protein requirements were lower than previously assumed, cultural beliefs in the power of meat persisted, and administrators needed to consider the effect of meat reduction on the morale of the normal soldier. It was believed that only exceptionally wilful and strong men such as the members of the SS would be able to fight on a vegetarian diet.[97] Thus the dietary schemes of the German Army mirrored not only the integration of seemingly useful nutritional science into the bureaucratic knowledge of institutions, but also the social order within a militaristic society in which the soldier held an exceptional position and was often looked at as a "combat machine."

This changed after the Second World War. Not surprisingly, the regulation of food rations followed established lines, as many former members of the army were in leading positions in the Bundeswehr, the new West German Army, which was founded in 1955.[98] Already at the beginning of the twentieth century, the system of fixed rations had been discontinued, and no definite weights were set for individual foods. Although the quality of the diet was calculated and checked regularly, quartermasters were not bound to a fixed schedule, but only to a fixed daily expenditure that had been calculated on the basis of nutritional physiology and food prices. Members of the former Military Academy, as well as nutritionists who had served as experts and advisers for the nutrition plans of the National Socialist army, now gave advice to the successor government and set new nutritional guidelines, following their former practical and scientific experiences.[99] Researchers and directors from low-status institutions used the political change to try to garner lucrative research contracts and increase the status of their institutions, which had struggled to continue without the research contracts they had received from the National Socialist state.[100] The medical department and administration of the Bundeswehr were, however, not satisfied with the work that the contract researchers delivered.[101] They realized that the researchers wanted to use the army as a research site, whereas the medical department wanted simple and manageable guidelines and believed that the military doctors were proficient enough in the field. Thus they rejected new research contracts, but calculations of the nutrient content were used to check the adequacy of the new food schedules as well as for regular checkups. Unlike the Wehrmacht, the Bundeswehr was not regarded as an army of warriors to be groomed to extraordinary strength and health. It was also not conceptualized as the health model for the rest of the population, and food was no longer used in an ideological manner to display Germany's physical strength. The new food schemes followed those of the citizens. The Bundeswehr was seen as an army of citizens that should get the citizen's food, but nothing special.[102]

The process I have analyzed above not only involves the impact of scientific and technological changes on army food and the army as a site for the production of new scientific and technological knowledge. It also sheds light on how social and political ideals are embodied in physiological and technological food standards. While influenced by science, they also closely follow social and political changes. Food is not only about the intake of calories and nutrients, but also relates to almost every aspect of human existence.

Notes

1. Friedrich II., König von Preussen, *General-Principia vom Kriege, applicieret auf die Tactique und auf die Disciplin derer Preußischen Trouppen* (Berlin: Schneider, 1753).

Reprinted in *Gesammelte Werke Friedrichs des Grossen in Prosa*, ed. and trans. Jost Isaak Markus (Berlin: Levent, 1837), 534.

2. *Besichtigungsbuch des königlichen Garnisonslazaretts zu Koblenz (1826–1912) fortgeführt als Besucherbuch des Bundeswehrzentralkrankenhauses (1968–1987)*, ed. Joachim Schnierstein and Friedrich Hermann (Bad Ems: Weidhellverlag, 1988).

3. Friedrich von Seelhorst, *Das Heerwesen des Preussischen Staates: Enthaltend die Grundsätze der allgemeinen Militärverpflichtung, die Armee Organisation und diejenigen militärischen Verwaltungszweigen und Verhältnisse, bei denen besonders das Civil mit dem Militär concurriert. Ein Handbuch* (Erfurth: Friedrich Wilhelm Otto, 1841), 246–48.

4. Ibid., 254.

5. The peacetime light ration consisted of two pounds of bread, 113 grams of meat, and either 88 grams of rice or 117 grams of grits or 234 grams of beans. The heavy ration for times of increased performance was fixed at 227 grams of meat and 117 grams of rice per head per day, plus the proportionate amounts of beans and grits. Ibid., 255.

6. C. J. Prager, *Das preußische Militär-Medicinal-Wesen in seiner gegenwärtigen Gestalt, systematisch dargestellt* (Berlin: August Hirschwald, 1864), 150.

7. Peter Lummel, "Food Provisioning in the German Army of the First World War," in *Food and War in Twentieth-Century Europe*, ed. Ina Zweiniger-Bargielowska, Rachel Duffett, and Alain Drouard (Surrey: Ashgate, 2011), 13–26; Rachel Duffet, *The Stomach for Fighting: Food and the Soldiers of the Great War* (Manchester: Manchester University Press, 2012).

8. Heinrich Hartmann, "Maßnehmen am Europäer: Wissenschaft und Militarismus im Spiegel der Musterungen, etwa 1890 bis 1914," in *Themenportal Europäische Geschichte* 2007, http://www.europa.clio-online.de/2007/Article=276 (accessed February 14, 2013); and Heinrich Hartmann, *Der Volkskörper bei der Musterung: Militärstatistik und Demographie in Europa vor dem Ersten Weltkrieg* (Göttingen: Wallstein, 2011).

9. This idea is most often connected to Max Rubner, though the term is older. See Armin von Lippe-Weissenfeld, *Die rationelle Ernährung des Volkes: Mit besonderer Berücksichtigung der Beköstigung in Schulen, Seminarien, Arbeitshäusern und Armenhäusern* (Leipzig: Wigand's, 1866). For a general outline, see Dietrich Milles, "Working Capacity and Calorie Consumption: The History of Rational Physical Economy," in *The Science and Culture of Nutrition, 1840s–1940s*, ed. Harmke Kamminga and Andrew Cunningham (Amsterdam: Rodopi, 1995), 75–96.

10. For Liebig's theory, see various essays in this volume and Mark R. Finlay, "Early Marketing of the Theory of Nutrition: The Science and Culture of Liebig's Extract of Meat," in Kamminga and Cunningham, *Science and Culture of Nutrition*, 48–74. For Moleschott, see especially Harmke Kamminga, "Nutrition for the People or the Fate of Jacob Moleschott's Contest for a Humanist Science," in Kamminga and Cunningham, *Science and Culture of Nutrition*, 15–47.

11. Justus von Liebig, *Chemische Briefe*, 4th rev. and impr. ed., 2 vols. (Leipzig: Winter, 1859), 195.

12. Ibid., 79.

13. Ibid., 284–95.

14. Ibid., 294–95.

15. Ibid.

16. Carl Kirchner, *Lehrbuch der Militärhygiene* (Erlangen: Enke, 1869), preface. Unless otherwise noted, all translations from the German and French are by UT.

17. Ibid., 4.

18. Winfried Baumgart, *The Crimean War, 1853–1856* (London: Arnold, 1999); Orlando Fighes, *Krimkrieg: Der letzte Kreuzzug* (Berlin: Berlin Verlag, 2011).

19. "Reglement über die Naturalverpflegung der Truppen im Frieden vom 13. Mai 1858," in *Heerwesen und Infanteriedienst der Königlich Preussischen Armee*, ed. August von Witzleben, 2 vols., 10th ed. (Berlin: A. Bath, 1858), 1: 274–76.

20. "Verordnung, betreffend die Einführung Preußischer Militärgesetze im ganzen Bundesgebiete," *Bundesgesetzblatt des Norddeutschen Bundes* 10 (1867): 125–30.

21. "Gesetz über die Naturalleistungen für die bewaffnete Macht im Frieden, 13. Februar 1875," *Deutsches Reichsgesetzblatt* (1875): 52–53.

22. Physiologists used this argument. See Carl Voit, "Anforderungen der Gesundheitspflege an die Kost in Waisenhäusern, Casernen, Gefangen- und Altersversorgungsanstalten, sowie in Volksküchen. Bericht des Ausschusses über die dritte Versammlung des deutschen Vereins für öffentliche Gesundheitspflege zu München," *Deutsche Vierteljahrsschrift für öffentliche Gesundheitspflege* 8 (1876): 7–57.

23. Adolphe Quetelet, *Sur l'homme et le développement de ses facultés, ou Essai de physique sociale*, 2 vols. (Paris: Bachelier, 1835).

24. J. Forster, "Hygiene der Massenernährung," in *Handbuch der Hygiene und Gewerbekrankheiten, 2. Teil: Sociale Hygiene, 1. Teil: Größere Gemeinwesen, 1. Hälfte*, ed. Hugo von Ziemssen (Leipzig: F. C. Vogel, 1880), 380–92; Wilhelm Schumburg, "Hygiene der Einzelernährung und Massenernährung," in *Handbuch der Hygiene*, ed. Theodor Weil, 2nd ed., vol. 3, part 3 (Leipzig: Johann Ambrosius Barth, 1913), 424–29.

25. Alexander Ochwadt, *Beiträge zur Militär-Hygiene im Kriege und im Frieden* (Berlin: Hirschwald, 1868); Carl Kirchner, *Lehrbuch der Militärhygiene* (Erlangen: Enke, 1869); Carl Kirchner, *Lehrbuch der Militärhygiene*, 2nd ed. (Stuttgart: Enke, 1877); Prager, *Das preußische Militär-Medicinal-Wesen*; H. Hoffmann, W. Hoffmann, and H. Schwiening, *Lehrbuch der Militärhygiene* (Berlin: A. Hirschwald, 1910); Hans Bischoff, *Lehrbuch der Militarhygiene*, vol. 5 (Leipzig: Hirschwald, 1913); H. Schwiening, *Lehrbuch der Militärhygiene* (Berlin: Verlag Hirschwald, 1913).

26. Voit, "Anforderungen."

27. Ernst von Engel, "Die physische Beschaffenheit der wehrpflichtigen Bevölkerung im Königreiche Sachsen," *Zeitschrift des statistischen Bureaus des Königlich Sächsischen Ministeriums des Innern* 8 (1864): 4–7; Otto Ammon, "Die Körpergröße der Wehrpflichtigen im Großherzogtum Baden in den Jahren 1840–64, dargestellt auf Grund der Rekrutierungslisten für Gemeinden, Amtsbezirke und Kreise," *Beiträge zur Statistik des Großherzogtums Baden* 5, no. 2 (1894): 3–27; Otto Ammon, *Anthropologische Untersuchungen der Wehrpflichtigen in Baden* (Hamburg: Verlags- und Druckerei-AG, 1890); Carl A. Meinert, *Armee- und Volksernährung. Ein Versuch Professor C. von Voit Ernährungstheorie für die Praxis zu verwerthen*, 2 vols. (Berlin: Mittler & Sons, 1880), 2: 345–47. Similar statements can be found in the numerous articles on the bodily condition of workers. See Fridolin Schuler, Über die Ernährung der Fabrikbevölkerung und ihre Mängel (Zürich: Herzog, 1883).

28. Wilhelm Hildesheim, *Die Normal-Diät: Physiologisch-chemischer Versuch zur Ermittelung des normalen Nahrungsbedürfnisses des Menschen behufs Aufstellung einer*

Normal-Diät. Mit besonderer Rücksicht auf das Diät-Regulativ des neuen Reglements für die Friedens-Garnisons-Lazarethe und die Natural-Verpflegung der Soldaten sowie auf die Verpflegung der Armen (Berlin: Hirschwald, 1856), 3. See also: Meinert, *Armee- und Volksernährung*, 2: 345–46.

29. Hildesheim, *Normaldiät*, 2. See also Schumburg, *Hygiene*, 424.

30. Ulrike Thoms, *Anstaltskost im Rationalisierungsprozess: Die Ernährung in Krankenhäusern und Gefängnissen im 18. und 19. Jahrhundert* (Stuttgart: Steiner, 2005), 350.

31. Ibid.

32. Voit, "Anforderungen," 28.

33. Carl Voit et al., *Untersuchung der Kost in einigen öffentlichen Anstalten:* Für Aerzte und Verwaltungsbeamte (Munich: R. Oldenbourg, 1877); Voit, "Anforderungen"; and Elizabeth Neswald, "Nutritional Knowledge between the Lab and the Field: The Search for Dietary Norms in the Late Nineteenth and Early Twentieth Centuries," chapter 1 of this volume.

34. Voit, "Anforderungen," 32.

35. Voit, *Untersuchung*, 4–5.

36. Ibid., 26.

37. Hans Lichtenfelt, "Ernährungsfragen," *Centralblatt für allgemeine Gesundheitspflege* 31 (1908): 13–23; Max Rubner, *Volksnährungsfragen* (Leipzig: Akademische Verlagsanstalt, 1908), see especially the chapter on the economic effects of the diet of the poor, 43–45; and Schumburg, *Hygiene*, 424.

38. "Verordnung Nr. 70: Feststellung des Nährwerthes der Speisen durch die Ober-Militärärzte. Berlin, 8. März 1879," *Armee-Verordnungsblatt* 13 (1879): 80.

39. The report was published in 1880. *Ernährung des Soldaten: Bericht der über die Ernährungsfrage des Soldaten niedergesetzten Special-Commission* (Munich: Hübschmann'sche Buchdruckerei, 1880).

40. Elmar Verner McCollum, *A History of Nutrition: The Sequence of Ideas in Nutrition Investigations* (Boston: Houghton Mifflin, 1957), 4, 63.

41. Nan Mellinger, *Fleisch: Ursprung und Wandel einer Lust* (Frankfurt: Campus, 2000); Ulrike Thoms, "Vegetarianism, Meat and Life Reform in Early Twentieth-Century Germany," In *Meat, Medicine, and Human Health in the Twentieth Century*, ed. Christian Bonah, David Cantor, and Matthias Doerries (London: Pickering & Chatto, 2010), 145–59.

42. Anon., Über *die rationelle Ernährung des Soldaten: Vor einem Pr. Officier der Artillerie* (Potsdam: von Stein, 1858).

43. Meinert, *Armee- und Volksernährung*; Engelbrecht, "Die Verwendung von Fischen zur Verpflegung des Soldaten," *Der Militärarzt* 55 (1905): 10–11, 54–58, 72–74.

44. Johannes Ranke, *Grundzüge der Physiologie des Menschen mit Rücksicht auf die Gesundheitspflege und das Bedürfnis des Arztes* (Leipzig: Wilhelm Engelmann, 1868), 162.

45. Voit, "Anforderungen."

46. Hildesheim, *Normaldiät*.

47. See Corinna Treitel, "How Vegetarians, Naturopaths, Scientists, and Physicians Unmade the Protein Standard in Modern Germany," chapter 2 of this volume.

48. Max Rubner, "Die Beziehungen zwischen dem Eiweissbedarf des Körpers und der Eiweissmenge der Nahrung," *Archiv für Anatomie und Physiologie, Physiologische Abteilung* (1911): 61–66. For Rubner in general, see Corinna Treitel, "Max Rubner and the Biopolitics of Rational Nutrition," *Central European History* 41 (2008): 1–25.

49. Thoms, "Vegetarianism, Meat and Life Reform."

50. Paul Schenk, "Bericht über die Verpflegung der im 'Olympischen Dorf' untergebrachten Teilnehmer an den XI. Olympischen Spielen 1936 zu Berlin," *Die Ernährung* 2 (1937): 1–24; A. Bickel, "Eiweiss: Die Art der Eiweißernährung als Grundlage körperlicher Leistungssteigerung," *1, Tagungsbericht der Arbeitsgemeinschaft Ernährung der Wehrmacht,* ed. E. Piesczek and Wilhelm Ziegelmayer (Dresden: Steinkopff, 1942), 25–45.

51. Kirchner, *Militärhygiene,* 27.

52. Schumburg, *Massenernährung,* 425–30.

53. Ibid., 434–35.

54. Grützmacher, "Die Selbstbewirtschaftung der Verpflegung in den Garnisonslazaretten," *Deutsche militärärztliche Zeitschrift* 43 (1914): 481–85.

55. Andreas Lang, *Lebensmittelchemiker in Uniform: Die Geschichte der Lebensmittelchemie als Teil der Militärpharmazie* (Munich: Lang, 2006).

56. See the annual bibliographies in *Deutsche militärärztliche Zeitschrift.*

57. See Ochwadt, *Beiträge,* 66; Seelhorst, *Heerwesen,* 255; Thoms, *Anstaltskost,* 173.

58. Thoms, *Anstaltskost,* 190; Fritz Roeder, *Die Naturalienbeschaffung für den Verpflegungsbedarf des bayerischen Heeres (seit 1884): Nach amtlichen Quellen bearbeitet* (Stuttgart: Cotta, 1909), 26–28, 141–43; Fritz Roeder, "Die militärische Verpflegungswirtschaft im Frieden," *Annalen des Deutschen Reichs* (1910): 1–18, 133–56, 241–63, 368–83, 598–617, 859–73, 918–30; ibid. (1911): 54–68, 298.

59. L. Derlin, "Aus Küche und Magazin," *Zeitschrift für Krankenanstalten* 5 (1909): 345–52, 375–89, 415–24.

60. Institutions also imitated the procedure for negotiating favorable offers and prices. Thoms, *Anstaltskost,* 173.

61. Wilhelm Hermann and Willo Rall, *Kommißbrot: Kriegs- u. Soldatenlieder,* 3rd ed. (Ulm a.d. Donau: Höhn, 1914/15); Daniel Kirn, *Soldatenleben in Württemberg 1871–1914: Zur Sozialgeschichte des deutschen Militärs* (Paderborn: Schöningh, 2009), 154–58.

62. Thoms, *Anstaltskost,* 152–54.

63. The normal mixture was three-quarters of rye flour with a 12 percent extraction and a quarter of wheat flour with an 8 percent extraction of bran.

64. Wenzeslaus Plagge and Georg Lebbin, *Untersuchungen über das Soldatenbrot: Im Auftrage des Königlichen Kriegsministeriums (Medizinal-Abtheilung)* (Berlin: Verlag von August Hirschwald, 1897).

65. Fritz Bein, *Handbuch der Soldatenverpflegung, Gemeinschaftsverpflegung, Truppenverpflegung,* 3rd. rev. ed. (Frankfurt: Bernard & Graefe, 1970), 12.

66. Johann Friedrich Hausmann, *Einfaches Mittel, die Beköstigung der vor dem Feinde stehenden Heere und die Stärkung der verwundeten und erkrankten Krieger zu erleichtern* (Göttingen: Vandenhoeck & Ruprecht, 1815). See also the idea for a preserved meat soup from the chemist Hermbstaedt, in Hermbstaedt, "Resultate der von mir angestellten Versuche über die Zubereitung nahrhafter Bouillon aus frischen und schon gekochten Knochen [1804]," Acta des Kabinets König Friedrich Wilhelms III. Varia in Armensachen 1801–4 (Versorgung von Waisenpp. Hermstaeadts Versuche

betr. Bouillon aus Knochen), I. HA, Rep. 96A, Tit. 8m, p. 5, Geheimes Staatsarchiv Preußischer Kulturbesitz, Berlin.

67. Militär-Ökonomie-Departement, "Zur Verwendung eines Fleisch-Mehl-Präparates zu Menage-Zwecken, Berlin 16.1.1874," *Armee-Verordnungs-Blatt* 8 (1874): 6–7.

68. Meinert, *Armee- und Volksernährung.*

69. J. Stinde, *Special Catalog für den Pavillon Carne pura: Allgemeine deutsche Ausstellung auf dem Gebiete der Hygiene u. des Rettungswesens: Collectiv-Ausstellung: Die rationelle Ernährung des Soldaten und Arbeiters* (Berlin: Mittler, 1882).

70. Ibid. See also Villaret, "Von der Hygiene-Ausstellung," *Berliner Klinische Wochenschrift* 21 (1884): 14–15, 46–48, 75–78, esp. 46–47; Wilhelm Roth, "Allgemeine Deutsche Ausstellung auf dem Gebiet der Hygiene und des Rettungswesens zu Berlin im Sommer 1883," *Deutsche Vierteljahrsschrift für öffentliche Gesundheitspflege* 16 (1884): 166–71; Kirchenberger, "Carne Pura Eine neuzeitliche Fleischconserve und ihre Verwertbarkeit im Felde," *Neue militärische Blätter* 26 (1885): 224; Wilhelm Roth, "Jahresbericht über die Leistungen und Fortschritte auf dem Gebiete des Militärgesundheitswesens," *Militärsanitätswesen* 11 (1884): 54–58.

71. Finlay, "Early Marketing."

72. "Die Erbswurst-Fabrik in Berlin," *Dinglers Polytechnisches Journal* 198 (1870): 181–82. Broxner, "Über Fleischconservirung für den Armeegebrauch," *Dinglers Polytechnisches Journal* 210 (1873): 150–53; Volkmar Leonhard, "Abgewogen und trocken gemischt: Zur Meldung 'Tütensuppe wird 125,'" *Berliner Zeitung,* November 17, 1995.

73. Volkmar Leonhard, "Scheller, Friedrich Heinrich Rudolf," in *Neue Deutsche Biographie,* vol. 22 (2005): 650–51, http://www.deutsche-biographie.de/pnd139524134.html (accessed March 3, 2014). For a positive review of Maggi products, see the 1909 report of the two apothecaries Varges and Rabenhorst and the physician Dufeldt: J. Varges, Rabenhorst, and Dufeldt, "Zur Truppenernährung im Kriege und Frieden," *Deutsche Militärärztliche Zeitschrift* 38 (1909): 793–814.

74. Thoms, *Anstaltskost,* 492–95; Georg von Viehbahn and Schubarth, *Amtlicher Bericht über die Allgemeine Pariser Ausstellung von Erzeugnisen der Landwirtschaft, des Gewerbefleisses und der schönen Kunst im Jahre 1855* (Berlin: Decker, 1856), 283; Martin Kirchner, *Grundriss der Militär-Gesundheitspflege* (Braunschweig: H. Bruhn, 1869), 99.

75. *Spandau einst und jetzt,* Supplement no. 19 of *Spandauer Volksblatt,* January 12, 1977; Joachim Jauch, *Wegweiser zu Berlins Straßennamen—Spandau* (Berlin: Luisenstaedtischer Bildungsverein, 1996).

76. Thoms, "Ernährung ist so wichtig."

77. Ibid.

78. See the picture in: *Zeitschrift für Heeresverpflegung* 5 (1940): 46. It is assumed that by this time Hitler was a vegetarian, but whether this affected the rations served when Hitler was with the troops is unknown. Ian Kershaw, *Hitler* (London: Penguin, 2009), 160.

79. See the title of the journal: *Zeitschrift für Gemeinschaftsverpflegung: Unterrichtsorgan für die deutschen Großküchenbetriebe* 1–22 (1937–42).

80. "Vitaminpolitik," *Zeitschrift für die Heeresverwaltung* 8 (1943): 78; Vitaminhaushalt im Kriege, *Zeitschrift für die Heeresverwaltung* 8 (1943): 138.

81. The physicians and physiologists at the Military Academy were more realistic. They did not follow the propagandistic exploitation of the vitamin craze. See Ulrike Thoms, "'Vitaminfragen—kein Vitaminrummel?' Die deutsche Vitaminforschung in der ersten Hälfte des 20. Jahrhunderts und ihr Verhältnis zur Öffentlichkeit," in *Wissenschaft und Öffentlichkeit als Ressource füreinander*, ed. Sybilla Nikolow and Arne Schirrmacher (Bielefeld: Transcript, 2007), 75–96.

82. See David F. Smith, "The Quest for a Nutritional El Dorado: Efforts to Demonstrate Dietary Impacts on Resistance to Infectious Disease in the 1920s and 1930s," chapter 5 of this volume.

83. Siegfried Matthes, "Sportliche Leistungsfähigkeit und Vitamin C," *Medizinische Welt* 14 (1940): 409.

84. Beat Bächi, *Vitamin C für alle!: Pharmazeutische Produktion, Vermarktung und Gesundheitspolitik (1933–1953)* (Zürich: Chronos 2009); Christoph Kopke, "Gladiolen aus Dachau: Das Vitamin-C-Projekt der SS," *Bulletin für Faschismus- und Weltkriegsforschung* 25–26 (2005): 200–219.

85. See Joachim Drews, *Die "Nazi"-Bohne: Anbau, Verwendung und Auswirkung der Sojabohne im Deutschen Reich und Südosteuropa (1933–1945)* (Münster: Lit-Verlag, 2004).

86. "Neuzeitliche Gesichtspunkte bei der Heeresverpflegung," *Die Deutsche Fettwirtschaft* 19 (1942): 167–68; "Volksernährung und Soldatenkost," *Zeitschrift für Volksernährung* 16 (1941): 58–59; Piesczek, "Neuzeitliche Gedanken auf dem Gebiete der Verpflegung," *Zeitschrift für die Heeresverwaltung* 5 (1940): 29–31; Hellweger, "Wechselwirkung zwischen Wissenschaft und Soldatenkost," *Zeitschrift für Heeresverwaltung* 8 (1943): 240–42.

87. Kurt G. Wagner, "Die Erfindertätigkeit auf dem Nahrungsmittelgebiet in Deutschland während des zweiten Weltkriegs," *Deutsche Lebensmittel-Rundschau* 45 (1949): 194–95, R. W. Pilcher, "German Wartime Food Processing and Packaging," *Food Technology* 1 (1947): 394–403.

88. The meal consisted of canned sausage on army bread as an appetizer, followed by tomato soup with rice and soy, mixed preserves (carrots, potatoes, pork), crispsbread with soft cheese, Scho-Ka-Kola, and German red wine. Wilhelm Ziegelmayer, "Der Führer läßt sich die Verpflegung der Festungstruppen vorführen [mit 2 Bildtafeln]," *Zeitschrift für die Heeresverwaltung*, 4 (1939): 212–14.

89. See the collection of articles in RH 12–23/1565, Federal Archives, Military Archive Freiburg.

90. Wilhelm Ziegelmayer, "Die Wehrmacht als Erzieher zur richtigen Verbrauchslenkung und gesunden Ernährung," *Zeitschrift für Volksernährung* 12 (1937): 13–15.

91. Ulrike Thoms, "Physical Reproduction, Eating Culture and Communication at the Workplace: The Case of Industrial Canteens in Germany 1850–1950," *Food & History* 7 (2009): 119–56.

92. See the remarks by the physiologist Otto Friedrich Ranke in his war diary from November 11, 1940, RH 12–23/1644, Federal Archives, Military Archive Freiburg.

93. Karl Becker, *Untersuchungen über den Eiweissstoffwechsel bei Soldaten* (Würzburg: Böttner, 1937).

94. Schenk, "Bericht über die Verpflegung." It is important to note that the importance of high-performance was acknowledged for the case of sports, but not for the army, where "only" a strong and robust body was needed.

95. See the protocol of the meeting predating the third "Osttagung," RH 12–23/247, Federal Archives, Military Archive Freiburg.

96. Martin Kehrig, *Stalingrad: Analyse und Dokumentation einer Schlacht* (Stuttgart: Deutsche Verlags-Anstalt, 1974), 300, 338, 500–502.

97. Becker, *Untersuchungen über den Eiweissstoffwechsel*, 46.

98. See, for example, Fritz Bein, who published the first comprehensive book on the food of the Bundeswehr: Fritz Bein, *Handbuch der Soldatenverpflegung: Aufbau und Organisation der Verpflegungswirtschaft im Standort* (Frankfurt am Main: Bernhard & Graefe, 1958).

99. Konrad Lang and Otto F. Ranke, *Stoffwechsel und Ernährung* (Berlin: Springer, 1949).

100. This is especially the case for the nutrition branch of the former Kaiser Wilhelm Institute for the Physiology of Work at Dortmund, which later became the Max Planck Institute for Nutritional Physiology, where Heinrich Kraut tried to organize research contracts. The inquiries mentioned are a result of his efforts.

101. Willi Wirths, "Die Kosten einer vollwertigen Ernährung für die Bundeswehr," *Archiv für Hygiene und Demographie* 143 (1959): 21–39; Willi Wirths, "Ernährungsphysiologische Auswertungen von Speisenplänen [*sic*] des Bundeswehrstandortes Andernach," *Archiv für Hygiene und Demographie* 142 (1958): 453–70; Willi Wirths, "Ernährungsphysiologische Auswertung der Verpflegung in Bundesgrenzschutzstandorten," *Internationale Zeitschrift für angewandte Physiologie einschl. Arbeitsphysiologie* 17 (1958): 316–32.

102. See *Wehrmedizin: Ein kurzes Handbuch mit Beiträgen zur Katastrophenmedizin*, ed. Ernst Rebentisch (Munich: Urban & Schwarzenberg, 1980), 10–12.

Chapter Five

The Quest for a Nutritional El Dorado

Efforts to Demonstrate Dietary Impacts on Resistance to Infectious Disease in the 1920s and 1930s

DAVID F. SMITH

Introduction

In a sense, any scientist who embarks on a research program exploring particular connections between diet and health, and who aspires to somehow alter diets in accordance with expected findings, has started a process of setting standards. And, frequently, the links between research and action are by no means simple and linear: research first, followed by policymaking or propaganda. Nutrition scientists are often, for example, publicly enthusiastic about the value of specific nutrients, before beginning new research that they hope will enhance the importance of these nutrients—and themselves. This essay explores an episode in which two groups of nutrition scientists attempted to demonstrate connections between nutrition and health, each focusing on their own favored nutrients. In the concluding section, it will be suggested that this affair illustrates the way in which the priorities of nutrition science are often set. The "activist" dimension of nutrition science, the impulse to set standards, generally means that research priorities reflect the health or social problems that are considered important at the time in wider public, political, medical, and scientific circles.

The context for the story explored in this chapter is Britain during the interwar period. During the First World War, nutrition scientists in Britain had organized and achieved some measure of consensus, largely focused on the need to maintain the efficiency of the military and civilian population via the application of energy and protein standards. Despite resistance from government and civil servants, they had gained a degree of influence on wartime food policy. But soon after peace returned, their hopes to institutionalize a role in policymaking dissipated when the state largely withdrew from the management of food supplies.[1] Researchers who attempted to make their reputations and careers in nutrition science and its applications now lacked the previous benefits of operating in a prolonged national emergency. One way to enhance the profile and power of the field in this situation was to demonstrate that nutrition could address the most significant and intractable problems of the day, such as morbidity and mortality from infections among humans and farm animals. This paper will explore how this possibility influenced the programatic rhetoric of three of the key actors within British nutrition science—Frederick Gowland Hopkins, Edward Mellanby, and John Boyd Orr—and the research programs of two of them (Mellanby and Orr). The vitamin research program came first, and Hopkins was the doyen of vitamin research in the United Kingdom, as well as Mellanby's mentor. We will therefore consider these three actors in turn, beginning with Hopkins and then proceeding to Mellanby and Orr. The concluding section will discuss the significance of the ultimately unsuccessful turn toward infectious disease in the interwar period.

Frederick Gowland Hopkins: Vitamins Pioneer

The story of Hopkins's role in the discovery of vitamins is well-known, beginning in 1906 when he highlighted the dietary need for small quantities of certain organic substances. He then published a paper in 1912 reporting that the growth of rats failed when fed purified carbohydrate, protein, and fat, but resumed when a small quantity of milk was added. He introduced the phrase "accessory food factors" for the unknown growth factors, and, in an overt priority claim, referred to his 1906 remarks and other oral presentations. This strategy proved highly successful, since in 1929 he shared a Nobel Prize for physiology and medicine for the discovery of vitamins with the Dutch scientist Christiaan Eijkmann.[2]

Hopkins became the first professor of biochemistry at Cambridge in 1914 but did little further research on vitamins, despite pleas from Walter Fletcher, secretary of the Medical Research Committee (later Council, MRC).[3] However, in 1918 Hopkins became chair of the MRC's Accessory Food Factors Committee and the most prominent British spokesman for the "vitamin" concept. Although his primary interest was in the development of biochemistry, his reputation depended greatly on his association with nutrition, and especially vitamins. He soon began claiming that vitamins could be the key to health problems beyond deficiency diseases—especially susceptibility to infections.

The expansive vision relied on the idea of health impacts of low-vitamin rather than vitamin-deficient diets. This approach appeared in a February 1919 paper on "The Practical Importance of Vitamins," in which Hopkins referred to the low vitamin intake of children subsisting on white bread and margarine, and remarked: "In spite of all this, beri-beri or pellagra or any diseases like them are unknown in this country; and scurvy is . . . very rare. But disturbances in health may exist without arriving at the extreme stage when the appearance of a severe set of symptoms leads to the recognition of actual disease." He was more explicit when speaking about rickets: "The case of rickets . . . stands out. Rickets is very common in this country. . . . It is . . . a factor of supreme importance. . . . The child who is rickety is much more prone to other ailments—much more vulnerable in all respects."[4]

Elsewhere, it became clear that this "vulnerability" referred to susceptibility to infections and sometimes specific diseases. The Accessory Food Factor Committee's 1919 *Report on the Present State of Knowledge,* prepared under Hopkins's supervision, referenced over two hundred papers,[5] and appealed to an assumed medical consensus about the benefits of a liberal diet in tuberculosis: "For many years the value of a generous dietary in combating diseases such as tuberculosis has been universally recognised, and it is a curious fact that many of the foodstuffs which enter so largely into the composition of these dietaries are those which are particularly rich in . . . accessory substances."[6] The section on the eye disease xerophthalmia, which involves a failure of tear production, and which was by then regarded as a vitamin deficiency, quoted the Danish paediatrician C. E. Bloch, who had called attention to "the frequency with which other diseases, such as diarrhoea, bronchitis, pneumonia, pyuria, discharges from ears and nose . . . were found associated in the patients . . . showing a lowered resistance to infection."[7]

Over the next few years Hopkins made less mention of these low-vitamin states, known as "partial," "relative," "subclinical," or "latent" deficiencies, and instead concentrated on the core of vitamin theory and supported Mellanby in a controversy over the role of vitamins in rickets, which will be discussed shortly.[8] However, in 1926, when the controversy was largely settled in Mellanby's favor, Hopkins returned to the theme. Writing on "The Criteria of an Efficient Diet" in *The Practitioner,* he explained that although deficiency diseases were rare in Britain, it was important to realize that "deficiency is relative, and that dietaries may be consumed which . . . involve impairment of health and diminished resistance to infection."[9] Similarly, in 1931 Hopkins's article in the first number of *Nutrition Abstracts and Reviews* showed the "vitamins and infections" thesis was central to his credo. He remarked that partial deficiencies "may greatly increase the liability to infection by bacteria and other parasites. Facts such as these are already established."[10] It seems that by the early 1930s, Hopkins felt able to present the existence of partial vitamin deficiencies and their involvement in infectious diseases as matters of general medical and scientific consensus. As we will see, however, this consensus was, at best, temporary.

Edward Mellanby, Vitamins and Infections

By 1931, Edward Mellanby, Hopkins's former pupil and colleague, was focusing specifically on vitamins and infections. This built on his rickets research, which began at the invitation of the MRC in 1914, when he was a lecturer at King's College of Household and Social Science in London.[11] He studied puppies, and the MRC Report for 1916–17 outlined his preliminary results: he could apparently produce or prevent rickets by manipulating the diet, indicating that "the primary cause of rickets" was "a deficiency of an accessory factor."[12] But in 1918 controversy erupted between Mellanby and a group in Glasgow led by the regius professor of physiology D. N. Paton and the pediatrician Leonard Findlay.[13] The Glaswegians attacked Mellanby's position on the basis of their social and dietary investigations. They suggested that rickets was connected with inadequate exercise, lack of general hygiene, poor housing, ineffective maternal care, and, possibly, "non-specific infection."[14]

The Glaswegians complained that Mellanby had not published his full data and cast him as an irresponsible laboratory worker, unaware of clinical complexities.[15] But the Accessory Food Factors Committee accepted Mellanby's position, and after summarizing his results, their report added that "the causative factor of rickets may be the secret of immunity and non-immunity to many of the children's diseases which result in the high death rate associated with urban conditions."[16] In a lecture to the Royal College of Surgeons, Mellanby claimed that "the rachitic condition need not be at all advanced before the animal's whole behavior is transformed. It . . . is far more liable to be affected by distemper and broncho-pneumonia and is very susceptible to mange. The low resistance . . . is impressive."[17]

In 1921, Mellanby presented his full results and arguments as to why rickets was a vitamin deficiency and alternative theories could be disregarded. Citing authors viewing rickets as an infection, he argued that they were "mixing cause and effect,"[18] since his own position was that vitamin deficiency caused both rickets and lowered resistance to germs. However, Mellanby's report failed to settle the controversy, and a vigorous exchange between Mellanby and Findlay occurred at the 1922 British Medical Association (BMA) annual meeting. This time Mellanby did not mention susceptibility to infection, while Findlay moved further toward an infective theory, suggesting that "some virus" might be responsible for rickets.[19] Even after the MRC published three further reports on rickets that supported Mellanby,[20] the Glasgwegians remained unconvinced.[21]

This was a time of rapid accumulation of knowledge of vitamins. In 1922 McCollum's group at Johns Hopkins University elucidated the process whereby the conjunctiva (the membrane covering the inner surface of the eyelid and the white part of the eyeball) becomes dry and scaly in vitamin deficiency (keratinization).[22] They differentiated between two fat soluble vitamins—vitamin A, required for healthy conjunctiva, and the antirachitic factor (vitamin D).[23] For a time some workers remained unconvinced of this distinction, including

Mellanby, who in 1924 still spoke alternately of "fat soluble vitamin" (singular) and "fat soluble vitamins" (plural).[24]

In 1926, Mellanby presented the main defects in the English diet as a lack of fat soluble vitamins and excessive consumption of cereals. He discussed diet and respiratory infections in animals and the possible significance for "catarrhal" children. He also declared that defective diets of pregnant and lactating women were probably "responsible for some, and possibly much, of the illness and mortality of young infants." He thought that "new teachings" in infant feeding were "partly responsible for the recent decrease in infant mortality," and added that such teachings should now be applied to maternal feeding. This would, he claimed, improve the health of pregnant women and eliminate some of their "unfortunate experiences."[25]

By this time Mellanby was a university professor of pharmacology in an English provincial city, Sheffield, and honorary physician to the city's Royal Infirmary. No longer a mere laboratory worker, he detailed therapeutic diets that he had deployed himself and showed photographs of his rickety patients before and after treatment.[26] Despite the reservations of his Glaswegian rivals, by the mid-1920s Mellanby had achieved widespread recognition as an effective and productive medical researcher. In moving on to research focused on nutrition and infection, and links with maternal mortality and morbidity in particular, he embarked on a topic of widespread social and political concern, which therefore promised to consolidate and enhance his professional position.

Research politics, however, made it difficult for Mellanby to obtain research funding for the precise project he favored. When he proposed an MRC study of "the proper feeding of 500 pregnant women to see the effect on all the mishaps of pregnancy," Fletcher told him that the Council was "in a tight fix about money" and that the proposal suggested "enormous expenditure," which they "could not undertake but in proprietary should not undertake."[27] This alluded to an agreement that the MRC would be responsible for basic nutrition research, while the Ministry of Health would cover applied dimensions. But Fletcher was aware of the disinterest in nutrition of the chief medical officer, George Newman, which became a bone of contention between the two men.[28]

Mellanby agreed about the neglect of nutrition by the state, and at the 1927 BMA conference argued for a "Board of Nutrition" to advise the Ministry of Health. He claimed that "a sane and forceful" nutrition policy would lead to "as revolutionary a change in . . . general health" as had followed the state's involvement in public hygiene. And "correct feeding," he asserted, was even more fundamental. It was possible to achieve "good health and perfect development" in unhygienic conditions as long as good food was eaten, but perfect hygiene would not prevent bad health if the diet was defective:

> Nothing has been more prominent in recent work . . . than the part played by correct feeding in increasing the individual resistance to infection. It is true that our knowledge of this problem is of an elementary nature, but the subject is one of active interest . . . and further facts of great importance will no doubt

> come to light. . . . I need only allude to the recent accumulation of facts showing the importance of vitamin A in increasing the resistance of the animal to inflammatory conditions of the respiratory passages and lungs.[29]

Mellanby was preaching to the authorities and the public about nutrition and infection at a time when the research accomplished on the subject was of the most preliminary nature. In lieu of the feeding experiment he had proposed, Mellanby and his assistant, H. N. Green, embarked on animal experiments and small-scale clinical studies and supplementation trials, their first publication appearing in 1928. They now distinguished between vitamin A and the antirickets factor and expressed the intention of demonstrating the anti-infective properties of vitamin A. They discussed histological changes accompanying vitamin A deficiency and the high mortality of vitamin-A deficient animals. Much previous work was complicated by multiple deficiencies, so Mellanby and Green's animal experiments explored vitamin A–deficiency alone. Postmortem examinations showed that of ninety-three deficient rats, ninety-one showed evidence of infection. No such evidence occurred in the control animals. The authors were quick to point to practical implications. It was "difficult to avoid the conclusion that an important, and probably the chief function of vitamin A . . . is an anti-infective agent, and that a large number of common infective conditions are due to a deficiency of this substance.[30] Conditions such as "inflammatory processes of the nasal sinuses, middle-ear disease, pneumonia, [and] ulcerative conditions of mouth and eyes" might be linked to vitamin A, and it was widely acknowledged that low vitamin A intake was "common . . . among civilised man," especially in the diet of the poor.

Mellanby and Green identified puerperal septicaemia as a problem worth investigating and addressed this subject in their next publication. Mentioning an ongoing trial testing vitamin A supplements as a preventative measure, they reported on the use of vitamin A in the treatment of five puerperal septicaemia cases—all of which recovered. While admitting this did not demonstrate that vitamin A was a specific treatment for septicaemia, Mellanby and Green claimed that the results indicated that "animal experiments pointed correctly to the hypothesis that vitamin A plays a part as an anti-infective agent" and in increased resistance of the body. They called for trials for other diseases and suggested that if "vitamin A should prove to have anti-infective qualities of a curative nature . . . it must also be of inestimable value in its prophylactic effect."[31]

By this time the "vitamins and infection" theme was already reaching the public via the advertising copy of the pharmaceutical and health food industries. The susceptibility of rachitic children to pneumonia featured in cod liver oil advertising as early as 1925. And in 1930, a manufacturer urged consumers to take cod liver oil because "science has discovered that the lowered resistance to disease . . . is a direct result of the scarcity in our winter diet of the twin Vitamins A and D."[32] Similar messages appeared in popular books by scientists, such as R. H. A. and Violet Plimmer's *Food, Health and Vitamins.*[33]

In Mellanby's March 1930 BMA Hastings lecture on "Diet and Disease," the anti-infective properties of vitamins featured prominently. Doctors, he said, had long recommended special diets during illness because they were pleasant and easily digested. Now, he remarked, "the view is to feed so as to prevent illness." When turning to the "influence of diet on the resistance of the body to bacterial infection," he summarized the evidence and reinforced his case with graphs showing higher respiratory tuberculosis and bronchitis mortality in poorer social classes—which he assumed to result from lower anti-infective vitamin intake among the poor.[34] Here Mellanby was tuning into rising concerns about the impacts of the prevailing economic conditions on health, which would intensify during the decade that followed.

The supplementation trial, reported in October 1931, has been the subject of some historical interest: Irvine Loudon considers it a step in the development of controlled clinical trials,[35] whereas Richard Semba regards this work as neglected and not fully appreciated for sixty years.[36] Of 275 pregnant women receiving vitamin A and D supplements, 19.2 percent developed puerperal pyrexia (fever), compared with 30.9 percent of 275 controls. Mellanby differentiated between appropriate action in terms of social class. The paper outlined the kind of diet that should be taken by better-off women and advocated cheap supplements such as cod liver oil for poorer women.[37] He assumed that better-off women could be taught to make better food choices, but for poorer women he proposed what amounted to a "technical fix." This was not, however, unchallenging to the health authorities: setting up a mass supplementation scheme was not a simple matter or without cost. But any hope of implementing such a scheme depended on the corroboration of Mellanby and Green's findings.

Mellanby and Green's view that vitamin A possessed general anti-infection properties was supported by some studies, such as that of J. B. Ellison, assistant medical officer of the London County Council Fever Hospital, which showed that vitamin A therapy reduced the mortality of children with measles.[38] A trial of vitamin A in the treatment of pneumonia among mine workers in South Africa also produced promising results, which were not, however, confirmed by a further study.[39] Additional negative results were reported. For example, a study on Royal Air Force apprentices found no significant differences in infections between supplemented and control groups.[40]

The 1932 revision of *Survey of Present Knowledge*, compiled by the Accessory Food Factors Committee, which was now chaired by Mellanby, was, however, very positive about Mellanby and Green's research and used their work to reinforce the reality of partial deficiencies.[41] They had shown "how wide is the margin between the doses of vitamin A which will just maintain a rat in life, if it is not attacked by infection, and the dose which will wholly prevent those infections. The latter dose is about four times as great as the former. . . . This example serves to show that a latent deficiency disease is a real thing and not an imaginary concept."[42] In 1933, Mellanby succeeded Fletcher as secretary of the MRC, and the following year published a book, *Nutrition and Disease: The Interaction of Clinical and Experimental Work*, which included a review of "Nutrition and Infection." Acknowledging that he might be accused of ignoring negative results, he continued:

> In excuse I may frankly admit that my object is to force open this closed door behind which, I believe, is the secret of the correlation of nutrition and susceptibility to infection, and with this object in view, I am prepared to use every available weapon. . . . On account of the positive evidence described, negative results only show that our knowledge is still very imperfect, but not that the problem is an unprofitable one to pursue.[43]

But the ascription of general anti-infective or resistance-boosting powers to vitamin A had long met with skepticism in several quarters, especially among epidemiologists and bacteriologists. After Mellanby's Hastings Lecture, *The Lancet* included an "annotation" referring to the work of the bacteriologist W. W. C. Topley and the statistician Major Greenwood.[44] Topley and Greenwood had introduced infections into groups of mice, but found no difference in the mortality rates of those receiving and not receiving a vitamin A supplement. The journal concluded that the "relation of diet to infection" was "far too large and complex a matter to be the subject of experimental enquiry." All that could be asked was, "Does a certain diet alter the resistance of a certain species of animal to a certain microbe administered to it in a certain way."[45]

A. H. G. Burton, medical officer of health for Ilford, argued from immunological principles that it was unlikely that any food factor could "effect a prophylactic action without the stimulus provided by an antigen." His experiments involved pregnant women taking a vitamin A supplement and used a skin test (the Dick test) to assess susceptibility to streptococci. He concluded that there was no evidence that

> the administration of vitamin A in pregnancy has any effect in increasing the resistance of the body to streptococcal infection. Whether or not it has any effect in raising the general resistance is unknown and impossible to determine. The term "general resistance" is a loose one and we have no evidence that, if a person is not actually immune to a specific infection, that "general resistance" will prevent him from contracting that infection.[46]

There was also opposition to Mellanby's position among some researchers who were pursuing careers in nutrition research focused on vitamins. Leslie Harris, director of the MRC Dunn Nutritional Laboratory, was anxious about the impact of extravagant and premature claims of commercial suppliers of vitamins. In September 1932, he attacked the "anti-infective" characterization of vitamin A in *The Lancet.* Already, he noted, vitamin A preparations were marketed as able to treat "septicaemias and acute infections," and increase "general immunity." But Harris reasoned that infections linked with vitamin A deficiency were localized and associated with the keratinization of membranes, and that therefore vitamin A's anti-infective powers were "limited in scope."[47] He renewed this attack in the *British Medical Journal* in 1933, quoting negative and inconclusive trials.[48]

In a November 1933 issue of *The Lancet,* which contained a lecture by Mellanby titled "Nutrition and Child-Bearing,"[49] an editorial reviewing "Vitamin

A and Infection" also appeared. Its author conceded that in pregnant women, native workers in South Africa, and children with measles, vitamin A status might influence morbidity. However, it also concluded that the published studies suggested that common human respiratory infections were not analogues of the infections of severely deficient experimental animals.[50] In summary, those who were skeptical about the anti-infection properties of vitamin A based their positions mostly on negative trials, immunological principles, and the nonapplicability of animal experiments to humans.

Soon after Mellanby became MRC secretary, he toned down his enthusiasm for the vitamin A–infection connection. In the MRC *Report* for 1934–35, a prominent section entitled "Nutrition: The Application of Modern Knowledge" made no mention of the subject.[51] In the *Report* for 1935–36, Mellanby included a section on "The Prevention and Treatment of Childbed Fever," which declared that there were two necessary measures. The first was strict hygiene, and the second was simply "an ample consumption of milk, green vegetables and other protective food." And if puerperal sepsis did occur there was a further line of defence: "the treatment which evidence suggests is now available." He did not mean vitamin A therapy, but the new class of antibacterial drugs, the sulphonamides.[52] In June 1936, Leonard Colebrook, director of the MRC's laboratories at Queen Charlotte's Hospital, London, published the first of five papers demonstrating the effectiveness of sulphonamides in treating puerperal fever.[53] Semba regards the advent of sulphonamides and later antibiotics as responsible for the neglect of the potential of vitamin A for reducing the risk of puerperal sepsis.[54]

By the 1940s, mainstream medical opinion had moved against the idea that vitamin A possessed any specific anti-infective action. *A Textbook of Dietetics*, published in 1940, commented: "Claims have been raised . . . that vitamin A has an anti-infective action. . . . It is now realised, however, that this susceptibility to infection is the result of the keratinisation of the various epithelial structures, and that vitamin A has no direct effect in increasing resistance to infection."[55] It should be noted, however, that although the notion of vitamin A as "anti-infective" was effectively dead, the idea of "partial deficiency" remained very much alive. In the opening paper at the first Nutrition Society conference in October 1941, Leslie Harris mentioned fourteen impacts of partial deficiencies of five vitamins, including "poor dark adaptation," "incipient xerosis," and "sub-optimal growth" for vitamin A.[56]

By the 1940s, Mellanby had explicitly reconsidered his position. In 1944, he declared that "nothing seems more certain than that nutritional defect is at least part of the aetiological basis of many of the more common illnesses, and yet, in most cases, this is only a conviction without satisfactory proof." The extent of "specific anti-infective action" of dietary factors remained for future investigation. He continued,

> Some investigators on nutrition have already had experience in the search for this El Dorado, and in consequence regard the problem with more respect. Nothing could have been more promising than the indications of

> a specific anti-infective action of vitamin A in young rats. . . . In endeavouring to extend these facts to human beings two points were not realized. The first, that rats hold a special place among animals in their susceptibility to infection when deprived of vitamin A. . . . The second, that it seldom happens that human beings are deprived of vitamin A to the extent produced experimentally in the rat.[57]

The flurry of scientific and medical enthusiasm for the anti-infective properties of vitamin A that had arisen during the interwar period was now over. But during that period there had been another nutrition-infection research program focusing on minerals rather than vitamins, which will be described in the next section.

John Boyd Orr, Minerals and Infection

In 1913, the Development Commission, a body charged with stimulating rural development, established an animal nutrition laboratory near the United Kingdom's most northerly university city, Aberdeen, Scotland. Throughout his career as its director, the Glasgow medical graduate John Boyd Orr always sought to avoid the potential for scientific as well as geographic marginalization by developing distinctive research programs and seeking additional funding vigorously. As a result of one early success, the laboratory was named the Rowett Institute, after a generous benefactor.[58] Orr's initial distinctive research program emphasized minerals and deemphasized vitamins in nutrition, this focus apparently beginning in 1920 with investigations into the influence of light and ventilation on the health and growth of pigs. Pigs were kept in dark, ill-ventilated pens, partially lit pens, or in well-lit pens with outside runs. The first group developed rickets, the second a lesser degree of malnutrition, and the third were in poor condition and grew slowly.[59] Subsequent experiments explored whether modifying the ration could prevent rickets in confined pigs. Rickets still occurred when blood meal, turnip, Marmite, and cod liver oil were added, but was prevented by a salt mixture. A 1922 paper argued that since grain-based rations were deficient in calcium as compared with sows' milk, the supplement's action was probably via its calcium content. This gave no support to "the suggestion . . . that rickets is due to a deficiency of an accessory factor."[60] In his opposition to the vitamin theory of rickets, Orr was therefore aligned with the research group at Glasgow led by D. N. Paton, his former teacher.

Further experiments showed that cod liver, linseed, and olive oils all enhanced the assimilation of calcium and phosphorus in piglets on grain-based rations, suggesting that the effect was due to oil per se rather than vitamins.[61] In 1924 Orr proudly told his management committee that "the Institute had become identified with minerals metabolism and was the only Institute in Britain doing organised work in this branch of Science."[62] Other experiments pointed to the practical unimportance of vitamins. Vitamin-rich supplements did not benefit fattening pigs or egg-laying fowls; "bent-leg" in sheep occurred in both grain- and pasture-fed animals and was prevented by mineral supplements.[63]

The first indication of interest in links between minerals and infections appears in remarks about tuberculosis in dairy cattle in a paper published in 1923. The information available was "scanty," but Orr claimed that it suggested that animals on ill-balanced rations succumbed earlier to tuberculosis than those on mineral-rich rations. He concluded: "The influence which long-continued deficiency of mineral matter . . . may have upon the incidence of disease, due to microbic infection, is well worthy of consideration. . . . It is very probable that a long-continued wrong balance of minerals . . . may produce such a condition that infective organisms, normally kept from entering the blood stream, are allowed to pass through and produce acute disease."[64] Orr included a discussion along these lines in *Veterinary Record*,[65] and in *Scottish Journal of Agriculture* he used the hypothetical association between the quality of the rations and the susceptibility to tuberculosis to argue against the wholesale slaughter of dairy cows testing positively for tuberculosis. Bovine tuberculosis and how to deal with it was much debated among health authorities, agriculturalists, and politicians at this time. Orr suggested a slaughter policy would be worthwhile only after improving the nutrition of dairy cows.[66] In 1930, in *Transactions of the Highland and Agricultural Society*, he mentioned other possible links between nutrition and infection. Losses from infections, he declared, were enormous, including "not only deaths, but losses caused by not-fatal diseases, such as mastitis, contagious abortion, and sterility. . . . In the past we have attempted to prevent or cure disease by a direct attack upon the micro-organisms. . . . The question now being considered is whether, in addition . . . defence against diseases could be increased by raising the resistance of the animal through its nutrition."[67] Orr also addressed these ideas to medical audiences. He spoke on "The Importance of the Mineral Elements in the Maintenance of Health" at the 1924 BMA conference, remarking: "The results of modern work show that a faulty diet is not only the direct cause of many diseases, but is also a potent predisposing cause of many infectious diseases."[68] When speaking on "The Importance of Mineral Elements in the Nutrition of Children" at a public health congress, he alluded to "low resistance to disease" several times.[69] In *The Practitioner*, he referred to associations between mineral deficiency and respiratory tract infections, which were notably among the conditions Mellanby associated with lack of vitamins. In tuberculosis, Orr observed, there was usually a negative calcium balance, and he claimed that the administration of calcium as a curative measure had produced favorable results.[70]

The opportunity to move beyond programatic rhetoric and suggestive evidence to focused research on nutrition-infection links arose after the formation of the Empire Marketing Board in 1926. This was created as a means of encouraging imperial trade and development without erecting tariff barriers: via advertising and research.[71] The board appointed a research grants committee chaired by Walter Elliot, a junior Scottish officer minister, Glasgow medical graduate, and farmer. Elliot was a strong supporter of Orr's Institute, where he had conducted research part time. The Empire Marketing Board provided grants for projects in which connections between nutrition and infection were the central theme, including a study of native diets and health in Kenya, supplementation experiments with farm animals in Kenya and Scotland, and a survey of the mineral content of pastures throughout the world.[72] The grants were provided on the recommendations of two subcommittees of the Committee for Civil Research chaired by Elliot: the Subcommittee on the Mineral Content of Pastures and the Dietetics Subcommittee.

The Kenyan native study was published by Orr and J. L. Gilks, director of medical and sanitary services in Kenya, as an MRC Report, *The Physique and Health of Two African Tribes* (1931). It compared the diets, physique, and health of the largely carnivorous Masai and the largely vegetarian Kikuyu. Constipation and arthritis were common among the former, and pulmonary and intestinal infections among the latter. Studies on the etiology of tropical ulcer and on hospital, prison, and reformatory diets were reported, including experiments on the influence of dietary supplements on blood calcium and calcium balance. The authors expected to demonstrate an impact of mineral intake on susceptibility to infections, but the report ended weakly. The concluding summary stated that they did "not feel justified in attempting a detailed discussion of the results obtained or in attempting to draw definite conclusions therefrom." Nevertheless, they asserted that "the possibility that diet may influence the susceptibility to certain infectious diseases raises one of the most important problems in nutritional research." They praised the Empire Marketing Board for funding "long-range research" that could "hasten the improvement of the physical condition of the native and increase his importance as an economic factor," promoting the development of the empire.[73]

In Scotland, a hill farm project developed from Elliot and Orr's interests in the mineral content of pastures. Attempts to collect mortality for sheep grazing on different pastures proved difficult, but it appeared that mortality was high on hill grazings, where pastures were low in minerals, especially calcium. During 1926–28 tests were conducted at hill farms on the effects of supplementary feeding. Systematic data collection proved impossible, but the testimony of the shepherds suggested that supplements had improved mortality rates.[74]

The Empire Marketing Board therefore provided a grant for the purchase of Garrachoran farm in Argyllshire to allow detailed observations, including tests on the immunological reactions of the blood of the sheep, under controlled conditions. The project was overseen by Orr, J. J. R. Macleod, a regius professor of physiology at Aberdeen, and T. J. Mackie, a professor of bacteriology in Edinburgh who carried out the serology. The sheep were weighed regularly and their blood tested for calcium, phosphorus, and immunological reactions. The same tests were carried out on sheep removed to Aberdeen and grazed on better pastures, and the results were compared. The tests covered haemolytic action of the sheep serum toward rabbit erythrocytes, bacteriolytic action on three different bacteria, and the agglutinating effects on two further bacteria.

In May, when the serum calcium level of the hill sheep was lowest, all the reactions were weaker than those of the sheep kept in Aberdeen. The next step was an experiment at the Institute, in which sheep kept on a basal diet of similar quality to hill pastures were given various feed supplement. Blood analyses were carried out, and in 1931 the findings appeared in *The Lancet*. The results raised as many questions as they answered, as the serological measures peaked and varied in puzzling ways. The final conclusion admitted that "many of the data" were "difficult to interpret," but claimed that they pointed to "the urgent need for extended and detailed studies."[75]

While this work was underway, the hill farm and its stock were divided into four by fences, and the sheep were numbered and weighed. Supplementary feeding started in October 1930. The first group received maize meal, the second a mixture including calcium, phosphorus, salt, and cod liver oil, designed to bring the mineral intake up to that of good pasture, the third both supplements, and the fourth no supplement. Eighteen to twenty animals from each group were tested via a subcutaneous injection of *B. welchi* exotoxin, the serology producing just one short paper published in 1932. This showed that at one level of dilution of the toxin a higher proportion of the unfed group than the fed groups showed skin reactions, whereas none of the group receiving both rations reacted. At other levels of dilution, the differences were unclear, but the paper concluded that the results could be regarded as "evidence that dietary deficiencies increase susceptibility to the action of a bacterial exotoxin."[76]

Other results appeared in 1932 in *Transactions of the Highland and Agricultural Society*. In a paper entitled "Restoring the Fertility of Scottish Sheep Grazings," Orr argued that the long-term loss of minerals from Highland soils, coupled with the increasing nutritional needs of the sheep, the consequence of selective breeding, were probably increasing the death rate on certain grazings. The Garrachoran experiments showed the beneficial effects of feeding on birth rate and the survival of ewes, and in terms of profits, the mineral mixture gave the best outcome. Although these were results of practical importance, they did little to advance the "nutrition and infection" research program.[77]

The Institute's collected works for 1930–33 included a preface by Macleod remarking that if good results continued at Garrachoran, there was every reason to hope that their application would restore the prosperity of sheep farming in the West of Scotland.[78] However, the experiments did not go well. The financial crisis of 1931 precluded the renewal of some of the grants that expired in 1932, and the Empire Marketing Board was disbanded in 1933. Some of the Garrachoran work continued, supported by the Development Commission, but after six years the mortality rates of the ewes and lambs, the average weight of the lambs at weaning, and the average weight of fleeces of the different groups were almost identical. A paper published in 1939 concluded that mineral supplements alone could not remedy the poor productivity of the Highland sheep industry.[79]

The long-range human work in Kenya was also abandoned owing to financial stringency. As for the animal work in Kenya, it centered on a farm provided by the Kenyan government. The Empire Marketing Board paid two researchers, who worked under the Rowett Institute's supervision, with the expenses otherwise covered by the profits. In these conditions, though the research led to some practical findings, by the time it passed out of the hands of the Rowett in 1932, it made little contribution to the "nutrition and infection" theme.[80]

In the mid-to-late 1930s, Orr adopted a more pluralistic approach that acknowledged the value of vitamins and refocused the research of the Rowett. After his 1934 Chadwick lecture, which urged a government food policy that would deploy agricultural surpluses in the interest of improving human health, he became increasingly concerned with relationships between the economic problems of agriculture and human nutrition, summarized by the phrase "the marriage of health and agriculture." He was eventually appointed first Director-General of the Food and Agricultural Organisation of the United Nations.[81] Orr's argument for scientific agricultural and food policies was based on analysis of variation in diet and nutritional status in relation to income. His famous report, *Food, Health and Income* (1936), included graphs powerfully illustrating gradients in the consumption of nutrients across income groups, compared with estimates of optimum requirements. But the "nutrition and infection" theme only formed a minor part of the book: there was one short paragraph on "Incidence of Infective Disease in Children."[82] Nevertheless, "nutrition and infection" remained a part of Orr's rhetorical armory. In 1940, for example, in a paper on "Trends in Nutrition," he argued that at times of movement of populations there was an urgent need to increase the resistance of people to infectious diseases by "improving their state of nutrition."[83] But Orr's minerals-focused "nutrition and infection" research program had certainly failed to meet his expectations.

Discussion and Conclusions: Nutrition, Infections, and Strategic Interests of Nutrition Science in the Interwar Period

First, it should be noted that it is not the aim of this paper to point to the prescience or otherwise of our actors, as Loudon and Semba do in the case of Mellanby's work on vitamin A.[84] In view of these authors' studies, Mellanby's work has received recent attention, but Orr's research on nutrition and infection has been neglected. Even James Howie, who worked on nutrition and infection at the Rowett Institute after the Second World War, failed to mention Orr's efforts when reviewing the subject for a volume celebrating fifty years of the Institute in 1963.[85] Second, as Hopkins pointed out, connecting nutrition and infection was by no means new with the work of our actors. For example, in 1902, in *Food and the Principles of Dietetics*, Robert Hutchison remarked that underfeeding lowered resistance to disease. As an example, he cited the epidemics following the Irish potato famine and declared that "the tubercle bacillus seems to find a specially-favourable soil in ill-nourished persons."[86] Similarly, in a 1905 lecture to the Royal College of Physicians, W. H. Alchin commented:

> It is generally supposed . . . that the underfed person is less resistant to the ill-effects of pathogenetic organisms. Perhaps this may be explained in great part by the absence of those protective materials which in a perfectly normal state circulate in the blood current or may be readily developed therein, and among these there is some reason to include the proteids of the blood serum . . . which . . . depend for their maintenance in the blood on the proteid food.[87]

So before our actors were making claims and experimenting in this area, there seems to have been a widespread view in, and probably beyond, medical circles that good feeding, and particularly plentiful protein, improves resistance to disease. Our actors, however, made more specific claims, which they attempted to demonstrate in a variety of settings: the laboratory, clinic, community, and in agriculture.

Hopkins and Mellanby, on the one hand, and Orr, on the other, seemingly adopted different approaches to nutrition. Orr was keen not only to downplay the role of vitamins (in line with the position of his Glaswegian associates) but also to pursue the role of minerals, to provide identity and direction for his Institute. He was so determined to enforce this stance that his vitamin-enthusiastic head of biochemistry, R. H. A. Plimmer, soon left.[88] But since Orr's focus was on deficiencies of nutrients other than those that had previously dominated nutrition science (carbohydrate, fat, and protein), there remains a sense in which his work was part of the same shift in approach as the "vitamin revolution": both Mellanby and Orr were concerned with deficiency diseases, and more with the quality than quantity of food. And since Hopkins, Mellanby, and Orr made similar rhetorical use of the assumed nutrition-infections connection and attempted to unravel the connection, this suggests possible common strategic interests.

Before proceeding, it should also be noted that connections between the germ theory and nutrition science have been discussed previously by historians. In 1971, Aaron Ihde and Stanley Becker argued that the success of the germ theory and its hold over the medical profession was one factor that "delayed" acceptance of the concept of "essential organic micronutrients" in the late nineteenth and early twentieth centuries. They also emphasized the role of American agricultural chemists in the emergence of the notion of "vitamins," suggesting that they were distant from and unhampered by medical concepts.[89] Charles Rosenberg told a similar story in a paper that aimed to demonstrate the inadequacies of an "internalist" approach to the history of science.[90] These authors owed much to the writings of the vitamin pioneers, particularly Elmer McCollum's *History of Nutrition* (1957).[91] Their emphasis on "delay" and "resistance to discovery" was criticized, however, by Naomi Aronson in 1986. She argued that the idea of "resistance" to the discovery of vitamins was constructed by vitamin pioneers to advance their claims in priority disputes and in the pursuit of disciplinary and institutional interests.[92]

The focus of this paper, however, has been a slightly later period than that addressed by Ihde and Becker. It is set in a period not of emergence, but of consolidation of the "vitamin" concept. But it does demonstrate a degree of competition between nutrition and the germ theory, which was not, as Aronson would have it, simply a retrospective construction of vitamin pioneers. In order to speak to the great human and animal health issues of the day, Hopkins, Mellanby, and Orr were prepared to raise the possibility of nutrition competing with, and even assuming greater importance than, bacteriology in the prevention and treatment of infections. But this rhetoric (and the research programs devised by Mellanby and Orr) can be explained along the lines of Aronson—in terms of actors pursuing professional, disciplinary, and institutional interests.

In Hopkins's case, the pursuit of his priority claim in the discovery of vitamins was linked to his interest in establishing an autonomous discipline of biochemistry in Britain and developing a department of biochemistry at Cambridge.[93] His identification with the discovery of vitamins could only help his ambitions to win the necessary financial and institutional support that would allow him to pursue his basic research program. By the mid-1910s, consensus had formed around the view that scurvy and beriberi were vitamin deficiencies, but, as Hopkins admitted, these were very rare in Britain. Pointing to "partial deficiencies" and links with diseases other than frank deficiencies, such as infectious diseases, could only add value to the vitamin discovery. Infections were the cause of much concern in connection with widely recognized social problems such as infant, child, and maternal mortality, and loss of worker productivity.

As we have seen, when rickets was first identified by Mellanby as a vitamin deficiency, Hopkins referred to connections between subclinical rickets and infections, but when the vitamin theory of rickets became controversial, he concentrated more on the core of the vitamin theory. Once the vitamin theory of rickets was effectively settled, however, Hopkins again began to give a prominent place to partial deficiencies and their connections with infections.

The rickets controversy in Britain demonstrates that with regard to this disease, which was widespread and economically important, the vitamin pioneers did face significant resistance: Mellanby needed to engage in a prolonged controversy before a broad consensus formed around the vitamin theory of rickets. It is also noteworthy that those who opposed the vitamin theory also seemed drawn to an infection theory of rickets. In contrast to Aronson's view, there was an element of competition between the germ theory and the vitamin and deficiency disease concepts.

Mellanby was less interested than Hopkins in pursuing the development of biochemistry as a fundamental science and was more consistently concerned with practical applications. After being criticized as an out-of-touch laboratory scientist, he engaged in clinical as well as laboratory research when he had the opportunity to do so at Sheffield. In an environment in which bacteriology was generally recognized as successful in explaining disease and in influencing government public health policies, but only partially successful in terms of prevention and much less successful in term of treatment, the claim that good nutrition could build resistance to infections and treat infectious disease was enticing. The claim was that food and nutrition were equally or more important than germs and bacteriology. Mellanby's claims were general in scope, but his focus on pregnant woman allowed him to speak to the seemingly intractable problem of maternal mortality that was much debated in the late 1920s.[94] It should be noted also that the anti-infective properties of vitamin concentrates made sense not only as nutritional research but also as pharmacological research, which was of relevance since Mellanby's chair in Sheffield was in pharmacology.

Orr, as director of a research institute charged specifically with research in nutrition with a view to stimulating rural development, was naturally interested in the applied and policy dimensions of nutrition. Exploring links between nutrition and infectious diseases allowed Orr to speak to the concerns of medical, veterinary, and agricultural audiences, and to engage with some of the great stock farming and public health problems not only in the United Kingdom but also in the empire. For a time, this strategy helped Orr to win substantial funding for a broad research program.

Quite apart from the contradictory findings of those who attempted to follow up Mellanby's research and Orr's difficulty in arriving at definite and convincing conclusions, there were changes in the circumstances of both men during the 1930s that contributed to the decline of their research programs: Mellanby's appointment as secretary of the MRC and Orr's loss of Empire Marketing Board funding. Mellanby maintained some part-time personal research on less ambitious topics, while, as has been noted, Orr refocused the program of the Rowett Institute toward topics well-suited to the "hungry thirties." It is also relevant that since the early 1930s a new episode of engagement of nutrition scientists in policymaking had begun. Mellanby was a member of the Ministry of Health's Advisory Committee on Nutrition from its first meeting in 1931, whereas Orr joined the committee when it was reconstituted in 1935. And through the League of Nations, they were also involved in international policymaking.[95] The formulation of nutritional standards or guidelines remained highly problematic, and there were continuing sources of frustration for the nutrition scientists, but there was a sense in which nutrition had arrived. Nutrition was now recognized as a science with important contributions to make to health and economic well-being, and in this context the demonstration of the specific role of nutrition in infectious disease was less necessary and important.

In conclusion, although Orr and Mellanby favored different nutrients in their hypotheses, that they both developed research programs focusing on infection illustrates the marginalization and challenges felt by these nutrition scientists during much of the interwar period. More generally, the "nutrition and infection" research programs illustrate the ways in which the research priorities of nutrition science are shaped by predominant medical, scientific, and societal concerns in which they arise.

Notes

1. David F. Smith, "Nutrition Science and the Two World Wars," in *Nutrition in Britain*, ed. David F. Smith (London: Routledge, 1997), 142–65.

2. Frederick G. Hopkins, "The Analyst and the Medical Man," *Analyst* 31 (1906): 385–97; Frederick G. Hopkins, "Feeding Experiments Illustrating the Importance of Accessory Food Factors in Normal Dietaries," *Journal of Physiology* 44 (1912): 425–60; Mark W. Weatherall and H. Kamminga, "The Making of a Biochemist: II: The Construction of Frederick Gowland Hopkins' Reputation," *Medical History* 40 (1996): 415–36.

3. Mark W. Weatherall, "The Foundation and Early Years of the Dunn Nutritional Laboratory," in Smith, *Nutrition in Britain*, 29–52.

4. Frederick G. Hopkins, "The Practical Importance of Vitamins," *British Medical Journal* 1 (1919): 510.

5. Accessory Food Factors Committee, *Report on the Present State of Knowledge concerning Accessory Food Factors (Vitamines)*, Medical Research Council Special Reports 38 (London: His Majesty's Stationery Office 1919), 4, 49.

6. Ibid., 51.

7. Ibid., 77.

8. See, for example, Frederick G. Hopkins, "Discussion on the Treatment and Management of Diseases Due to Dietetic Deficiencies," *Proceedings of the Royal Society of Medicine* 13, Section of Therapeutics and Pharmacology (1920): 1–5; and "Recent Advances in Science in Relation to Practical Medicine and the Nutritional Requirement of the Body," *Lancet* 1 (1921): 1–7.

9. Frederick G. Hopkins, "The Criteria of an Efficient Diet," *The Practitioner* 114 (1926): 14.

10. Frederick G. Hopkins, "Nutrition and Human Welfare," *Nutrition Abstracts and Reviews* 1 (1931): 3–5.

11. Walter Fletcher to Edward Mellanby, July 31, 1914, FD1/43, National Archives, Kew (hereafter NA).

12. Medical Research Committee, *Third Annual Report* (London, 1917), 28.

13. David F. Smith, "Nutrition in Britain," unpublished PhD thesis, University of Edinburgh, 1986, 62–82; and David F. Smith and M. Nicolson, "The 'Glasgow School' of Paton, Findlay and Cathcart: Conservative Thought in Chemical Physiology, Nutrition and Public Health," *Social Studies of Science* 19 (1989): 195–238.

14. D. Noël Paton and L. Findlay, "General Considerations," in Margaret Ferguson, *A Study of Social and Economic Factors in the Causation of Rickets*, Medical Research Council Special Reports 20 (London: His Majesty's Stationery Office, 1918), 98.

15. D. Noël Paton, L. Findlay, and A. Watson, "Observations on the Cause of Rickets," *British Medical Journal* 2 (1918): 625.

16. Accessory Food Factors Committee, *Report on the Present State of Knowledge*, 89.

17. Edward Mellanby, "An Experimental Investigation on Rickets," *Lancet* 1 (1919): 407.

18. Edward Mellanby, *Experimental Rickets*, Medical Research Council Special Reports 61 (London: His Majesty's Stationery Office, 1921), 70–72.

19. Edward Mellanby, "Discussion on the Etiology of Rickets: Opening Paper II," *British Medical Journal* 2 (1922): 849–53; Leonard Findlay, "Discussion on the Etiology of Rickets: Opening Paper I," *British Medical Journal* 2 (1922): 847–49.

20. Accessory Food Factors Committee, *Studies of Rickets in Vienna*, Medical Research Council Special Reports 77 (London: His Majesty's Stationery Office,

1923); Harold C. Corry Mann, *Rickets: The Relative Importance of Environment and Diet as Factors of Causation: An Investigation in London*, Medical Research Council Special Reports 68 (London: His Majesty's Stationery Office, 1922); Vladimir Korenchevski, *The Aetiology and Pathology of Rickets from an Experimental Point of View*, Medical Research Council Special Reports 71 (London: His Majesty's Stationery Office, 1922).

21. Leonard Findlay, "The Underlying Cause in the Pathogenesis of Rickets," *Journal of the American Medical Association* 83 (1924): 1473–79.

22. Shinnosuke Mori, "Primary Changes in the Eyes of Rats Which Result from Deficiency of Fat-Soluble A in Diet," *Journal of the American Medical Association* 79 (1922): 197–200.

23. Elmer McCollum, *A History of Nutrition* (Boston: Houghton Miffin, 1957), 281; Elmer V. McCollum, N. Simmonds, J. E. Becker, P. G. Shipley, and E. A. Park, "Studies on Experimental Rickets XXIII: The Production of Rickets in the Rat by Diets Consisting Essentially of Purified Food Substances," *Journal of Biological Chemistry* 54 (1922): 249–52.

24. Edward Mellanby, "Deficiency Diseases, with Special Reference to Rickets," *British Medical Journal* 1 (1924): 895–900.

25. Edward Mellanby, "Diet and Disease: With Special Reference to Teeth, Lungs, and Pre-natal Feeding," *British Medical Journal* 1 (1926): 515–19. The reference to cereals arose from Mellanby's studies of their antagonistic effect upon the antirachitic factor. Edward Mellanby, *Experimental Rickets: The Effects of Cereals and Their Interaction with Other factors of Diet and Environment in Producing Rickets*, Medical Research Council Special Reports 93 (London: His Majesty's Stationery Office, 1925).

26. Mellanby, "Deficiency Diseases, with Special Reference to Rickets," 895–900.

27. Edward Mellanby, "Addendum to Memorandum on Proposed Extension of Researches in Human Nutrition," January 25, 1927, FD1/4368, NA; Walter Fletcher to Edward Mellanby, February 7, 1927, FD1/44, NA.

28. See Walter Fletcher to George Newman, October 22, 1931, FD1/1375, NA, and other letters in the same file.

29. Edward Mellanby, "Duties of the State in Relation to the Nation's Food Supply," *British Medical Journal* 2 (1927): 633–36.

30. Harry N. Green and E. Mellanby, "Vitamin A as an Anti-infective Agent," *British Medical Journal* 2 (1928): 693.

31. Edward Mellanby and H. N. Green, "Vitamin A as an Antiinfective Agent: Its Use in the Treatment of Puerperal Septicaemia: Preliminary Communication," *British Medical Journal* 1 (1929): 986. Later work on the use of vitamin A in puerperal septicaemia achieved a mortality rate of seven in twenty-seven cases, but was only reported in MRC, *Annual Report 1930–31* (London: His Majesty's Stationery Office, 1932), 66.

32. Rima D. Apple, *Vitamania: Vitamins in American Culture* (New Jersey: Rutgers University Press, 1996), 26, 39.

33. Robert H. A. Plimmer and V. G. Plimmer, *Food, Health and Vitamins* (London: Longmans, Green, and Co., 1928). This book went through nine editions from 1925 to 1942.

34. Edward Mellanby, "Diet and Health," *British Medical Journal Supplement* 21 (March 1931): 85–92.

35. Irvine Loudon, "An Early Medical Research Council Controlled Trial of Vitamins for Preventing Infection," *Journal of the Royal Society of Medicine* 100 (2007): 195–98.

36. Richard D. Semba, "Vitamin A as 'Anti-infective' Therapy 1920–1940," *Journal of Nutrition* 129 (1999): 783–91. See also Richard D. Semba, *The Vitamin A Story—Lifting the Shadow of Death* (Basel: Karger, 2012), 132–50.

37. Harry N. Green, D. Pindar, G. Davis, and E. Mellanby, "Diet as a Prophylactic Agent against Puerperal Sepsis," *British Medical Journal* 2 (1931): 595–98.

38. Joseph B. Ellison, "Intensive Vitamin Therapy in Measles," *British Medical Journal* 2 (1932): 708–11. Semba regards this as an important and pioneering study: Richard D. Semba, "On Joseph Bramhall Ellison's Discovery That Vitamin A Reduces Measles Mortality," *Nutrition* 19 (2003): 390–94.

39. Samuel Donaldson and J. Tasker, "Preliminary Notes in the Treatment of Pneumonia with Vitamin A," *Proceedings of the Transvaal Mine Officers Association* (1930): 64–68; Alexander J. Orenstein, "Vitamin A in the Treatment of Pneumonia," *South African Medical Journal* 6 (1932): 685–89.

40. MRC, *Annual Report 1929–30* (London, 1931), 17; MRC, *Annual Report 1930–31*, 81.

41. Accessory Food Factors Committee, *Vitamins: A Survey of Present Knowledge*, Medical Research Council Special Reports 167 (London: His Majesty's Stationery Office, 1932), 30–31.

42. Ibid., 227.

43. Edward Mellanby, *Nutrition and Disease: The Interaction of Clinical and Experimental Work* (London: Oliver and Boyd, 1934).

44. William W. C. Topley, M. Greenwood, and J. Wilson, "The Effect of Diet in Epidemic Infections in Mice," *Journal of Pathology and Bacteriology* 34 (1931): 163–76.

45. "Diet and Infection," *Lancet* 1 (1931): 766–67.

46. Albert H. G. Burton and A. R. Balmain, "Vitamin A and Streptococcal Antitoxic Immunity," *Lancet* 1 (1930): 1063–66.

47. Leslie J. Harris, J. R. M. Innes, and A. S. Griffith, "On the Pathogenesis of Avitaminosis A," *Lancet* 2 (1932): 614–17, quote on 615.

48. Leslie J. Harris, "A Note on Vitamins in Practical Experience," *British Medical Journal* 2 (1933): 231–33.

49. Edward Mellanby, "Nutrition and Child-Bearing," *Lancet* 2 (1933): 1131–37.

50. "Vitamin A and Infection," *Lancet* 2 (1933): 1155–56.

51. MRC, *Annual Report 1934–35* (London: His Majesty's Stationery Office, 1936), 9–12.

52. MRC, *Annual Report 1935–36* (London: His Majesty's Stationery Office, 1937), 25.

53. Irvine Loudon, "The Use of Historical Controls and Concurrent Controls to Assess the Effects of Sulphonamides, 1936–1945," *James Lind Library Bulletin: Commentaries on the History of Treatment Evaluation*, 2002, http://www.jameslindlibrary.org/illustrating/articles/the-use-of-historical-controls-and-concurrent-controls-to-assess (accessed April 15, 2014).

54. Semba, "Vitamin A as 'Anti-infective,'" 789.

55. L. S. P. Davidson and I. A. Anderson, *A Textbook of Dietetics* (London: Hamish Hamilton, 1940), 37–38.

56. Leslie J. Harris, "Assessment of Level of Nutrition in Man," *Proceedings of the Nutrition Society* 1 (1944): 7–8.

57. Edward Mellanby, "Nutritional Science in Medicine," *British Medical Bulletin* 2 (1944): 202–4.

58. David F. Smith, "The Agricultural Research Association, the Development Fund, and the Origins of the Rowett Research Institute," *Agricultural History Review* 46 (1998): 47–63.

59. David F. Smith, "The Early Institutional and Scientific Development of the Rowett Research Institute," in *To the Great Support and Advancement of Health*, ed. Alexander Adam, D. F. Smith, and F. Watson (Aberdeen: Aberdeen History of Medicine Publications, 1996), 45–53; Rowett Institute, *First Report* (Aberdeen: Rowett Institute, 1922), 79–80.

60. Walter E. Elliot, A. Crichton, and J. B. Orr, "The Importance of the Inorganic Constituents of the Food in Nutritional Disorders I: Rickets in Pigs," *British Journal of Experimental Pathology* 3 (1922): 10–19, quote on 18.

61. Alfred D. Husband, W. Godden, M. B. Richards, "The Influence of Cod-Liver Oil, Linseed Oil and Olive Oil on the Assimilation of Calcium and Phosphorus in the Growing Pig," *Biochemical Journal* 17 (1923): 707–19.

62. Research Subcommittee, October 2, 1924, Joint Committee Minutes, Rowett Research Institute Archives, University of Aberdeen Special Collections.

63. John B. Orr and A. Crichton, "The Requirements of the Pig for 'Vitamin A' and 'Vitamin C,'" *Journal of Agricultural Science* 14 (1924): 114–25; John B. Orr and H. Maciver, "The Nutritive Requirements of Poultry," *Scottish Journal of Agriculture* 7 (1924): 264–66; Walter Elliot, "Investigation on the Mineral Content of Pasture Grass and Its Effect on Herbivora: I General Report," *Journal of Agricultural Science* 16 (1926): 59–64; Walter Elliot and A. Crichton, "Report on the Effect of the Addition of Mineral Salts to the Ration of Sheep," *Journal of Agricultural Science* 16 (1926): 65–77.

64. John B. Orr, "The Importance of Mineral Matter in Nutrition," *Transactions of the Highland and Agricultural Society of Scotland* 35 (1923): 1–27.

65. John B. Orr, "The Influence of Nutrition on the Incidence of Disease," *Veterinary Record* 4 (1924): 943–55.

66. John B. Orr, "The Chemical and Physiological Properties of Milk, and Their Bearing on Problems of the Dairy Industry," *Transactions of the Highland and Agricultural Society* 36 (1924): 40–64.

67. John B. Orr, "The Influence of Diet on Susceptibility to Disease," *Transactions of the Highland and Agricultural Society* 42 (1930): 34.

68. John B. Orr, "The Importance of the Mineral Elements in the Maintenance of Health," *British Medical Journal* 2 (1924): 504–8.

69. John B. Orr, "The Importance of Mineral Elements in the Nutrition of Children," *Journal of State Medicine* 32 (1924): 421–30.

70. John B. Orr, "Mineral Metabolism and Disease," *The Practitioner* 115 (1925): 32–39.

71. Michael Worboys, "Science and British Colonial Imperialism," unpublished PhD thesis, University of Sussex, 1979, chapter 6.

72. John B. Orr and H. Scherbatoff, *Minerals in Pastures and Their Relation to Animal Nutrition* (London: Lewis, 1929).

73. John B. Orr and J. L. Gilks, *The Physique and Health of Two African Tribes,* Medical Research Council Special Reports 155 (London: His Majesty's Stationery Office, 1931).

74. John B. Orr, J. J. R. Macleod, and T. J. Mackie, "Studies on Nutrition in Relation to Immunity," *Lancet* 1 (1931): 1177–82.

75. Ibid., 1182.

76. Thomas J. Mackie, A. H. H. Fraser, M. H. Finkelstein, and E. J. M. Anderson, "The Influence of Nutrition in Susceptibility to a Bacterial Toxin," *British Journal of Experimental Pathology* 13 (1932): 328–33.

77. John B. Orr, "Restoring the Fertility of Scottish Sheep Grazings," *Transactions of the Highland and Agricultural Society of Scotland* 44 (1932): 64–85.

78. John J. R. Macleod, "The Work of the Rowett Institute," in Rowett Research Institute, *Collected Works 3* (Aberdeen, 1933), 1–13.

79. Allan H. H. Fraser, "Economic Aspects of the Scottish Sheep Industry," *Transactions of the Highland and Agricultural Society* 51 (1939): 39–57.

80. Walter E. Eliott, Seventh Report of the Committee on the Mineral Content of Pastures, October 1, 1931, CO758/2/5, NA.

81. John B. Orr, *The National Food Supply and Its influence on Public Health* (London: Chadwick Trust, 1934); Herbert D. Kay, "John Boyd Orr: Baron Boyd Orr of Brechin Mearns, 1880–1971," *Biographical Memoirs of Fellows of the Royal Society* 18 (1972): 43–81.

82. John B. Orr, *Food, Health and Income* (London: Macmillan, 1936), 43.

83. John B. Orr, "Trends in Nutrition," *British Medical Journal* 1 (1941): 73–77.

84. Loudon, "Controlled Trial"; Semba, "Vitamin A as 'Anti-infective.'"

85. James W. Howie, "Nutrition and Resistance to Infection," in *Progress in Nutrition and Allied Sciences* ed. David P. Cuthbertson (London: Oliver and Boyd, 1963), 357–66.

86. Robert Hutchison, *Food and the Principles of Dietetics* (London: Edward Arnold, 1902), 54–55.

87. William H. Allchin, "The Lumleian Lectures on Nutrition and Malnutrition, Lecture 3," *Lancet* 1 (1905): 1321.

88. David F. Smith, "The Use of 'Team Work' in the Practical Management of Research in the Inter-War Period: The Case of John Boyd Orr at the Rowett Research Institute near Aberdeen," *Minerva* 37 (1999): 259–80.

89. Aaron J. Ihde and S. L. Becker, "Conflict of Concepts in Early Vitamin Studies," *Journal of the History of Biology* 4 (1971): 1–33.

90. Charles Rosenberg, "On the Study of American Biology and Medicine: Some Justifications," *Bulletin of the History of Medicine* 38 (1964): 364–66.

91. McCollum, *History of Nutrition.*

92. Naomi Aronson, "The Discovery of Resistance: Historical Accounts and Scientific Careers," *Isis* 77 (1986): 286–306.

93. Weatherall and Kamminga, "Making of a Biochemist."

94. Ministry of Health, *Interim Report of the Departmental Committee on Maternal Mortality and Morbidity* (London: His Majesty's Stationery Office, 1930).

95. David F. Smith, "The Social Construction of Dietary Standards: The British Medical Association—Ministry of Health Advisory Committee on Nutrition Report of 1934," in *Food, Eating, and Nutrition as Social Problems: Constructivist Perspectives,* ed. Donna Maurer and J. Sobal (New York: Transaction, 1995), 279–304; Paul Weindling, "The Role of International Organizations in Setting Nutritional Standards in the 1920s and 1930s," in *The Science and Culture of Nutrition, 1840s–1940s,* ed. Harmke Kamminga and A. Cunningham (Amsterdam: Rodopi, 1995), 319–32.

Chapter Six

"Not a Complete Food for Man"

The Controversy about White versus Wholemeal Bread in Interwar Britain

Ina Zweiniger-Bargielowska

Introduction

In June 1927 the New Health Society (NHS) issued a "Wholemeal Manifesto" that claimed wholemeal flour was "superior in nutritional value and vitamin content" to its white counterpart, which was "not a complete food for man." The manifesto maintained that the daily requirement of vitamin B could only be "ensured by the use of wholemeal flour" in the working-class diet, which relied heavily on bread. Published in the mass-circulation *Daily Mail*, which welcomed this "striking and convincing confirmation" of its long-standing campaign for wholemeal bread, the manifesto was signed by "thirteen distinguished medical men and scientists." The signatories included the NHS president Sir William Arbuthnot Lane and leading members of society, namely, the eugenicist Caleb Williams Saleeby, the radiologist Alfred Jordan, the physician S. Henning Belfrage, and the biochemist Robert Plimmer.[1] Lane attributed "many of the ills of civilization" to "wrong habits of feeding" in a series of articles published in the *Daily Mail* the previous autumn, in which he highlighted the importance of vitamins to health and advocated wholemeal bread.[2] The *Journal of the American Medical Association*, which reported on the "bread controversy," noted that in support of his arguments Lane invoked the "accumulated intelligence of those who have made dietetics a life study—Gowland Hopkins, Plimmer, Hindhede, McCollum, McCarrison and others."[3]

Using the NHS's "Wholemeal Manifesto" as a jumping-off point, this chapter explores the debate about different types of bread and flour in Britain during the interwar years. Claims about the poor nutritional value of white bread and advocacy of wholemeal can be traced back to the nineteenth century, but the issue received renewed attention in the wake of the discovery of vitamins and the launch of health education pressure groups such as the NHS in the 1920s. The bread controversy focused on chemical properties and nutritional benefits, but these were framed within a wider cultural perspective. There was no general shift in favor of brown bread among nutritionists in interwar Britain, as suggested by Uwe Spiekermann.[4] Rather, this chapter highlights that doctors, nutrition experts, and scientists continued to debate the merits of different types of bread and flour. This debate was conducted not only in scientific, technical terms, but also with regard to stages of civilization, Western culture, and modernity. Lane, whose idiosyncratic opinions had caused controversy in the medical profession for decades, could be dismissed as a crank, but the NHS counted many prominent physicians and scientists among its members and supporters. Ultimately, scientific opinion was divided, and a belief in the cultural superiority of white bread as more civilized and preferable in peacetime colored the conclusions of a study on the topic sponsored by the Medical Research Council.

The New Health Society

The NHS was one of several health education pressure groups founded in Britain after the First World War that also included the People's League of Health and the Sunlight League. These organizations, which were part of a wider life reform movement, had similar aims and shared an overlapping membership. They combined anxiety about racial degeneration, heightened by wartime casualties and revelations of high rejection rates among men called up, with a belief in the cultivation of health as a moral and civic duty.[5] Life reform was of course not confined to Britain, and similar organizations flourished on both sides of the Atlantic.[6] Lane founded the NHS in 1925 with the aim to "convert what is a rapidly degenerating community, in other words a C 3 nation, into an A 1 nation composed of healthy, vigorous members, whose bodies will be able to avoid and combat disease" and whose lives were distinguished by "physical health and moral happiness." The classifications A 1 or "fully fit" and C 3 (unfit for combat) were based on military medical examinations and became a metaphor for fitness in debates about public health throughout the interwar years. The society saw the bowels as central to health and considered chronic intestinal stasis or constipation as the root cause of "all the troubles in civilised life."[7]

Lane, who formulated his idiosyncratic views on chronic intestinal stasis in the 1890s, was a pioneering surgeon.[8] He made his name in orthopedic and cleft palate surgery, but his most controversial innovation was colectomy, that is, removal of the colon, as the ultimate remedy for constipation. Lane operated only in the last resort, but he performed hundreds of colectomies in the early twentieth century. The operation was discredited in the wake of a debate on alimentary toxemia conducted by the Royal Society of Medicine in 1913.[9]

Subsequently, Lane faced widespread condemnation and ridicule, and he abandoned the operation by the 1920s. This did not put an end to his obsession with stasis, and he now advocated increased consumption of dietary fiber to combat constipation.[10] Although medical opinion was divided on the dangers of constipation, according to James Whorton, at the "level of popular belief and behavior, constipation phobia was entering its golden age" during the 1920s.[11] Thus, Lane and the NHS considered wholemeal bread as nutritionally superior because of its higher content of both vitamins and fiber.

Lane's endeavor to counter extensive "physical, mental and moral unfitness," which he saw as a "natural reaction" to the "morbid condition of civilization," drew on economic and biological arguments: "Firstly, sickness, physical or moral, is expensive to the community, as is of necessity its cure; and secondly, the persistence of the conditions which lead to such sickness will ultimately produce a deterioration of the racial health." Lane believed that the "*fundamental causes of disease*" were "faulty habits" and that the elimination of disease was not dependent on therapeutic medicine, but rather required a "complete revolution in our diet and habits."[12] The ill effects of civilization were evinced by the "Lilliputian race that swarms on the pavements of large cities like beetles on the floor of a cellar."[13] By contrast, "natives living in their natural surroundings, eating their simple diet and performing their functions normally," were "quite free from all the diseases of the gastro-intestinal tract peculiar to civilization."[14] For Lane "natives" were "vastly more far-seeing . . . *from a eugenic standpoint* than are the members of a civilised community."[15] He considered health reform as imperative for Britain's future as an imperial nation because "great empires stand and fall by the health of their peoples."[16] The "solution of the national health problem" was "health education," and Lane proclaimed his "chief and constant aim . . . to spread amongst the people a knowledge of the simple laws of health."[17]

The NHS, which was primarily financed by Lane, was run by prominent physicians, scientists, and public figures.[18] Former prime minister H. H. Asquith was a founder-member, and David Lloyd George and Ramsay MacDonald served on its council.[19] With a membership of several thousand and a monthly journal, *New Health*, edited by Lane, the society embarked on an ambitious program of health education discussed fully below, which included public lectures, exhibitions, a film, and articles in the popular press. Lane's high public profile brought him into conflict with the ethical committee of the British Medical Association (BMA), which prohibited individual publicity that could be construed as "indirect advertising."[20] Lane's embrace of modern mass media was considered unethical by the BMA, which had long campaigned against advertisements of quack remedies. In correspondence with the BMA's ethical committee in 1925, Lane threatened to resign, and, indeed, the launch of the NHS in December of that year coincided with the expiration of his BMA membership.[21] Press reporting about Lane's campaigning culminated in BMA lawyers issuing a writ for libel against the *Star*, a mass-circulation daily newspaper, but the case was ultimately dropped. Lane was never brought before the General Medical Council, the statutory body regulating the medical profession, and he remained on the medical register until 1932.[22]

The NHS's objectives included spreading "knowledge of the newer discoveries of science" on the "preservation of health and prevention of disease" and teaching the "advantages of right food, fresh air, sunshine and exercise." It campaigned for better food quality, sought to influence caterers, and hoped to cooperate with local authorities, schools, churches, trade unions, and women's organizations.[23] The society's advice is summed up in a poster of ten "health rules," which recommended increased consumption of wholemeal flour and bread, milk, fruit, vegetables, and "strict moderation" with regard to "flesh foods." This was intended to raise the intake of vitamins and dietary fiber, crucial in the battle against constipation and the promotion of "internal cleanliness." A minimum of two daily bowel movements could be achieved by means of a "suitable diet" and "regular habits." The health rules further included exposure to fresh air and sunlight along with advocacy of "loose" clothing, personal cleanliness, and exercise.[24]

Bread Reform and the "Standard Bread" Campaign of 1911

The debate on the nutritional deficiencies of white bread has a long history. White flour and bread, which had been a luxury of the well-to-do in the eighteenth century, became a dietary staple accounting for over 90 percent of consumption in the wake of the rapid expansion of roller-milling in last quarter of the nineteenth century.[25] A Bread and Food Reform League, which aimed to educate the working class on the health benefits of wholemeal bread, was established in the 1880s. With bread a principal item of the working-class diet, the League warned against the "white loaf's threat to national fitness and dental health."[26] This call was taken up by cooperative mills and the nutritional advantages of wholemeal were promoted, for example, by the Women's Cooperative Guild.[27] The leading brands, Allinson's wholemeal and Hovis wheat germ bread, were launched in the late nineteenth century. T. R. Allinson, an Edinburgh trained physician, published a best-selling pamphlet on the health benefits of wholemeal bread, and he began to market "Allinson Unadulterated Wholemeal Bread" in 1885. The bread sold well in the health food market and it became Britain's best-selling wholemeal loaf in the interwar years.[28] The Hovis Bread Company, established in 1898, produced a patented flour that included a high concentration of wheat germ normally removed in the milling process of white flour. The bread was baked in local bakeries and the brand was widely advertised by the company and promoted on billboards, delivery vans, and bread tins. With the claim that Hovis combined the benefits of wholemeal with the palatability of white bread, the company expanded rapidly and accounted for about 7 to 8 percent of national flour production by 1939.[29]

In 1911 the *Daily Mail* embarked on a campaign promoting so-called standard bread, which contained at least 80 percent of the whole wheat, in view of the "inferior nourishing qualities of white bread."[30] The *Daily Mail*, launched in 1896, pioneered prominent display advertising and appealed to a female readership with human interest journalism. This formula proved highly successful, and in the early twentieth century, the *Daily Mail* was Britain's most popular newspaper, although by the eve of war this popularity was eclipsed by its rival, the *Daily Express*.[31] The campaign, in Mark Weatherall's words, aimed to "sell bread, sell newspapers, and sell science."[32] It was backed by Frederick Gowland Hopkins, Cambridge professor of biochemistry and corecipient of the Nobel Prize for the discovery of vitamins in 1929. Hopkins supported "standard bread" because of the greater presence of previously "unrecognized food substances." Hailed by the *Daily Mail* as a "Revolution in the Science of Food," Hopkins's new theory of the nutritional significance of what he later called "accessory food factors" was first published in a mass-circulation newspaper rather than a scientific or medical journal.[33] Hopkins discussed his research in teaching and public lectures, but his motives for publishing in the *Daily Mail* cannot be established fully. According to Weatherall he may well have been influenced by the fact that medical opinion, rather than that of a "mere laboratory scientist," was considered authoritative on questions of nutrition at this time.[34]

Reporting on the campaign, the *British Medical Journal* warned that "exaggerated claims would lead to reaction and renewed indifference," noting that the "public was beginning to tire of the crusade." In the words of a "prominent weekly," the campaign was "the silliest nonsense that has possessed the British public for years." Millers and bakers were critical, and experiments suggested that white bread allowed for a greater assimilation of protein by the body. According to the *British Medical Journal* this was reassuring for "those who prefer to continue the use of well-made white bread prepared from good wheat."[35] Leonard Hill, lecturer on physiology at the London Hospital Medical School, countered this criticism of "standard bread" and endorsed Hopkins's controversial theory based on experiments in which he fed rats on either standard or white flour for several weeks. Hill, who became director of the Department of Applied Physiology at the National Institute of Medical Research in 1914, served on the NHS's Medical and Scientific Committee in the 1920s.[36] For Hill, the fact that the rats fed on white bread and flour had "done far the worse" was "astonishing." They suffered disproportionately from cold weather, twice as many died, and they were more likely to resort to cannibalism. There were considerable differences in weight, and the "white-fed rats [were] far less lively and less sleek in appearance." Hill concluded that there was "something essential to growth" in the standard flour that was absent from the white flour. This hypothesis was strengthened by a second experiment in which rats fed with wheat germ added to white flour did as well as the standard flour group. In view of these "striking" results, Hill argued that "children of the poor" ought to be fed standard and not white bread.[37]

Hill's article sparked off a debate about the relative merits of the different types of bread in the *British Medical Journal*. Researchers from the Liverpool School of Tropical Medicine, who conducted similar feeding experiments on pigeons, confirmed Hill's findings.[38] By contrast, Douglas Chalmers Watson, an Edinburgh-based physician and author of a popular manual on diet, maintained that Hill's experiment was misleading because mice fed on either type of bread in combination with milk did equally well, which suggested that the "value of standard bread in ordinary dietetics" had been "exaggerated."[39] A general discussion on food warned against taking dietary "principles to a ridiculous extreme," of which the "standard bread" campaign was a "case in point." The article noted that white bread contained higher levels of protein than standard bread, and it welcomed Watson's intervention, which "opportunely" reminded doctors that "after all white bread [was] not a poison."[40] In response, Hill acknowledged that the choice of bread "matters little" to those who could afford milk or meat, but in view of his observations of East End children who often ate bread with nothing on it, he implored the government to "use all its powers to make standard or wholemeal bread the food of the children of the poor."[41] Hopkins's controversial theory was not generally accepted before the war. There was a division within scientific and medical opinion between those who emphasized basic nutrients such as protein and others who acknowledged the importance of the nutritional deficiencies of white bread. "Standard bread" was fiercely opposed by bakers and millers, who denounced it as a "passing fad" or "craze" stirred up by the press, and the campaign fizzled out at the end of the year.[42] Although the campaign garnered considerable attention, and brands such as Allinson's and Hovis were expanding, these remained niche products, and white bread retained its role as a dietary staple of the working class.

The "standard bread" campaign has to be understood against the background of a wider political debate about liberalism and government regulation, free trade, and tariff reform.[43] After the abolition of the Corn Laws in 1846, wheat imports expanded rapidly as prices tumbled, and by 1914 imports accounted for the bulk of consumption.[44] Frank Trentmann posits the cheap white loaf as a powerful symbol of the advantage of free trade, whereas the *Daily Mail* supported the unsuccessful tariff reform campaign in support of import duties. The limited appeal of wholemeal or standard bread underlines the deep cultural resonance of white bread, which stood for "civilized life," "liberty, and comfort," in contrast with the association of brown or rye bread with "poverty and dirt."[45] White bread symbolized "nationalist representations of the superiority of British civilization" defined against "barbaric conditions" in protectionist Germany, where a "coarse black" rye loaf predominated.[46]

This argument draws attention to the fact that wheat was of course not the only bread grain. Whereas oatmeal was consumed extensively in Scotland, in England a cultural preference for wheat had become firmly entrenched by the nineteenth century.[47] It is worth pointing out that the bread controversy focused entirely on what kind of wheat flour was to be eaten rather than alternative grains. This predilection was, if anything, reinforced during the First World War. From November 1916, the government mandated a so-called war bread distinguished by a higher extraction rate and the inclusion of different cereals. The extraction rate rose from 81 to 92 percent between February 1917 and spring

1918, when "war bread" contained up to 30 percent of other cereals such as barley, oats, or rye, as well as soya and potato flour.[48] Despite some successful feeding experiments and a proclamation by the Ministry of Food of the "Passing of the White Loaf" in spring 1918, the bread was not popular, and people returned to their long-standing preference for white bread when the regulations were abolished after the war was over.[49]

Vitamins, Diet, and Health

Lane tapped into this long-established discourse on the health benefits of wholemeal bread, which acquired new impetus in the wake of the discovery of vitamins and new scientific research on the relationship between diet and health. Research of what Hopkins called "accessory food factors" was pioneered before the First World War, but the term "vitamin" was not adopted until the 1920s. Building on the prewar discoveries, nutrition research shifted from an earlier focus on quantitative chemistry and the ratio between protein, carbohydrates, and fats to a new emphasis on food quality during the interwar years. A healthy diet now needed to be not only adequate in terms of calories and protein, but also had to contain sufficient vitamins. This enhanced the significance of expensive foods such as fruit, vegetables, and milk. The Medical Research Council (MRC), established in 1920, became the major source of funding for research on vitamins under the leadership of Walter Morley Fletcher and Edward Mellanby. Mellanby, whose work on rickets led to the identification of vitamin D, and Hopkins were central figures in the field. The MRC's first external research laboratory, the Dunn Nutritional Laboratory at Cambridge, founded in 1927, focused on vitamin research. Other important centers included the Rowett Institute, Aberdeen, under John Boyd Orr. The empire became a key site of nutrition research based on human populations rather than the animal experiments typical in Britain. The close link between diet and health was confirmed by Orr's studies of dietary variations between tribes in East Africa and by Sir Robert McCarrison, a physician in the Indian Medical Service, who focused on Indian diets.[50] The nutritional significance of vitamins was generally accepted in the 1920s, but this was rather less the case with regard to dietary fiber, and the question of the nutritional adequacy of the typical working-class diet remained hotly contested.[51]

Lane frequently cited the work of McCarrison and Mikkel Hindhede, who were among the most prominent critics of conventional Western diets and advocates of wholemeal bread in the 1920s. The former was a member of the NHS, and the latter served on the society's council.[52] McCarrison's studies of "isolated races" in the Himalayas, first published in the early 1920s, noted their exceptional vitality and longevity as well as absence of gastrointestinal diseases and cancer. McCarrison examined the relationship between diet, health, and physique in India. Comparing the diverse diets throughout India, he argued that the "level of physical efficiency of Indian races" was "above all else, a matter of food." In rat experiments, McCarrison replicated various diets, including that of the poorer classes in England. These demonstrated the superiority of the Sikh diet of wholemeal flour, dairy produce, pulses, vegetables, and a little meat. The rats flourished, possessed glossy coats, and "lived happily together." By contrast, rats fed on a diet typical of the poorer classes in England, consisting of white bread, margarine, tinned meat, boiled vegetables, tea, and sugar, showed little weight gain. They were "stunted," "badly proportioned," and lacked gloss in their coats. The rats were also "nervous," "apt to bite the attendants," and "lived unhappily together." After sixty days they "began to kill and eat the weaker ones amongst them," at which point they were segregated. Postmortem examinations showed a prevalence of pulmonary and gastrointestinal diseases that resembled those frequent in Britain. Similar patterns of disease were also observed among the poor in Madras who lived mainly on white rice.[53] McCarrison's work was extensively cited by Lane, despite the fact that the emphasis on dietary diversity undermined Lane's idealized portrayal of a generic superior native culture.[54]

Lane drew a lesson from Danish war rationing supervised by Hindhede, a controversial scientist and nutritional reformer, who was a well-known advocate of a low-protein, high carbohydrate diet.[55] Hindhede was charged with formulating a nutrition policy in response to the German blockade of Denmark, introduced in 1917 despite Denmark's neutrality. The blockade, which cut off imports of fertilizer and grain, devastated domestic agriculture and threatened food supplies. In response, Hindhede advised reducing livestock and particularly pigs, which made the wheat bran and grains normally fed to the animals available for human consumption. Meat consumption was cut drastically, while fiber intake increased, and the decline in protein intake was compensated with extra milk. This rationing regime resembled the frugal diet of small farmers in Western Denmark, whose "excellent health" had long been extolled by Hindhede as evidence of "nature's call for simplicity" in contrast with the "conventional modern diet." Wartime rationing not only prevented hunger, but actually resulted in a reduction of mortality rates, in contrast with rising rates in neighboring countries. Hindhede subsequently celebrated the experience as Denmark's "year of health," which validated his theories of the detrimental effect of what he considered an "unnatural way of life" exemplified by a diet of excessive protein and refined foods.[56] For Lane it was "impossible to exaggerate" the significance of this episode. It provided clear evidence that by altering a nation's diet, "disease may be rapidly reduced" and a nation "can be transformed from a C 3 to an A 1 type."[57]

The Countermanifesto

The medical profession continued to be divided on the bread question. As Sir George Newman, the Chief Medical Officer, put it in his annual report for 1926, there was "still room for differences of opinion in regard to the relative advantages of white bread and brown bread."[58] In response to the NHS's wholemeal manifesto, the prominent physician Sir Thomas Horder vehemently denounced the society's message in a lecture published in the *Lancet* in July 1927. He warned against the zeal of "evangelical dietists" and rejected suggestions of a link between a conventional Western diet and disease. He dismissed Lane's claim that "colonic stasis" was responsible for cancer and other diseases, because there were "no established facts at all which justify the notion—I will not distinguish it by the term hypothesis." Horder maintained that the "common mixed diet of most households" contained sufficient vitamins and, therefore, the higher vitamin B content of wholemeal bread was of "very minor importance." He further noted that although white flour contained little vitamin B, this was compensated for by the addition of yeast in white bread. Maintaining that too much "cellulose" irritated the bowel, he saw wholemeal bread as a deterrent to digestion and claimed that excessive evacuation did more harm than good. Horder alleged an "absence of clear thinking" on the part of wholemeal advocates whose "ill-informed enthusiasm" had suspended "considered judgment." He hoped to see a "health society which spread a less confusing and a more comforting gospel; it might be called the Society of Common Sense."[59]

Horder and a group of like-minded scientists, including V. H. Mottram, professor of physiology at London University, and Gladys Hartwell, lecturer on physiology at King's College of Household and Social Science, wrote a joint letter, published in the next issue of the *Lancet*. This letter effectively amounted to a countermanifesto or "counterblast," as the *Journal of the American Medical Association* put it.[60] The signatories of the *Lancet* correspondence wished to "place on record" their belief that statements about the causal relationship between white bread and disease, including cancer, were "unwarranted, there being a complete absence of scientific data to justify them." The signatories accepted that vitamin B was "essential to health" and that it was "practically absent from white flour." However, vitamin B deficiency was "difficult for a European" because the vitamin was present in many other foods. They further highlighted the difference between white flour and bread with regard to vitamin B content, as a result of the addition of yeast, and emphasized the higher calorific value and palatability of white bread. The signatories questioned the supposed advantages of additional "roughage" in wholemeal bread. Not only did "most people obtain all the 'roughage' they require from other foodstuffs," but too much was "definitely harmful." In sum, the "case for wholemeal bread" had been "overstated" and good quality white bread was a "wholesome and nutritious food." There were "no good reasons for thinking" that the adoption of wholemeal bread "would make for material improvement in the national health and physique."[61]

These views were echoed by the overwhelming majority of doctors who responded to a questionnaire by the National Association of British and Irish Millers mailed to one thousand doctors in 1927. The association aimed to supply the public with "good flour," but did not wish to dislocate milling processes designed to produce white flour on the basis of claims that were "probably unsupported by the medical profession as a whole." The questionnaire was intended to obtain "representative and authoritative medical opinion" on the different types of bread. Doctors were asked whether they agreed with Lane's claim that white bread was the "curse of our age," to assess the health value of different types of bread, and to state their own preference.[62] Among respondents 76 percent rejected Lane's claim. Four out of five considered white bread a "good and nutritious food in a mixed diet," and they refuted the argument that the bread was "likely to lower the standard of national health." Not surprisingly, 89 percent ate white bread themselves.[63]

Horder's comments and the countermanifesto unleashed a torrent of correspondence and stimulated further research. Robert Plimmer and S. Henning Belfrage, signatories of the NHS's wholemeal manifesto, defended the society's case. Plimmer maintained that the additional fiber did not "adversely affect normal digestion."[64] The question "really at issue" was the vitamin B content. The yeast added to produce bread was not sufficient to compensate for the vitamin's absence in white flour, much of which was consumed in the form of cakes or puddings, which did not contain any yeast. He drew attention to research by McCarrison and others that demonstrated a link between vitamin deficiency and digestive and heart troubles. For Plimmer the "crux of the food question" was that the working-class diet dominated by white flour, sugar, chocolate, fat, and meat simply did not contain enough vitamin B. Wholemeal bread and flour were the "easiest and cheapest way" to make up the shortfall.[65] Belfrage similarly argued that Horder's notion of a mixed diet was beyond the reach of millions on low incomes whose diet was "neither wholesome nor sufficiently varied" to ensure against deficiency. Maintaining that the "correct balance" of nutrients was found in "nature's unspoilt product," Belfrage further rejected the implication that wholemeal bread was a "novelty" and stressed that white bread was the "innovation."[66] These arguments were countered by another correspondent who welcomed Horder's "sanity," "clearness and common sense" with regard to the bread question and colonic stasis and deplored the "campaign of propaganda in connexion with that nebulous idea."[67] For the *Journal of the American Medical Association* the "spectacle of eminent physicians and physiologists unable to agree on such an apparently simple question" was "not edifying for the public."[68] Regardless of these misgivings, the controversy continued in the following months and, indeed, years.

A study of the nutritive value of bread with special reference to its vitamin B content by W. Cramer and J. C. Mottram, who were based at the Imperial Cancer Research Fund Radium Institute, London, published in November 1927, noted that the discovery of vitamins had added a "new factor around which the recent controversy has centred."[69] Based on chemical analysis and rat experiments, they concluded that white bread, even with the addition of yeast, was "so deficient in vitamin B that it has ceased to be a supply of this vitamin in our dietary," whereas wholemeal or germ bread of the Hovis type was "rich" in the vitamin. For Cramer and Mottram, the question of vitamin intake had to be considered "in relation to the diet as a whole." If bread accounted for the bulk of a diet generally poor in vitamin B, the nutritive value of white bread was "definitely inferior," amounting to a "serious dietetic defect."[70]

Horder's fellow signatories Hartwell and V. H. Mottram maintained that they were misquoted by Cramer and J. C. Mottram. The latter rejected this accusation in reference to the "manifesto" Hartwell and V. H. Mottram had signed.[71] V. H. Mottram now acknowledged a "slight superiority" of wholemeal over white bread, but this was "no basis" for the current agitation and, therefore, there was "no reason to discard" white bread as part of a "good mixed diet." Nevertheless, he accepted that under conditions of "severely restricted" food choice, when bread was the "main source of energy," brown should "be necessarily preferred" to white.[72] Not surprisingly, Leonard Hill endorsed Cramer and J. C. Mottram's "valuable" study, and he drew attention to his prewar research that endorsed the results.[73] Likewise, Belfrage welcomed the study as "extremely valuable."[74] The ongoing debate about the relative merits of different types of bread is discussed further below, but first of all it is necessary to explore the NHS's wholemeal campaign.

The NHS's Wholemeal Campaign

The NHS embarked on a multimedia education campaign promoting wholemeal bread and flour, ranging from the popular press and books to exhibitions and a specially commissioned film. Under the headline "Secrets of Good Health," Lane published a series of articles in the *Daily Mail* in autumn 1926. He welcomed the "innumerable" efforts by the press to educate the public. These efforts had contributed to a growing realization of the "vital importance" of health, since the "misery and dissatisfaction that exist so generally" were due to "lowered vitality." Lane attributed this misery to ignorance and, in a later article, he declared that doctors' "most important function" was to teach the "laws of health." This "absolutely essential duty" far transcended "all attempts to alleviate suffering and disease."[75]

Lane deplored the rise of "manufactured, over-refined and preserved foods" and the simultaneous decline of "fresh and natural food" as an "evil of our civilization." He advised reduced consumption of meat and advocated vitamin-rich fruit, vegetables, dairy produce, eggs, and wholemeal flour.[76] Drawing "lessons from savages" who evacuated after every meal, he stressed the need for "drainage of waste products." Lane blamed "civilised" habits and diet for the "White Man's burden" of constipation. This could be countered by a fiber-rich diet coupled with "beneficial exercises" such as those recommended in Fred Hornibrook's best-selling *Culture of the Abdomen*.[77] Published with the encouragement of Lane, who saluted the book as of the "greatest service to the public," Hornibrook's system aimed to cultivate the "muscles of the abdomen and the organs of digestion and excretion" by means of rhythmic abdominal exercises based on "native" dances.[78] *Sex and Exercise* by Ettie Rout, Hornibrook's wife, which adapted the system to women, also sold well, and both manuals remained in print until the early postwar years. Rout was a founder-member of the NHS and the couple were among the society's leading popular writers.[79]

Lane's articles attracted "extraordinary attention" and the *Daily Mail* reaffirmed its long-standing commitment to "vigorous" public health campaigning in view of the "enormous number of C 3 subjects examined during the war." By spreading "knowledge of the ways to maintain health," the paper aimed to contribute to "securing an A 1 people."[80] *New Health* hailed Lane's articles as of "vital importance to our movement" because they had "excited" a "great deal of public interest" and generated an "immense correspondence" that expressed "keen appreciation." With Lane's fees paid directly to the society, the articles also provided a "very handsome donation." In response to numerous requests for copies, they were republished as *Secrets of Good Health* in 1927.[81]

Lane's advice was echoed by Robert Plimmer and his wife Violet Plimmer in *Food and Health,* first published in 1925, one of the most successful popular nutrition manuals of the interwar years. The book was later renamed *Food, Health and Vitamins,* and it remained in print until the 1940s.[82] The Plimmers contrasted the recent rise of increasingly refined, processed, and "artificial" foods eaten by "civilised man" with the diet of "natives" who lived on wholemeal flour, fruit, vegetables, dairy produce, and a little meat. The fitness of "natives" was demonstrated by their "splendid physique" and the fact that they did "not suffer from the diseases of civilization" such as constipation, cancer, and diabetes. The book included a brief history of the discovery of vitamins and highlighted the devastating effect of deficiency diseases. The Plimmers explained the principles of food selection with the concept of a "square meal," which provided a balanced combination of carbohydrates, protein, and fat as well as vitamins and minerals. The quality of the diet depended on the "squareness" of meals, represented in a diagram that listed healthy, vitamin-rich items such as wholemeal flour, milk, butter, eggs, fresh fruit, and vegetables. In another diagram, unhealthy items including white flour and bread were placed outside the square. To "produce an A 1 stock" everyone must eat "square meals" and avoid foodstuffs "outside" the square. These dietary principles were translated into weekly shopping lists and menus that provided balanced and economical meals.[83]

Violet Plimmer also offered "practical" advice in *New Health.* She suggested making "one change" at a time to "convert" the "ordinary poor diet" into a "healthy" one by substituting wholemeal for white bread and replacing processed foods with fresh fruit and vegetables.[84] Ettie Rout was the society's other leading expert on wholemeal cookery. She wrote extensively on the nutritional advantages of wholemeal bread and flour, publishing numerous recipes in *New Health.*[85] In her book *Whole-Meal: With Practical Recipes,* Rout held up wholemeal as a "natural" food and provided instructions for cooking and baking. The book was written in response to Lane's "urgent request" and published simultaneously with the NHS's wholemeal manifesto.[86] Rout published another cookery book, *Native Diet: With Numerous Practical Recipes,* which was written at the request of the society and drew on ostensibly "native" customs. Lane welcomed the book as a "great service for civilised humanity" because the "underlying principles of native life" provided "much valuable knowledge" of healthful habits such as steaming rather than boiling food to preserve vitamins. *Native Diet* made extensive use of high-fiber vegetables and fruit to stimulate bowel movement and it introduced unfamiliar foods such as artichokes and protein-rich soybeans as an ideal meat substitute.[87]

The promotion of wholemeal bread took center stage at the NHS's stall at the *Daily Mail*'s Ideal Home Exhibition in 1927, which was organized by Rout.[88] The health benefits of wholemeal were particularly important for children, according to a poster displayed at the society's stall that maintained: "You would not give your children skimmed milk. Why give them 'skimmed bread'?"[89] This annual exhibition at Olympia, established in 1908, tapped into lower-middle-class women's consumer aspirations and desires. The spectacle of the exhibitions, which presented the "ideal" home as the center of a modern, efficient way of life, dovetailed neatly with the health and hygiene message of the NHS.[90] Hailing the event as "one of the most wonderful exhibitions held," *New Health* took pride in the society's stall in 1927. This helped to promote a "greater realisation" that "there can never be an 'ideal home' unless those dwelling within it possess that greatest of all treasures—good health." By positing "Ideal Homes—blessed with Ideal Health" as "inseparable," the society claimed to have fostered the development of a "personal health conscience."[91] Based on the "keen interest" and "number of new members enrolled," *New Health* considered the 1929 stall as yet another success. The magazine welcomed that people were "becoming alive to the desirability of acquiring an elementary knowledge concerning their personal health."[92]

The NHS also staged its own New Health Exhibition, held at the Royal Horticultural Hall, Westminster, in 1928. The *Daily Mail* hailed the exhibition as an "important milestone in the history of public health effort."[93] It featured stalls by health education societies, lectures by leading NHS activists, films on health subjects, and presentations of modern dance.[94] A second exhibition in 1929 built on the success of the first and a third was planned for 1930. However, it was never held, and in the face of straightened finances and economic downturn the society's activities were significantly curtailed in the early 1930s.[95] These exhibitions depended on commercial exhibitors such as the well-known brands Allinson's and Hovis Bread, Grape Nuts breakfast cereal, and Ryvita crispbread. Exhibitors also presented a range of wholemeal cereal bars and biscuits, dried fruit and nuts, fruit juices, health teas, and vitamin supplements.[96]

New Health accepted that the "academic principles" of healthy living and "commercial enterprise must find a point of contact." Lane applauded "how rapidly the ideals of New Health have opened new avenues of manufacturing and trading enterprise, which now—happily for the health and well-being of the community—are being extended more and more widely."[97] *New Health* considered the exhibitions as a "most significant and successful attempt to effect a link between the public, anxious to follow the health principles," and the "commercial organizations which endeavour to put these principles into a concrete form." The exhibitions gave a "graphic illustration" of the extent to which the "health idea" had been taken up by a wide range of producers, as "no reader of the advertisements in the daily press and the periodicals can have failed to notice."[98]

Allinson's and Hovis Bread were advertised extensively in *New Health* as well as the popular press. Allinson Wholemeal Bread, made with "only the finest quality Empire wheats," promised "New Freedom from all Health worries" to "sedentary workers" who required "protection against constipation." Wholemeal was rich in not only vitamins and minerals but also "roughage," "Nature's sure method of relieving and preventing constipation and its attendant disorders."[99] The market-leader Hovis Bread was "very rich in vitamins" but more "palatable" and "easy to digest" than wholemeal. With the "vital life and health-giving elements of the Wheat in *ideal proportions*," Hovis promised "100% Efficiency."[100] The leading breakfast cereal brands Shredded Wheat, Kellogg's, and Post's were also advertised widely. These "ready-to-eat" breakfast cereals, which originated in the United States in the late nineteenth century, had become an established part of the British diet by the 1930s as a result of "vigorous promotion." Indeed, cereal foods accounted for 10 percent of total food advertising expenditure in 1938.[101] For example, Post's Bran Flakes were promoted as a "delightful" and "deliciously palatable . . . remedy" for constipation, rich in minerals and vitamins. Shredded Wheat was the "Golden Key to Vitamin B," Kellogg's All-Bran "never fails," and Grape-Nuts gave the "Joy of Health."[102]

The NHS commissioned the film *Health Is Wealth* (1929), which provided a "further stage" in the society's endeavor toward "greater popularization" of its message. The "popular and striking" medium of film was perceived as an ideal tool to teach the "large mass of the population" the lessons that needed to be learned to "raise our general standard of health and national efficiency." According to *New Health*, the film provided the first attempt to bring together the "range of activities covered by the Public Health Services" with the "prevention of disease through individual effort." *Health Is Wealth* consisted of four reels, which could be shown separately. The first two portrayed public health work and healthcare provision, and they drew attention to the extent of "preventable wastage of life, health, efficiency, happiness" and "money." The second two reels approached health from the perspective of "individual welfare and responsibility, particularly with regard to the inculcation of sound habits of life and diet." The dangers of constipation and its link with "diseases of civilization" were covered in the final reel, which advised increased "roughage" and regular evacuation.[103] The film's production costs contributed to a deficit in the society's finances in 1930, but it was hoped that much of this would be recuperated by future rental income. There is no evidence of a general release, but *Health Is Wealth* was screened, for example, during "health weeks" and at the New Health Exhibition of 1929.[104]

The Bread Controversy Reignited

The bread controversy was reignited in the wake of an MRC study of the carbohydrate content of foods by R. A. McCance and R. D. Lawrence, biochemists at King's College Hospital, London, published in April 1929.[105] The MRC sponsored this research because "accurate information" about the "values" of carbohydrates was "still surprisingly scanty and inaccessible." This included a "critical discussion" of the role of dietary fiber, which would shed light on the "longstanding debate upon the relative merits of brown and white bread."[106] Noting that fiber was part of human and domestic animal diets from the "earliest times" and used by "all nations in times of stress," McCance and Lawrence maintained that its "value in nutrition . . . has never been defined." Generally, human beings were "not well fitted by nature for high cellulose diets," but "normally" ate some cellulose in vegetables, fruit, and "especially brown bread."[107]

McCance and Lawrence claimed that the debate about the "relative merits" of white and wholemeal bread was informed "more by psychological bias than by experimental facts." They argued that "cranks of all kinds" had advocated the latter with "ever recurring waves of enthusiasm." They noted the "tendency . . . for civilized peoples, finding white bread more appetizing, to depart further and further from the whole-meal flour of their ancestors."[108] This preference persisted in the face of campaigns on both sides of the Atlantic exhorting a largely unresponsive public to eat wholemeal bread since the mid-nineteenth century. The discovery of vitamin B provided a "fresh impetus to the whole-meal bread agitation." Although the vitamin question was now agreed on, it "remains to be proved . . . that the chronic indigestion and constipation of civilized populations has its origin in a vitamin B deficiency." They speculated that if vitamin deficiency was the "cause of so much constipation," which could be cured by wholemeal bread, this would "hardly have failed to attract the attention of physicians."[109] This argument apparently confuses wholemeal advocates' case that the extra fiber rather than vitamins was critical in the battle against constipation.

McCance and Lawrence reaffirmed established opinion that white bread was a "better source of energy" and more digestible. Wholemeal was rich in vitamins and contained more protein, but this did "not rank with animal or other vegetable proteins." Finally, with regard to wholemeal bread's role as a cure for constipation, the authors argued that its laxative properties were no greater than other materials, suggesting that there was "no reason why those who prefer to eat white and use other laxatives should not do so."[110] In conclusion, McCance and Lawrence called on nutritionists to be "cautious in advising whole-meal bread generally." There was a need for more research on its effect, particularly with regard to women and children. Appetite was another key consideration, and "no one who dislikes a food of unproved value should be forced to eat it." In "time of peace" adults, "if they have the choice, will never eat whole-meal bread unless they like it."[111]

Better Health, the journal of the Central Council for Health Education, subsequently weighed up the pros and cons of white and wholemeal or brown bread. The MRC study had "given us some facts" to "appraise the relative merits" of the different types of bread. *Better Health* acknowledged the advantages of wholemeal bread, but nevertheless endorsed the MRC study's conclusions because "being part of and not the *entire* diet, white bread wins hands down." In a "civilized community in ordinary times," bread was simply one of numerous foods eaten primarily for its starch; therefore, "the whiter the bread the better it is." *Better Health* acknowledged that man would "starve on white bread . . . *if bread were his sole article of diet*" and that in "time of scarcity" brown bread was "preferable." However, essential vitamins were available from "many other sources." Brown bread was "less digestible" and "less nutritious." Excessive fiber was "bad," particularly for children and pregnant women.[112]

For Gladys Hartwell and V. H. Mottram, the "brown versus white bread controversy" had "engendered more heat than light." They acknowledged the nutritional benefits of higher vitamin B content in brown bread, but also argued that this was "amply compensated" in an "ordinary mixed diet." Hartwell and Mottram drew attention to the "overwhelming instinct" of the working classes in favor of white bread, which could be seen as "mute and inarticulate evidence of its dietetic value." On the basis of yet more rat experiments in which the rats were fed on white or brown bread as part of a mixed diet resembling that of an English agricultural laborer, the authors noted that both sets had a similar growth pattern, which was "far behind the normal growth rate" of rats fed a middle-class diet. The choice of bread made little difference and, indeed, the coats of the rats fed on brown bread were in a worse condition than those of the rats fed on white bread. The rats also differed in their behavior, and the brown-bread fed rats were "highly nervous," "threatened to bite," and started to eat excreta. In conclusion, this experiment gave "but little support to the propaganda" advocating brown bread for the working class.[113]

This evidence was countered by Hill, who found that mice, fed on his version of an agricultural laborer's diet, were "fine-looking and well-breeding."[114] Lane rejected the criticisms of wholemeal as "incorrect" and "likely to mislead the general public to the detriment of the health of the nation." Drawing on Plimmer, McCarrison, and other authorities, Lane maintained that the absence of vitamin B from white flour was not compensated adequately in the "ordinary mixed diet." The chronic vitamin shortage was the root cause of the "common everyday troubles from which many people suffer."[115] In a public lecture in 1936, McCarrison himself reiterated his long-standing claim that "faulty nutrition" was the "principal cause of ill health." McCarrison attributed the high proportion of respiratory and digestive diseases to a diet deficient in vitamins, and he called for "better feeding," including the adoption of wholemeal bread to "achieve the end in view—the building of an A 1 nation."[116]

Evidence of consumption trends and popular attitudes clearly demonstrates that white bread was preferred by the overwhelming majority. Sir William Crawford and H. Broadley's late 1930s survey of eating habits showed that brown bread, which was significantly more popular among the higher income groups, accounted for only 8.6 percent of total consumption. In view of its nutritional superiority, the authors considered the "inability or reluctance" of the working class to purchase brown bread as "greatly to be regretted."[117] There was considerable opposition to raising the extraction rate of flour in the early years of the Second World War, but in the face of shipping losses a compulsory brown bread was finally introduced in spring 1942.[118] Despite the Ministry of Food's extensive propaganda campaign promoting so-called national wheatmeal bread, it was never popular. One correspondent described the loaf as a "nasty, dirty, dark, coarse, indigestible bread."[119] The grudging acceptance of the bread is demonstrated by a wartime social survey of a representative sample of over 2,800 people conducted in 1944. The survey found that three-quarters of respondents accepted the bread "under wartime conditions," but two-thirds preferred white bread, and a similar proportion did not want this bread to be continued after the war.[120]

The supply situation deteriorated after 1945. In the context of a world food shortage, extractions rates increased to unprecedented levels and bread was rationed between 1946 and 1948. Described by Winston Churchill as "one of the gravest announcements" that he had "ever heard . . . in time of peace," the policy was controversial; many doubted its necessity and worried about potential hardship. In the event, the ration was generous and consumption was barely affected.[121] In the face of extensive discontent, the Ministry of Food intensified its propaganda effort explaining and justifying bread rationing.[122] Against the background of hardship in Britain and elsewhere during the early years of the Cold War, American industrial white bread came to symbolize the "strength, stability, choice, and abundance on which world peace could rest." Harking back to earlier British notions of the cultural superiority of white bread, its American variant now represented the "idea of alimentary affluence in the West" defined against the "dark Soviet bread" on the Eastern side of the Iron Curtain.[123]

There is no evidence to suggest that attitudes to brown bread in Britain changed in the following decade. When flour was finally decontrolled in 1955, consumption of brown bread dropped close to zero in a matter of weeks and the white loaf again became the principal bread eaten in Britain. This habit began to shift only in the final quarter of the twentieth century, and from the mid-1970s onward brown bread consumption rose gradually. In the wake of renewed enthusiasm for dietary fiber, wholemeal bread became increasingly popular in the 1980s, and by the end of the decade brown and wholemeal bread together accounted for nearly 40 percent of total bread consumption.[124]

Conclusion

The NHS's campaign for wholemeal bread failed, just as the earlier "standard bread" campaign had met with limited, if any, success. The society's multimedia health education effort extolling the virtues of wholemeal bread, which ranged from books and magazine articles to film, exhibitions, and the popular press, did not alter consumption significantly. Indeed, even the much more extensive official propaganda promoting national wheatmeal bread during and after the Second World War largely fell on deaf ears. Consumer preference for white bread, established in the nineteenth century, was deeply ingrained, and the state was willing to interfere with the free market only in periods of national emergency. This reluctance stood in contrast with Germany, where the Nazi regime embraced wholemeal and rye bread as the "right fuel for an efficient and healthy Aryan race" in the 1930s.[125]

There was no general endorsement in favor of wholemeal bread. The scientific debate revolved around the value attached to dietary fiber and the question as to whether the remainder of the diet contained sufficient vitamin B regardless of the choice of bread. Although vitamins became part of scientific orthodoxy, the NHS's advocacy of the nutritional benefits of dietary fiber remained a minority position in the interwar years. Despite extensive research into the chemical properties of different types of flour and bread, numerous feeding experiments with animals, and lessons drawn from human experiences, scientific and medical opinion remained divided. Both camps used the latest research to justify their support for either white or wholemeal bread and none of the protagonists discussed in this chapter changed their stance on the issue.

This debate was not conducted in a vacuum and the bread controversy should be understood within a wider cultural and political context. Factors such as appetite and consumer freedom colored the conclusions of the MRC study, arguably the closest to an official pronouncement on the topic. The dominant scientific and medical position favored white flour and bread because it was perceived as an integral aspect of a superior British civilization, in contrast with a more primitive and poorer past, a darker loaf imposed by wartime hardship, or the coarse bread associated with Eastern European despotism and dictatorship. By contrast, wholemeal advocates extolled the supposed virtues of non-Western lifestyles and the more natural diet of earlier generations. This conclusion sheds new light on our understanding of nutrition science at a critical stage in the emergence of the discipline in the early decades of the twentieth century.

Notes

1. *New Health* (June 1927): 31–32.
2. *Daily Mail*, October 21, 1926, 8; *Daily Mail*, November 20, 1926, 6.
3. *Journal of the American Medical Association* 88 (April 23, 1927): 1334.
4. Uwe Spiekermann, "Brown Bread for Victory: German and British Wholemeal Politics in the Inter-War Period," in *Food and Conflict in Europe in the Age of the Two World Wars*, ed. Frank Trentmann and Flemming Just (Basingstoke, England: Palgrave Macmillan, 2006), 161, 163–64.
5. For a full discussion of the NHS and the wider debate about public health in interwar Britain, see Ina Zweiniger-Bargielowska, *Managing the Body: Beauty, Health, and Fitness in Britain, 1880–1939* (Oxford: Oxford University Press, 2010).
6. James C. Whorton, *Crusaders for Fitness: The History of American Health Reformers* (Princeton, NJ: Princeton University Press, 1982); James C. Whorton, *Inner Hygiene: Constipation and the Pursuit of Health in Modern Society* (New York: Oxford University Press, 2000); Mary Lynn Stewart, *For Health and Beauty: Physical Culture and the Female Body in France* (Baltimore, MD: Johns Hopkins University Press, 2001); Michael

Hau, *The Cult of Health and Beauty in Germany: A Social History, 1890–1930* (Chicago: University of Chicago Press, 2003).

7. *New Health* (February 1927): 35.

8. On Lane's career and influence, see Thomas B. Layton, *Sir William Arbuthnot Lane: An Enquiry into the Mind and Influence of a Surgeon* (Edinburgh: E. & S. Livingstone, 1956); Andrew A. G. Morrice, "Lane, Sir William Arbuthnot, First Baronet (1856–1943), Surgeon and Health Campaigner," in *Oxford Dictionary of National Biography*, vol. 32, ed. H. C. G. Matthew and Brian Harrison (Oxford: Oxford University Press, 2004), 442–44.

9. Ann Dally, *Fantasy Surgery, 1880–1930: With Special Reference to Sir William Arbuthnot Lane* (Amsterdam: Rodopi, 1996), 164–82.

10. Whorton, *Inner Hygiene*, 56–65.

11. Ibid., 79.

12. Sir William Arbuthnot Lane, *The Prevention of Diseases Peculiar to Civilization* (London: Faber & Faber, 1929), vii, ix–x (emphasis in original).

13. Sir William Arbuthnot Lane, "Women and the Race," in *The Golden Health Library: A Complete Guide to Golden Health for Men and Women of All Ages*, vol. 3, ed. Sir William Arbuthnot Lane (London: New Health Society, 1930), 868 (emphasis in original).

14. *New Health* (January 1926): 5.

15. *New Health* (June 1927): 28 (emphasis in original).

16. *New Health* (December 1931): 32.

17. Sir William Arbuthnot Lane, *Blazing the Health Trail* (London: Faber & Faber, 1929), vii.

18. Sir William Arbuthnot Lane, "Autobiography" (unpublished), printed in Dally, *Fantasy Surgery*, 318. Lane had a lucrative private practice. See Morrice, "Sir William Arbuthnot Lane," 443.

19. *New Health* (January 1926): 3–4.

20. Andrew A. G. Morrice, "'The Medical Pundits': Doctors and Indirect Advertising in the Lay Press 1922–27," *Medical History* 38 (1994): 255.

21. Ibid., 269–71.

22. Ibid., 275–78.

23. *New Health* (June 1926): i.

24. *New Health* (August 1929): 18.

25. John Burnett, *Plenty and Want: A Social History of Diet in England from 1815 to the Present Day* (London: Methuen, 1979), 16, 139–40.

26. Frank Trentmann, "Bread, Milk and Democracy: Consumption and Citizenship in Twentieth-Century Britain," in *The Politics of Consumption: Material Culture and Citizenship in Europe and America*, ed. Martin Daunton and Matthew Hilton (Oxford: Berg, 2001), 136.

27. Ibid., 137–38.

28. Whorton, *Inner Hygiene*, 214–15.

29. E. J. T. Collins, "The 'Consumer Revolution' and the Growth of Factory Foods: Changing Patterns of Bread and Cereal Eating in Britain in the Twentieth Century," in *The Making of the Modern British Diet*, ed. Derek J. Oddy and Derek S. Miller (London: Croom Helm, 1976), 29–31.

30. Mark Weatherall, "Bread and Newspapers: The Making of 'A Revolution in the Science of Food,'" in *The Science and Culture of Nutrition, 1840s–1940s,* ed. Harmke Kamminga and Andrew Cunningham (Amsterdam: Rodopi, 1995), 183.

31. Adrian Bingham, *Gender, Modernity, and the Popular Press in Interwar Britain* (Oxford: Oxford University Press, 2004), 3–4, 8–10, 22–34. On circulation figures, see David Butler and Gareth Butler, *British Political Facts, 1900–1985,* 6th ed. (London: Macmillan, 1986), 494.

32. Weatherall, "Bread and Newspapers," 181.

33. Ibid., 180, 187–88.

34. Ibid., 189, 191.

35. *British Medical Journal* 1 (1911): 643–44.

36. *New Health* (January 1926): 4.

37. *British Medical Journal* 1 (1911): 1068–69.

38. Ibid., 1151.

39. Ibid. See Douglas Chalmers Watson, *Food and Feeding in Health and Disease: A Manual of Practical Dietetics* (Edinburgh: Oliver & Boyd, 1910).

40. *British Medical Journal* 1 (1911): 1218–19.

41. Ibid., 1310–11.

42. Weatherall, "Bread and Newspapers," 196.

43. Ibid., 180.

44. Burnett, *Plenty and Want,* 133–34, 286–89.

45. Frank Trentmann, *Free Trade Nation: Commerce, Consumption and Civil Society in Modern Britain* (Oxford: Oxford University Press, 2008), 39, 214.

46. Ibid., 88, 95.

47. Burnett, *Plenty and Want,* 16; Collins, "Consumer Revolution," 26, 28.

48. Burnett, *Plenty and Want,* 277; Derek J. Oddy, *From Plain Fare to Fusion Food: British Diet from the 1890s to the 1990s* (Woodbridge, England: Boydell, 2003), 77, 92.

49. Trentmann, *Free Trade Nation,* 215–16.

50. There is an extensive literature on this research. See David Smith, ed., *Nutrition in Britain: Science, Scientists and Politics in the Twentieth Century* (London: Routledge, 1997); Harmke Kamminga, "'Axes to Grind': Popularising the Science of Vitamins, 1920s–1930s," in *Food, Science, Policy and Regulation in the Twentieth Century: International and Comparative Perspectives,* ed. David Smith and Jim Phillips (London: Routledge, 2000), 83–100; Oddy, *From Plain Fare,* 115–19; James Vernon, *Hunger: A Modern History* (Cambridge, MA: Belknap Press, 2007), 81–104.

51. Zweiniger-Bargielowska, *Managing the Body,* 284–93.

52. Dally, *Fantasy Surgery,* 226, 230; *New Health* (December 1928), inside cover.

53. Sir Robert McCarrison, *Nutrition and Health: Being the Cantor Lectures Delivered before the Royal Society of Arts 1936 Together with Two Earlier Essays,* 3rd ed. (London: Faber, 1961), 22–23, 29–30.

54. Lane, *Prevention of Diseases,* 53–56; Lane, *Blazing the Health Trail,* 31.

55. Svend Skafte Overgaard, "Mikkel Hindehede and the Science and Rhetoric of Food Rationing in Denmark 1917–1918," in *Food and War in Twentieth Century Europe,* ed. Ina Zweiniger-Bargielowska, Rachel Duffett, and Alain Drouard (Farnham: Ashgate, 2011), 202.

56. Ibid., 204, 210.

57. Lane, *Prevention of Diseases,* 56–57.

58. Ministry of Health, *On the State of Public Health: Annual Report of the Chief Medical Officer of the Ministry of Health for the Year 1926* (London: HMSO, 1927), 184.

59. Sir Thomas Horder, "MacAlister Lecture on Diet and Dietists," *Lancet* 2 (1927): 103–7.

60. *Journal of the American Medical Association* 89, no. 11 (1927): 893.

61. *Lancet* 2 (1927): 201.

62. *Journal of the American Medical Association* 88, no. 12 (1927): 938.

63. *Journal of the American Medical Association* 88, no. 17 (1927): 1334.

64. *Lancet* 2 (1927): 201–2.

65. Ibid.

66. Ibid., 203.

67. Ibid., 202–3.

68. *Journal of the American Medical Association*, 89, no. 11 (1927): 893.

69. *Lancet* 2 (1927): 1090–94; *Lancet* 2 (1929): 586.

70. *Lancet* 2 (1927): 1090–94.

71. Ibid., 1265.

72. Ibid., 1153–54.

73. Ibid., 1212.

74. Ibid., 1264.

75. *Daily Mail*, October 15, 1926, 9–10; *Daily Mail*, October 23, 1926, 13.

76. *Daily Mail*, October 19, 1926, 8; *Daily Mail*, October 21, 1936, 8.

77. *Daily Mail*, October 23, 1926, 7; *Daily Mail*, November 13, 1926, 6.

78. Frederick Arthur Hornibrook, *The Culture of the Abdomen: The Cure of Obesity and Constipation* (London: William Heinemann, 1924), v, 4, 15. A seventeenth edition was published in 1947.

79. Ettie A. Rout [Hornibrook], *Sex and Exercise: A Study of the Sex Function in Women and Its Relation to Exercise* (London: William Heinemann, 1925). A nineth edition was published in 1948. On Hornibrook and Rout, see Zweiniger-Bargielowska, *Managing the Body*.

80. *Daily Mail*, November 6, 1926, 6, 8.

81. *New Health* (November, 1926): 4; *New Health* (December 1926): 5, 25–26; Sir William Arbuthnot Lane, *Secrets of Good Health* (London: William Heinemann, 1927).

82. Robert H. A. Plimmer and Violet G. Plimmer, *Food and Health* (London: Longmans & Co., 1925); Robert H. A. Plimmer and Violet G. Plimmer, *Food, Health and Vitamins*, 4th ed. (London: Longmans & Co., 1929).

83. Plimmer and Plimmer, *Food, Health and Vitamins*, vii–viii, 3–6, 13–16, 90.

84. *New Health* (November 1926): 15–17.

85. *New Health* (May 1927): 14; *New Health* (September 1927): 52; *New Health* (March 1928): 62; *New Health* (December 1928): 29–31; *New Health* (July 1931): 17.

86. Ettie A. Rout, *Whole-Meal: With Practical Recipes* (London: William Heinemann: 1927), vii, 16.

87. Ettie A. Rout, *Native Diet: With Numerous Practical Recipes* (London: William Heinemann: 1926), v.

88. *New Health* (May 1927): 14.

89. Illustration in *New Health* (April 1927): 10.

90. Deborah S. Ryan, "'All the World and Her Husband': The *Daily Mail* Ideal Home Exhibition, 1908–39," in *All the World and Her Husband: Women in*

Twentieth-Century Consumer Culture, ed. Maggie Andrews and Mary M. Talbot (London: Cassell, 2000), 11; Bingham, *Gender, Modernity, and the Popular Press*, 97–100.

91. *New Health* (April 1927): 28.

92. *New Health* (April 1929): 70.

93. *Daily Mail*, November 10, 1928, 16.

94. *New Health* (October 1928): 47–48; *New Health* (November 1928): 63–64; *New Health* (January 1929): 35–40.

95. *New Health* (October 1929): 57–58; *New Health* (November 1929): 57–58; *New Health* (December 1929): 37–41; *New Health* (March 1930): 74; *New Health* (May 1930): 52.

96. *New Health* (January 1929): 37–40; *New Health* (December 1929): 38–41.

97. *New Health* (January 1929): 35; *New Health* (May 1929): 48.

98. *New Health* (January 1929): 37.

99. *New Health* (July 1928): 55; *New Health* (October 1928): 57; *New Health* (July 1930): 51.

100. *New Health* (November 1927): 76, *New Health* (January 1928): 60; *New Health* (August 1929): 58 (emphasis in original).

101. Collins, "Consumer Revolution," 33–38.

102. *New Health* (January 1928): 1–2; *New Health* (November 1928): 9; *New Health* (July 1930): 2.

103. *New Health* (October 1929): 38. According to my research, no copy of *Health Is Wealth* survives.

104. *New Health* (October 1929): 65–66; *New Health* (November 1929): 58; *New Health* (March 1930): 74; *New Health* (December 1930): 48; *New Health* (March 1931): 46.

105. R. A. McCance and R. D. Lawrence, *The Carbohydrate Content of Foods*, Medical Research Council Special Reports 135 (London: HMSO, 1929), 53–58.

106. Ibid., 3–4.

107. Ibid., 24–25, 35.

108. Ibid., 53–54.

109. Ibid., 54–55.

110. Ibid., 56–57.

111. Ibid., 58.

112. *Better Health*, August 1929, 214–15 (emphasis in original). On the Central Council for Health Education, a coordinating body founded in 1927 that brought together public health professionals, representatives of local authorities, and voluntary organizations, see Zweiniger-Bargielowska, *Managing the Body*, 185–87.

113. *Lancet* 2 (1929): 892–94.

114. Ibid., 1063.

115. Lane, *Blazing the Health Trail*, 19–24.

116. McCarrison, *Nutrition and Health*, 60, 72, 78.

117. Sir William Crawford and H. Broadley, *The People's Food* (London: Heinemann, 1938), 168–69.

118. Oddy, *From Plain Fare*, 138–40.

119. Richard Farmer, *The Food Companions: Cinema and Consumption in Wartime Britain, 1939–45* (Manchester: Manchester University Press, 2011), 37–38.

120. Ina Zweiniger-Bargielowska, *Austerity in Britain: Rationing, Controls, and Consumption, 1939–1955* (Oxford: Oxford University Press, 2000), 74.

121. Ibid., 83–84, 215–16. For a full discussion, see Ina Zweiniger-Bargielowska, "Bread Rationing in Britain, July 1946–July 1948," *Twentieth Century British History* 4 (1993): 57–85.

122. Farmer, *Food Companions,* 90–91.

123. Aaron Bobrow-Strain, "Making White Bread by the Bomb's Early Light: Anxiety, Abundance, and Industrial Food Power in the Early Cold War," *Food and Foodways* 19 (2011): 75, 86.

124. D. H. Buss, "The British Diet since the End of Food Rationing," in *Food, Diet and Economic Change Past and Present,* ed. Catherine Geissler and Derek J. Oddy (Leicester: Leicester University Press, 1993), 124–25. On new scientific research and increased enthusiasm for dietary fiber from the 1970s onward, see Whorton, *Inner Hygiene,* 228–37, 250–51.

125. Spiekermann, "Brown Bread for Victory," 149.

Chapter Seven

"Proscribing Deception"

The Gould Net Weight Amendment and the Origins of Mandatory Nutrition Labeling

Suzanne Junod

As a vehicle for conveying nutritional information to the individual consumer, the modern US food-package label has evolved steadily throughout the twentieth century, and its content and format are regularly revised to reflect and apply new knowledge in the fields of medical, nutritional, and regulatory science. Today, the most prominent feature of that label is the Nutrition Facts panel, which has, since it first appeared in 1994, become the most widely recognized graphic in the world.[1] Although the current food label focuses on nutrition and health, the roots of mandatory food labeling lay in the commercial landscape of the Progressive Era in American history.

In 1913 the first mandatory food labeling law was enacted—the Gould Net Weight Amendment to the 1906 Pure Food and Drugs Act—which required that all packaged foods have the "quantity of their contents plainly and conspicuously marked on the outside of the package in terms of weight, measure, or numerical count." The United States thereby became the first country in the modern world to enact mandatory food labeling in lieu of voluntary compliance with published standards, and paved the way for the twentieth-century adoption of mandatory nutrition labeling.[2]

In addition to its groundbreaking legal significance, the obscure Gould law is also historically important as a small yet compelling example of the critical role that standardization in many fields played in changing the commercial, social, and economic landscape of America during the Progressive Era (ca. 1890–1920).

In an era challenged by immigration, industrialization, and urbanization, the scope and scale of such change was unprecedented. Reforming activists drew support from a growing middle class, professionals began to transform many fields of endeavor, and in science and engineering, in particular, greater efficiency served as both goal and symbol of the Progressives' commitment to the nation's overall advancement.

Over time, the Progressives profoundly influenced local, state, and federal government agencies, originally in an effort to curb political corruption, but increasingly as a means of promoting order and efficiency. One key to their success was their reliance on new scientific knowledge, methodology, and tools. The Gould saga crosses paths with two important federal agencies undergoing significant change during the Progressive Era. The Bureau of Chemistry in the Department of Agriculture began as a federal scientific laboratory after the Civil War, but was given regulatory responsibilities with the passage of a federal food and drugs statute. The Bureau of Standards was a new Progressive-era agency created within the Department of Commerce and Labor in 1901 to work with the states "in securing uniformity in weights and measures law and methods of inspection."[3] Although officials in the Bureau of Standards coveted a federal statute, one was never enacted. Rather, national uniformity came only after a lengthy process of developing written specifications and tolerances adapted by all states.

Despite the fact that the Gould law mandates package labels with accurate weights, measures, and numerical counts, it was enacted to solve a pure food problem: short-weight packages. The short-weight problem was actually a key piece of unfinished business carried over from the fight for the first federal law governing foods and drugs moving in interstate commerce: the 1906 Pure Food and Drugs Act. This law bore the imprimatur of Dr. Harvey Wiley, chief of the Bureau of Chemistry in the Department of Agriculture, referred to as its "crusading chemist" and "father of the Pure Foods Act" for his efforts to secure the 1906 statute. Less than a decade later, as short-weight problems expanded, new legislation was proposed to amend the "Wiley Act." The Gould amendment drew less on the more celebrated health protection provisions of the 1906 statute and more on provisions intended to root out fraud. Ultimately, however, it rounded the circle of economic protection for consumers, securing for them the full benefits of the 1906 Act, while protecting producers from unfair and deceptive trade practices.

Omission of Net Weight Labeling Requirements from the 1906 Act

Testifying before the House Committee on Interstate and Foreign Commerce in 1911, a representative of the International Stewards' Association explained the origins of short-weighted food package problems:

> Packaged food products were a rather recent innovation in the early years of the 20th century. Previously, only choice or select goods had been packaged, with most food being sold in bulk. Select goods cost more, and the market for them was confined to those willing to pay a higher price for convenience and ease of handling. Would-be competitors could only place their goods on the market by underselling since the originators put up in an attractive package the finest goods that could be produced. A solution to this problem of market entry was the short weight package, which appeared to contain as much as the original high-quality package but which sold at a lower price.[4]

In 1906, however, such commercial perspective was lacking. When President Theodore Roosevelt signed the Pure Food and Drugs Act into law, it contained only a "paper tiger" provision addressing net weight labeling. Packaged foods were just beginning to compete with bulk goods in the marketplace, and most people still purchased such staples as vinegar and sugar from vats and barrels in dry-goods stores or ordered them from mail-order catalogues.[5] Concerns about short weight were focused on the accuracy of bulk and retail scales rather than packaged goods.

James R. Mann, the indefatigable House Republican Minority leader who championed the food and drug legislation, was the first to draw attention to the short-weight problem in Congress shortly before the 1906 law was passed. One of the most influential legislators from his election in 1897 until his death in 1922, Mann claimed to have "drafted more amendments to bills, which were adopted, than any other member of the House," and no one contradicted him. His colleagues accused Mann of possessing an "excess of knowledge"; he reportedly studied every significant bill and committee report, and participated in virtually all floor debates.[6] Although his influence was felt on almost every piece of legislation examined by the House Interstate and Commerce Committee, his name was attached to only two laws.[7] Nonetheless, his support was pivotal in securing passage of the 1906 Pure Food and Drugs Act. Speaker Joseph Cannon cited Mann's work on the 1906 statute as "one of the greatest triumphs of individual judgment, based on careful investigation, I have ever seen."[8]

Mann first attempted to engage Harvey Wiley on the subject of short-weight packages when Wiley testified at hearings in front of the Interstate Commerce Committee in February 1906. Mann remarked, "I understand it to be the fact that in the case of nearly all goods that are now put up in packages the manufacturers have quit putting on the amount of the article contained because they are reducing the amount and whereas they purport to sell a 2 pound or a 1 pound package they put in 30 ounces or 14 ounces or something like that." Wiley's response acknowledged that the existing law did not cover "false weights and measures," but he made it clear he was more interested in mandating ingredient statements on the packages of compounded articles. Mann tried again: "Should he not also put upon his package how much there is in it?" "Yes," Wiley agreed, "and what it is so that the consumer will know."[9]

The Senate pure food bill then under discussion, S88, was silent on the issue of net weight labeling.[10] After the House Commerce Committee hearings in February 1906, Wiley met with Mann, who included a mandated net weight statement on packaged product labels in his revised food and drug bill.[11] The first to protest Mann's net weight provision was Democratic Senator Charles L. Bartlett, whose minority report was submitted on March 14, 1906. He opposed not only mandatory net weight statements, however, but also the entire concept of federal food and drug regulation.[12] With momentum already building toward passage of a federal law, such obvious obstructionism was quickly swept away. Many businessmen had, over time, come to support a federal law, if for no other reason than conforming to the increasing number of state laws had become expensive. As one witness at the House hearings put it, "we want it [the federal law] so we can comply with it."[13] Canners, however, although they had supported the Wiley Act up to that point, considered its newly amended net weight provision carefully and quickly declared that they could not comply with such a "revolutionary" requirement.

Important support for Mann's net weight provision came from the Bureau of Standards, established in 1901 within the Department of Commerce and Labor. Louis A. Fischer, the Bureau's Chief of Weights and Measures, became the first federal official to advocate national weights and measures supervision in much the same way that Wiley had earlier advocated for a national pure food and drug law. In 1902, after directing scattered inspections of weighing and measuring devices and transactions in several larger cities in New York State, he concluded that the public was receiving little protection against short weight and short measure and that it was costing them over ten million dollars a year.[14] Fischer's investigations, bolstered by an increasing number of complaints to Washington, led the Bureau staff to convene a meeting of officials to discuss the supervision of weights and measures in "everyday" transactions in 1905. They recognized and supported Mann's efforts with regard to packaging provisions in the Pure Food and Drugs Act draft.[15]

In May 1906, Mann finally won over the reluctant Wiley to his cause. Wiley initially dismissed the net weight issue in a letter to Mann as "not a chemical question at all."[16] Mann responded by requesting that Wiley procure and test sample goods directly from the marketplace. On May 6, 1906, Wiley reported to Mann that he had tested a large number of samples of goods sold as "guaranteed as so much by weight or measure."[17] "In no instance," wrote Wiley, "have we found the guaranty correct." Wiley suggested that they talk about some of the more "flagrant misrepresentations" he had uncovered, concluding: "The more I look into it, the more I feel that your amendment is not only demanded for public protection, but is justified in every respect by reason and the practices of the trade."[18]

At the June hearings before the House Commerce Committee, Mann demonstrated, much to the delight of his colleagues, many of the "frauds and artifices practiced in the use of deleterious and unhealthful food adulterants." Included were manufactured glucose, masquerading as honey, "with an occasional dead bee to give verisimilitude"; pepper corns constructed from tapioca dyed with lampblack and sold for use as the "finest pepper"; and an extensive collection of artificial alcohols. Praised as a "splendid" demonstration of the need for action, Mann's presentation also employed Wiley's net weight samples and "ably demonstrated how the public are deceived by the use of short-weight and measures."[19]

Even with the support of Wiley and a few others, it was too late to engage many of the law's principal supporters, those who had exercised the most influence over key provisions of the emerging law. Women's groups, for example, were generally unaware that short-weight packaging was a problem, because packaged foods were relatively new. Most states had neither studied nor taken action on the problem, and there were no muckraking journalists bringing public attention to the issue. All that was required to defeat Mann's amendment was strong opposition from the canning industry.

Congressman James S. Sherman (R-NY), future vice president of the United States, and then president of a canning company, spoke on behalf of the canners. The short-weight provision, he said, was "unrelated" to the "health issue," the focus of the pending food and drug legislation, which most canners already supported. It was rather an economic issue affecting trade. He criticized the "vague" definition of a "package." Thousands of containers would be subject to regulation and the job would be overwhelming. Cans and bottles, moreover, were made according to standard sizes rather than weight capacity. Weighing each filled container would create difficulties for manufacturers and would "revolutionize" current trade practices. He recognized that there was an unavoidable loss of weight during canning, but overfilling to compensate would not benefit consumers and would harm the industry. "Besides," he quipped, "the housewife is not concerned with it [production losses]."[20] Sherman also denied there was demand for net weight branding, claiming that there were no widespread frauds.

Congressman Sherman's statement contradicts some of the available evidence. Wiley's marketplace investigations had indicated otherwise. Sherman opined that products were as often above as below weight, indicating that the real issue was imprecise manufacturing technology.[21] Wiley, however, identified no samples with larger than promised quantities. The state of Arizona, in fact, one of the few states with a short-weight regulation, had already ruled that variations would be considered unavoidable only if inspectors found there to be an equal number of packages overweight as underweight.[22] Sherman's amendment countered with a provision that eliminated the mandatory requirement for a net weight declaration on packages, proposing only that *if* a product was labeled with weight and measurements, the label had to be accurate. This was consistent with the other labeling provisions of the 1906 Act, which, except in the case of some dangerous drugs, gave producers two options: tell the truth or remain silent.[23] Some support for Sherman's amendment came from congressmen who objected to Mann singling out packaged goods. Both bulk products and packaged food, they noted, presented equal opportunities for fraud whether it be short weights in packaged goods or fingers on a scale

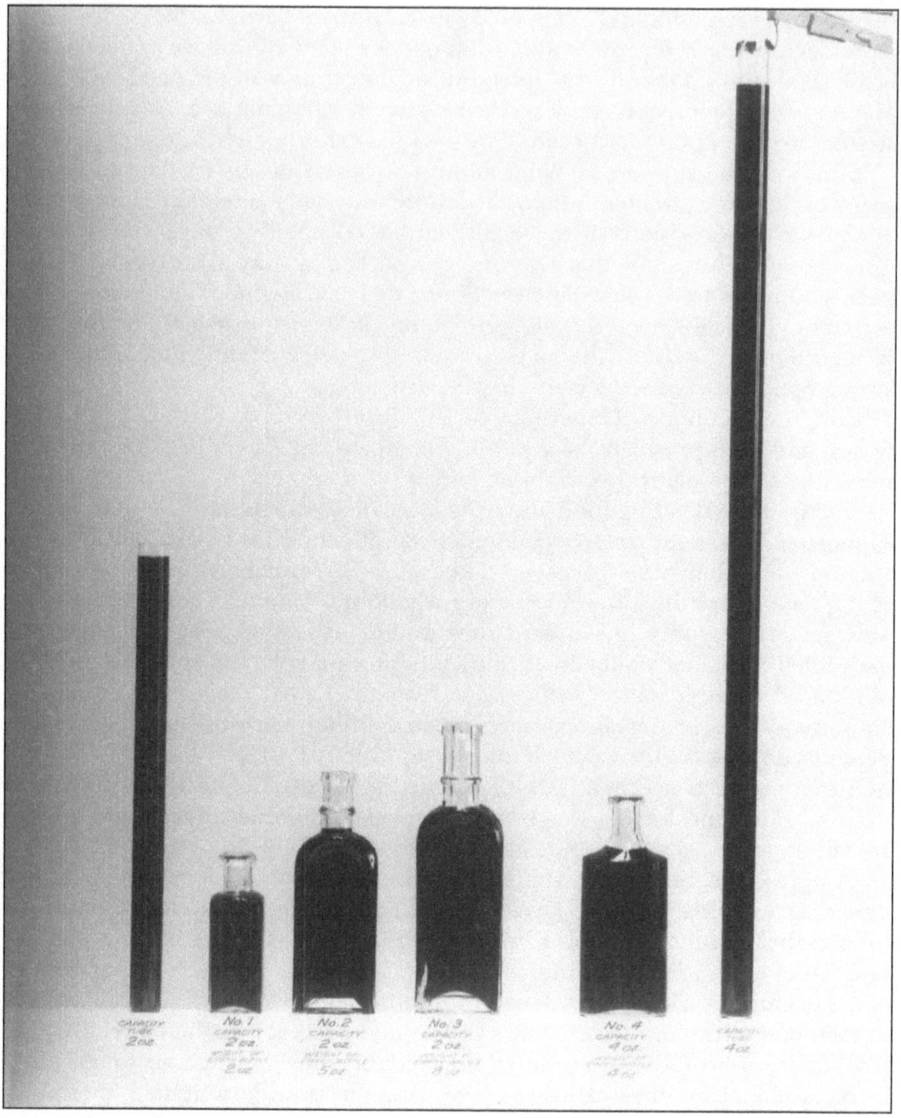

Figure 7.1. Bottles showing variations. One of several photos from an exhibit staged by the Bureau of Chemistry to explain the problems with commercial bottles. Capacity tubes on each side demonstrate how difficult it was for consumers to distinguish between two-ounce and four-ounce bottles without a net weight statement. The outside of the bottles bear little resemblance to the bottles' actual contents. National Archives and Records Center, RG 88, Prints and Photographs, and FDA History Office.

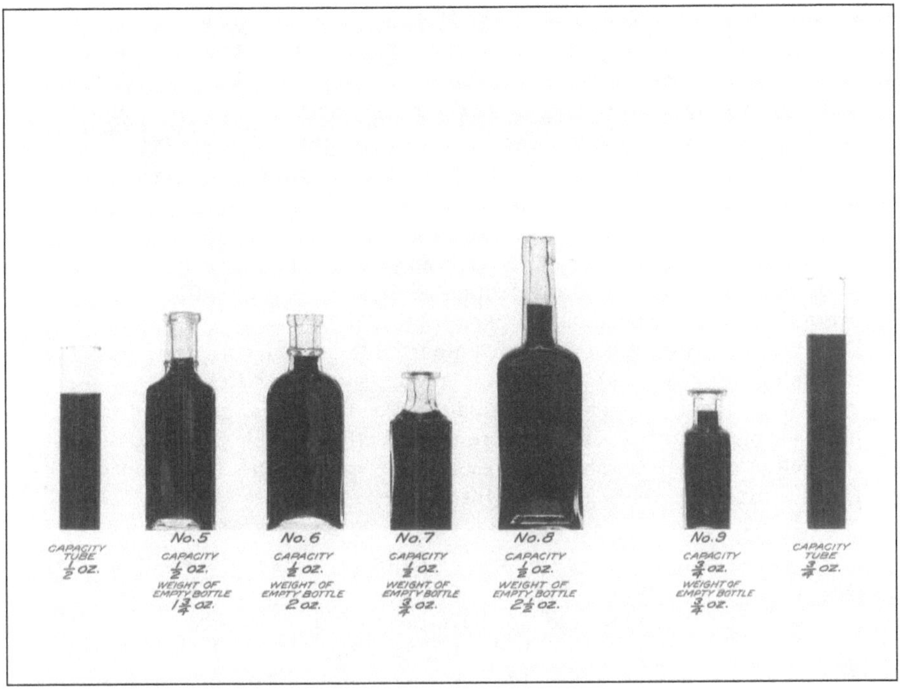

Figure 7.2. Bottles showing capacities. Bottles not only had different capacities, but their empty weight also varied greatly. Bottles 5–8 all had a capacity of half an ounce, but their empty weights were wide ranging. The smallest bottle (9) not only sported a greater capacity than all of the other bottles but its empty weight was also less. The consumer would have been deceived into thinking this to be the poorest value for the money, whereas it actually represented the best value. Net weight declarations, it was argued, would compensate for such inconsistent bottles. National Archives and Records Center, RG 88, Prints and Photographs and FDA History Office.

measuring bulk purchases. According to one weights and measures official, the most reprehensible short-weight issue was one he referred to as "selling by the "unknown," whether it be package, cup, pail, basket, jar, bottle, glass, tub, print, handful, or double handful.[24]

Joseph Howell (R-UT) felt that it was a "debatable question how far the Federal Government ought to enter upon this extensive and unlimited field where the end sought is purely a monetary one."[25] Sherman himself argued that Mann's provision would be unenforceable without uniform federal standards for weights and measure. This was a rather weak and somewhat disingenuous argument, however, since many states had already begun using standardized weights and measures in commercial transactions.

Some states had a stronger stake in the outcome of the debate than others. Impassioned testimony, for example, came from John Gill (D-MD). Maryland relied on canned seafood, which was notorious for both short-weighting and for "watering." Gill echoed Sherman's objections: that the issue was "totally irrelevant" to the pure food measure, which was "framed to protect men's stomachs . . . and their health and lives," that there had been no "public clamor," that the definition of "package" was vague, and the proposed law was unenforceable. With a rousing rhetorical flourish, he lamented the heavy burdens the provision would impose on the "agricultural and piscatorial classes."

> It requires them, directly and indirectly, to purchase labels, weights, and measures, and to employ additional labor. Are they not already sufficiently taxed? Is not their real and personal property subjected to State and county taxation? Does not Congress mullet ample tribute from them by levying tariff duties on their clothing, their food, and their implements? Does Congress not exact more from them through its internal-revenue tax on the grain and tobacco products of the land? Yet, insatiate, you seek further of their substance through this delusive weight and measure clause. Are you impelled by an uncontrollable desire to breed new trusts in this country?[26]

On June 23, 1906, Mann unsuccessfully sought to mollify critics with a new proposal that allowed labels to carry the "approximate" weight at the time the product was put up. Canners would not have been held responsible for weight loss due to shrinkage, evaporation, and other unavoidable production conditions. The proposed amendment would have permitted the use of customary-sized packages without a net weight label. Allowing cans to be marked as "standard size," Mann assured his colleagues, would protect honest canners from dishonest canners using slightly smaller containers.[27] Packages, under Mann's concept, could be branded with weight or measure, and stamped, recognizing them as the standard size they purported to be.[28]

In the end, the canner's campaign succeeded. Wiley had personally converted many of the canners to his side some years prior, but now, because of their objections to Mann's proviso, many threatened to withdraw support for the overall food and drugs law.[29] Mandatory package labeling was not included in the final bill, but the weak Sherman amendment passed 112 votes to 45 and was incorporated into the final 1906 statute.

Changes in the Commercial and Consumer Landscape

Implementing the expansive 1906 Pure Food and Drugs Act proved challenging. Wiley testified at the Mann hearings that there would be "relatively little additional expenses" involved in enforcing the new law. As soon as the food industry "understood and fully appreciated" the law, believed Wiley, "they will all conform to it."[30] But this proved not to be the case. The legal work proved far more prevalent, challenging, time-consuming, and transformative than Wiley ever anticipated. In spite of his assurances to Congress that enforcement could be carried out in collaboration with state food and drug officials, Congress required the creation of new federal inspectors to help implement the new law. Unfortunately, and perhaps by design, a federal inspector did not enjoy the police powers of his state counterpart, and had to rely, instead, "solely upon his own initiative" to obtain product samples and interstate shipping records.[31] When the initial group of federal food and drug inspectors reported for duty, Wiley told his assistant that he was "damned if he knew what to do with them" and envisioned them as mere "sample grabbers" securing problem products for the chemists.[32] A professional cadre of inspectors, however, soon proved indispensable. Interacting daily with food and drug purveyors, they were able to effect changes simply by their presence. Wiley had also been overly optimistic in thinking that Bureau chemists alone would be able to carry out the "real work" of enforcement by simply identifying violations. Especially in the early years, identifying problematic products in the laboratory often expanded an investigation—from one factory to one industry and from one product to a group of products. Empty imported cheese crates, for example, led investigators to examine American cheeses, which, they discovered, were being disguised as exotic imported cheeses. Upon closer examination, they also discovered substandard milk fat content and a shrinkage problem that led to short weights.[33]

From the outset, the Bureau's legal actions focused on industry-wide problems such as, for example, the poor sanitary practices that plagued the egg industry and the catsup business. By securing legal precedents against one company that could be used as a deterrent against others, the Bureau began to "clean up" the marketplace. Amidst a growing number of prosecutions for misrepresentations and false claims for foods and patent medicines, the Bureau of Chemistry discovered that short-weighted packaged foods were far more common than expected. Nearly one-third of all legal actions against misbranded food carried a secondary charge of short weight, despite the fact that weight statements were optional. Such violations proved most prevalent among canned goods, due largely to the extraordinary growth of the canning industry between 1900 and 1920. Productivity leapt as technology improved.[34] At the turn of the century, can makers could solder 1,500 cans a day. By 1910, assisted by new machines that could "peel, shell, clean, slice, chop and cook" foods, a single machine could turn out 35,000 cans a day. Processors employed more than sixty-eight thousand people and turned out over 3 billion cans of food yearly.[35]

Just prior to passage of the 1906 statute, the Second National Conference on Weights and Measures, held under the auspices of the Bureau of Standards, had endorsed Mann's proposal for national legislation requiring net weight statements on packaged goods.[36] Shortly thereafter, weights and measures officials reported new interest in short-weighted packages from retail grocers. At their third annual meeting in 1907, the deputy state sealer of weights and measures in Massachusetts, D. C. V. Palmer, reported making inroads with the Massachusetts Retail Grocers' Association after briefing them on the problem with short-weight lard and butter. Palmer thought that if the grocery trade had known more about the 1906 bill, the short-weight clause would have been retained: "The grocer sells the goods, exactly as he received them. He is the innocent party, therefore the grocers ought to support any movement which makes for honest weights and measures, and I know that in our State the grocers and merchants are awakening to the state of things."[37]

Conference participants nonetheless agreed that it was still difficult to educate the public about such fraud. Dr. Fritz Reichman, a New York weights and measures official, estimated that 99 percent of purchasers knew nothing of the issues. Stratton, director of the Bureau of Standards, also reported making "some headway" against the indifference of officials, but felt that many state and city officials were "not free from political influence," insisting that people would have to demand passage and enforcement of weights and measures laws and to insist that weights and measures officials be "scientific men." As to packaged products, opinions varied. An Iowa official felt that the desire for convenience overcame concerns about the weight of the contents, while a Rhode Island official disagreed, insisting that "people want full weight." A Bureau of Standards official pessimistically observed that the public "expects to be cheated" and "fears that if full weight is guaranteed, they will pay more."[38]

In the extensive historical literature centered on the 1906 Pure Food and Drugs Act and the founding of the US Food and Drug Administration, attention has focused on the more dramatic and compelling parts of the story. At the center is the imposing figure of Harvey Wiley, a populist hero and touchstone for personal and commercial honesty and integrity. His prejudices and predilections were well known and attracted tabloid-style attention beginning in 1902 with studies of food preservative safety on human subjects, dubbed the "poison squad" by the press. His face-to-face disagreement with President Roosevelt over the safety of saccharin was popularly portrayed as an affront to the chief chemist. His antipathy toward "cola" beverages culminated in his honeymoon spent at the government's trial against Coca-Cola.[39] The press had a field day covering the 1911 judicial matchup between Wiley, "the crusading chemist," against Asa Griggs Candler, the mogul of "medicated soft drinks." In terms of sheer entertainment value, it hardly mattered to the public that the jury was hung and failed to return a verdict.

Wiley has also been the subject of two biographies to date, with a third underway.[40] It is hard to overestimate Wiley's centrality in the pure food and drugs campaign narrative, but his imposing persona has made it difficult to shift the focus to more prosaic aspects of the revolutionary changes in food and drug production and distribution during his lifetime. After Wiley's departure from the Bureau in 1912, the historical narrative seems to wander as the work gets more scientific, the science gets more complex, legal challenges mount, and the early courtroom dramas fade into precedents for the legal casebooks.

Wiley, as noted, was far from prescient in anticipating the challenges of implementing the 1906 Pure Food and Drugs Act. Frequently missing from the narrative is a more detailed understanding of how early decisions on enforcement responsibilities, priorities, and regulatory roles were worked out within the Bureau of Chemistry and the impact of other influential individuals and

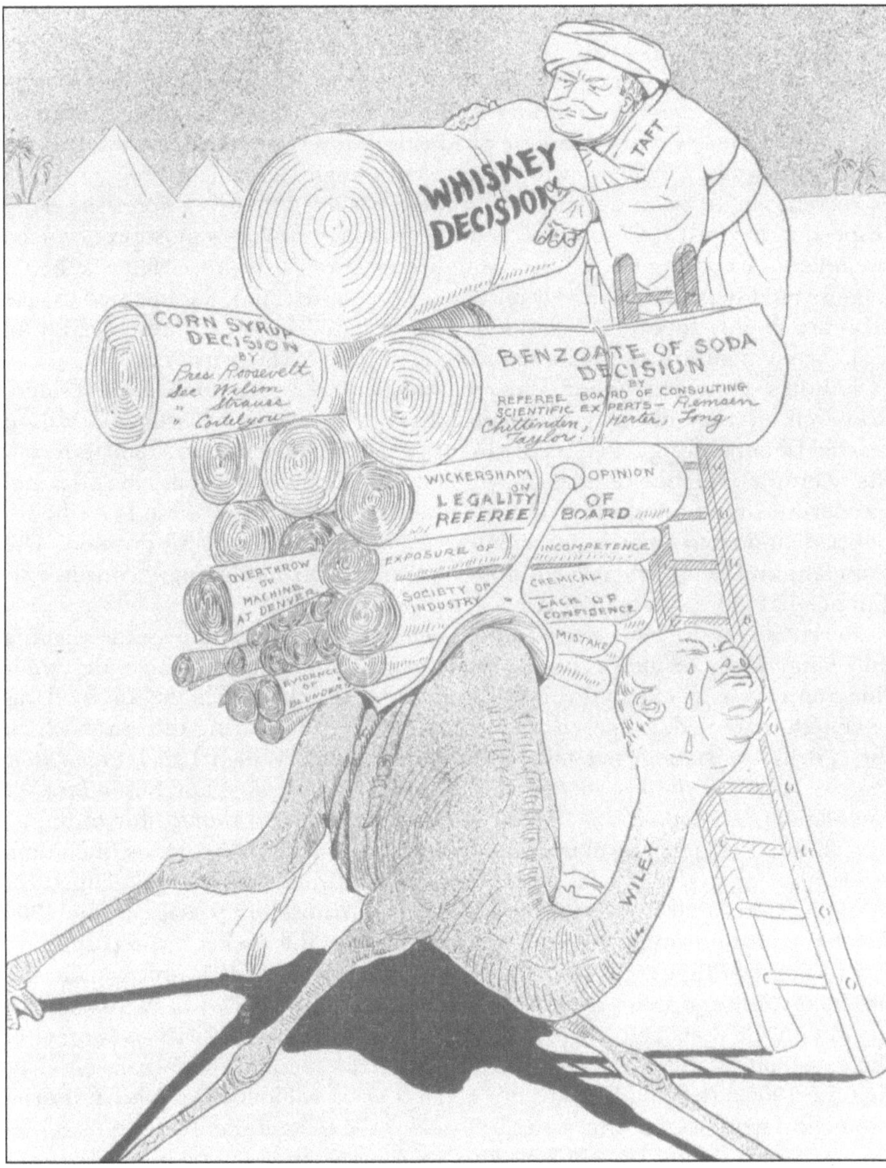

Figure 7.3. "The Last Straw that Broke the Camel's Back." Harvey Wiley, "father of the Pure Food and Drugs Act" and the Bureau of Chemistry's "crusading chemist," was no anonymous bureaucrat. To consumers, he was the very personification of the pure food movement, and he remained a populist hero to many until his death in 1930. Wiley is shown here, loaded down by dissenting decisions handed down by the Board of Food and Drug Inspectors and the Referee Board of Consulting Scientists. Both groups were appointed by the Secretary of Agriculture in an effort to curb what some interpreted to be Wiley's excessive zeal in enforcing the 1906 Pure Food and Drugs Act. *American Food Journal,* January 15, 1910, 15.

groups as an initial, workable regulatory system was established.[41] Net weight provisions, for example, according to the solicitors who were charged with its legal dissection, "presented unique problems in interpreting administrative laws and regulations."[42] Wiley's own influence was dually diluted in 1907 and 1908 as Secretary of Agriculture James Wilson established a Board of Food and Drug Inspection in April 1907 to act as a counterbalance to Wiley's most pronounced prejudices. According to Anderson, the Secretary of Agriculture "felt that he no longer could depend exclusively on Wiley, who, to his mind, was inclined to take arbitrary, highly theoretical positions that irritated business interests without making any significant contributions to the welfare of the consumer."[43]

Wilson's concerns about Wiley's objectivity were echoed by President Roosevelt after his disagreement with him over the safety of saccharin. Wilson reacted by appointing a Referee Board of Consulting Scientists in 1908 to review the scientific evidence on the safety of sulphur dioxide, benzoate of soda, and saccharin as food additives. Wiley opposed the use of all of these ingredients, but had submitted only vague scientific evidence to support his position. The president and Secretary Wilson, however, were confronting angry constituents and needed more surety than Wiley was providing.

Recent literature on early twentieth-century transformations, some relating only tangentially to the pure food movement, has begun to balance the Wiley "biography bias" by expanding understanding of the changes in the way food was obtained, marketed, prepared, and regulated (or not) during the era in which the "purity" movement was most influential. Pamela Walker Laird (*Advertising Progress: American Business and the Rise of Consumer Marketing*) and Susan Strasser (*Satisfaction Guaranteed: The Making of the American Mass Market*), for example, have studied changes in marketing and advertising of many goods, including foods, that altered the relationships between buyers and sellers.[44] Laird, for example, notes that it was during the period surrounding passage of the 1906 Act that goods previously marked with the name of the packer or preparer gave way to fictional figures such as the cheery Quaker Oats man, which made the producers ever more anonymous.[45] Mitchell Okun's *Fair Play in the Marketplace* focuses on the years before the federal pure food campaign.[46] His assessment of the early state statutes and the officials who implemented them makes it clear that the 1906 federal statute was not created *de novo*. Pioneering food and drug protection systems in several states influenced the federal statute more than previously known. James Harvey Young's *Pure Food: Securing the 1906 Pure Food and Drugs Act* characterizes the forces coming together to promote the federal law as "7Cs" (change, complexity, competition, crusading, coalescence, compromise, and catastrophe), of which Wiley constitutes only one—crusading chemist.[47] Another "C" was the coalition of pure food law supporters dominated by middle-class women's organizations.

Lorine Swainston Goodwin's *Pure Food, Drug, and Drink Crusaders, 1879–1914* examines the women organizing and working together at the state and local level to promote pure "food, drug, and drink," finding that they were a diverse group rather than exclusively middle-class clubwomen."[48] They had often already fought unpopular campaigns to force the cleanup their local environments, from swill stables and slaughterhouses to patent medicine sales fostering drug addiction and alcoholism. Goodwin's assessment of their motivation is important. She found no evidence that these women were involved out of any sense of "boredom," "feminist" concerns, or "status anxiety," as other scholars have speculated, claiming that they organized out of a sense of "necessity and responsibility."[49]

From this body of research it is clear that although scholars and observers (and Wiley himself) have correctly acknowledged the importance of women's activism in the passage of the 1906 Act, their view was not sufficiently inclusive. Wiley lectured in "top hat and tails" to middle-class clubwomen at their luncheons, and Alice Lakey personally supported him and instigated a letter-writing campaign to President Roosevelt, but they were not the only women to play significant roles.[50] Ordinary women, working in their own towns and communities, were also critical. Likewise, I would argue, so were all women who bought and served food in the midst of a commercial food revolution. Clubwomen and activists took a particular interest, but almost all women had an interest in the law and its success. It was essential to women, who were influenced profoundly by the changes in marketing and advertising. Effective shopping was a learned activity and the day-to-day decisions of women steered the early twentieth-century food industry—whether it was choosing convenience and the assurances that sanitary packaging provided, or choosing unpackaged goods that allowed the comparison of quality and price and careful budgeting. But shoppers could be easily confused as to the quality and quantity of foods they purchased by colorful labels and misleading claims (for example "benzoate free"). Organized women's groups, such as the Housewives' League, urged women to be their own (food and drug) inspectors.[51] It was unlikely, for example that the average consumer would notice when the traditional half-pound package of tea was reduced by an ounce or two—so long as the price remained constant. Likewise, comparing the value and quality of canned foods such as peas was problematic.[52]

One of the most insightful books on the changes in food procurement and consumption in the late nineteenth and early twentieth centuries is Harvey Levenstein's *Revolution at the Table*. Levenstein's compelling research on women and their response to what he describes as "the servant problem" makes it clearer why some middle-class women were more or less compelled to embrace, or at least accept, simpler recipes using prepackaged ingredients sold in smaller containers. The shortage of servants confronted middle-class women with the dilemma of how to feed their families and maintain their lifestyle, which included extensive entertaining. Experiments with "group cooking," in which middle-class women shared servants and ate in a common but separate house, were short-lived and largely unsuccessful. Most families preferred eating at home.[53] The problems were not just associated with cooking. These middle-class women spent much time planning menus and ordering supplies.[54] Those who abandoned or modified their lifestyle had to shop increasingly for themselves, making packaged goods even more attractive.

Levenstein's work and that of other recent scholars shifts the pure food narrative by documenting the myriad of ways in which a wider network of women took an active interest in pure food, starting locally but extending nationally. Women, whose self-identity was closely associated with their role as "guardians of the household," were motivated to seek changes in many arenas outside the home, including pure foods and drugs, and alcohol and drug abuse. For middle-class women, the club movement and servant shortages made them more aware of the conditions under which their food was purchased, packaged, and prepared.

A woman who had begun to rely on foods that had not been prepared in her presence was likely to insist, first and foremost, that the conditions under which her purchased food products were prepared mimicked as closely as possible the conditions in her own kitchen. Evidence abounds that much food in the early twentieth century was prepared, held, and sold under filthy conditions.[55] Some consumers worried about packaged goods simply because they could not see or smell them before purchasing.[56] At the height of the "purity movement," for example, many companies reassured customers by conducting tours of their facilities, displaying white-coated workers processing food in a spotless assembly line. There was also widespread support for "constituent labeling" to identify the major ingredients in a compound food (for example, crackers as opposed to flour). Although Wiley and many other pure food activists supported such mandatory labeling, they did not get it in 1906. The Bureau of Chemistry could cajole, but it could not compel ingredient labeling under the Pure Food and Drugs Act.[57] Home economists began to play an important role in helping women navigate the new commercial landscape as well as government and social organizations involved with consumer issues and concerns.[58]

Whether women purchased packaged foods because they were more sanitary, more portable, of higher quality, kept better, tasted better, or were marketed and labeled more enticingly, they did increasingly buy packaged goods.[59] Some of the earliest successes were condiments: relishes, jams, and jellies that enlivened the monotony of many family diets but were time consuming to prepare at home. Packaged cereals revolutionized the breakfast meal, making it lighter, simpler, and often healthier. Canned and bottled products became more affordable. The original bottled catsups, for example, often fermented and exploded, so producers resorted to preservatives such as benzoate of soda to stabilize them. Henry Heinz set a new preservative-free standard by using ripe fruit, prepared and packaged aseptically. Pure-food savvy consumers increasingly came to consider preservatives as *prima fascia* evidence of insanitary production. Heinz catsup, in turn, was one of the first American food products to be successfully exported to foreign markets.

The Resurrected Campaign for Net Weight Food Labeling

It is in the resurrected campaign for a federally enforced net weight label requirement that we see how important the choices made by consumers were in affecting change. In 1913 a new set of hearings was convened by the Senate

Committee on Manufactures. It was apparent that much had changed in the food industry. Key trade groups testified in support of net weight labeling. The movement away from "jobbers" and middlemen in the bulk grocery trade is reflected in the makeup of those testifying. Grocers and other retailers such as hotels were strongly represented, as were container manufacturers and trade associations from the confection industry.[60]

The testimony of Dana T. Ackerly, counsel to what was arguably the most powerful food organization in the country, the National Wholesale Grocers' Association (NWGA), was critical in the subsequent enactment of the Gould amendment. Founded in 1906, the NWGA was formed to offer strong endorsement to the 1906 statute and assist with its implementation. Ackerly testified that during the past year and a half, two-thirds of manufacturers who had previously sold by gross weight were now selling by net weight. He freely admitted that his organization did not come "to pose as altruists," but had rather recognized the problems that would be created if states began to act independently, as was already happening. "We very frankly admit that we do not see the absolute necessity of such a measure on package goods," he testified, "but there can be no denial of the existing public demand for it."[61] Sherman's housewives, joined by other institutional groups, it seems, had woken up and found that they minded not getting full weight and filled containers. Manufacturers, in turn, did not want to have to conform to conflicting state laws.[62]

The NWGA was undoubtedly motivated by the challenges faced by grocers as the marketplace for foods changed. National brands, trademarked packages, and a decline in demand for bulk goods changed the traditional role of many grocers. As Strasser points out, consumers needed less of the traditional advice and expertise provided by grocers when they asked for branded packaged products by name.[63] Piggly Wiggly was the first grocery chain to create self-service stores in 1912.[64] The other trade associations represented at the hearings all agreed that the net weight requirement was just good business. A metric measurement mandate was shelved for later consideration, and there were concerns about the establishment of "reasonable variations" and "tolerances" and the meaning of "small packages," but there was sufficient general agreement after the hearings to allow the Gould amendment to be reported out of committee and swiftly enacted into law on March 31, 1913. The fact that the amendment carried the name of "Gould" rather than "Mann" seems to be due to Mann's career-long reticence to put his name on laws, even those that he himself had advocated. In this case, it seems to have been a parting gift to the Democratic Representative Samuel W. Gould, who had failed in his reelection bid. The Gould amendment was passed on the last day of his only term in office, a permanent tribute to his service.[65]

The Gould Net Weight Amendment: A Transformative Law

Just prior to passage of the Gould amendment, Harvey Wiley left government service amidst a chorus of well wishes and a profusion of flowery tributes, heartfelt thanks, and cartoon caricatures en masse. When he left office, he was convinced that the 1906 law had been perverted by inadequate and ineffective enforcement, a position from which he never wavered. Though many expected him to take on a lucrative commercial position to support his new family, he soon announced that he had chosen to continue his advocacy for the "principles of pure food, pure drugs, and public health."[66]

In 1912, *Good Housekeeping Magazine* announced that it was establishing a Bureau of Foods, Sanitation, and Health in Washington DC and that the renowned Doctor Wiley would be its director. The headline read: "He Says He Will Be a Watchdog for the Nation's Housekeepers."[67] In his first article, Wiley declared that it would not be the bureau's "sole purpose" to impart instruction and scientific knowledge, but "also to arouse in the housekeepers of the country a living interest in the problems which concern the common welfare of the country, especially as influenced by domestic life."[68] The consumer, Wiley proclaimed, was his sole focus. "What is best for him, what is best for his pocketbook, and for his labor, are to me the controlling factors in reaching conclusions." One of Wiley's first, and most lasting, accomplishments was his creation of the renowned *Good Housekeeping* "Seal of Approval" to recognize products that met his strict standards for purity and honest advertising. Wiley also declared his intent to keep housewives informed about pending consumer legislation. First on his list, he said, was "protecting the patrons of the magazine against false weights," which "have cost the consumers of this country vast sums."

Although Wiley's biographers to date have not given any consideration to Wiley's postgovernment career at *Good Housekeeping*, it is clear that, through the magazine, he became a trusted source of information and provided a critical link to help guide housewives to make informed choices in the marketplace. The magazine was certainly not above a little showmanship in promoting him as their "star" critic "performing an unparalleled service for the American people," and Wiley himself remained ever the crusader and never minced words, but his most hard-hitting articles were not mere editorials. They were both educational and informative, containing careful critiques about specific problems well-illustrated and well-documented.[69] An article published by the *Saturday Evening Post* on May 4, 1912, around the time of Wiley's departure, was one of the first to publicly criticize any aspect of the "Wiley" law and did so by citing the absence of net weight labeling as its "one important defect."[70] Both reflective and reminiscent of the battlefield rhetoric employed by the muckraking journalists of the early twentieth century, the writer accused food producers of "getting even with Wiley" by short-weighting, since they could no longer profit through frank adulteration. This was allowing "a handier profit than that derived from using benzoate of soda and adulterants," which had been Wiley's signature issues.[71] Wiley's pure-food fight had started out as a fight for the health of the nation, but was moving forward as a commercial issue in the form of a fight against short-weight packages.

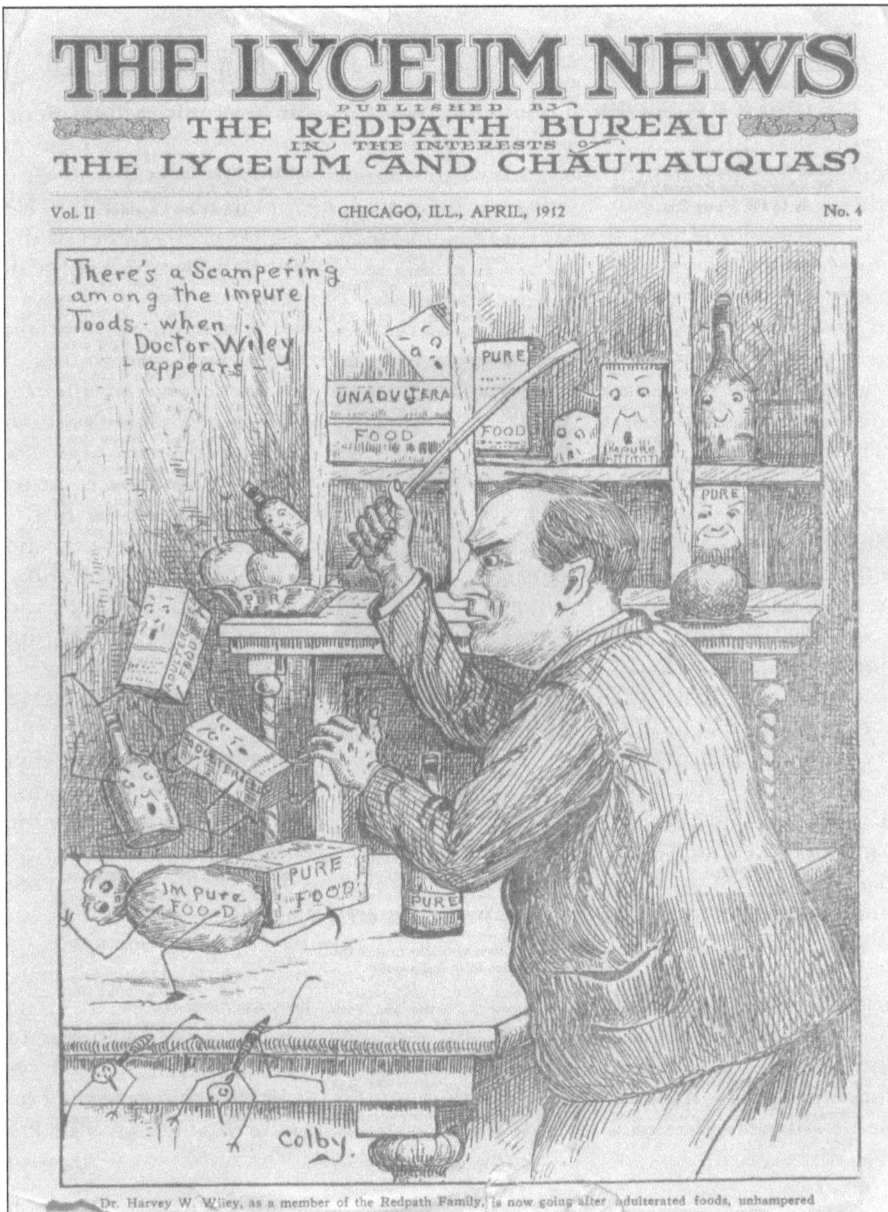
THE LYCEUM NEWS
PUBLISHED BY
THE REDPATH BUREAU
IN THE INTERESTS OF
THE LYCEUM AND CHAUTAUQUAS
Vol. II
CHICAGO, ILL., APRIL, 1912
No. 4
There's a Scampering among the impure Foods when Doctor Wiley appears
UNADULTERA
FOOD
PURE
FOOD
IMPURE
PURE
ADULTERATED FOOD
IMPURE FOOD
PURE FOOD
PURE
Colby.
Dr. Harvey W. Wiley, as a member of the Redpath Family, is now going after adulterated foods, unhampered

Figure 7.4. Harvey Wiley caricature. Wiley's departure to *Good Housekeeping Magazine* in 1912 inspired a host of responses, including this one depicting Wiley as the principled enforcer protecting the public from adulterated and misbranded foods and drugs. At *Good Housekeeping,* he refined and extended the use of the *Good Housekeeping* "Seal of Approval" to recognize products that met his strict standards for purity and honest advertising, transforming the seal itself into a recognized "brand" for the magazine. Colby, front cover illustration, *Lyceum News* 2, no. 4 (April 1912).

It fell to Wiley's successor, Dr. Carl Alsberg, then thirty-six years old, to implement the net weight amendment. Wiley had opposed his appointment, saying that the position should have been given to someone experienced in food-law enforcement.[72] Elements of the public were eager to see him seize the crusader's torch, but Alsberg was no crusader by nature or conviction. He was, first and foremost, a scientist who had served earlier in his career as the chief chemist for New York City's first Board of Health.[73] The contrast with his predecessor was obvious to everyone observing the transition of power in the Bureau of Chemistry. A colleague recalled that Alberg "never thought he was a crusading kind of administrator. He impressed you as someone who was very deliberate in arriving at his conclusions, but very strong in supporting those conclusions after they had been arrived at and he demanded first-class evidence."[74]

Alsberg's practical approach to the 1906 law was well received, partly because many of the original food-related issues of fraud embodied in the 1906 statute had already been addressed with regulation, inspection, and enforcement. While he made drug work a priority during his administration, he also paid attention to the emerging issues relating to consumer fraud and economic deception. Alsberg recognized the need for closer relationships both with industry and with state food and drug officials and tried to steer a much more centrist course than his predecessor. Yet he too was dedicated to seeing the law's ambitious reforms brought to fruition. Working with industry and acknowledging their challenges was a means toward this end, but it did not preclude effective enforcement actions. His clerk recalled that Alsberg "did not hesitate to enforce the law where it was warranted, being eager to catch and to have the courts penalize any food concern perpetrating fraud. If a supposedly reputable concern cheated, it was his delight to see them convicted on evidence dug up by his staff."[75]

In an article on Alsberg published in 1913, just after he took office, a reporter summarized a meeting between Alsberg and flavoring extract manufacturers over compliance with the Gould Net Weight Amendment.[76] The Bottle Manufacturers' Association had already acknowledged that prior to the 1906 Act, some companies had ordered short-weight bottles, but reassured Congress that since that time demand had been for full-measure bottles.[77] No such admission came from the extractors, and the audited meeting was Alsberg's opportunity to demonstrate his determination to work with industry.

Willsie, the reporter who witnessed the meeting, reported that a group of eight to ten extract manufacturers came "with a grip full of empty bottles, familiar to every housewife as the ten cent size, with some of the larger variety." They wanted to know "what leeway" the Bureau of Chemistry was going to allow them in labeling the amount of extract in their bottles, with each reporting "great difficulty" in procuring a uniform bottle: "We order the eight dram size. We get anything from 4.5 to 8, all looking exactly alike. We can't measure each bottle."[78]

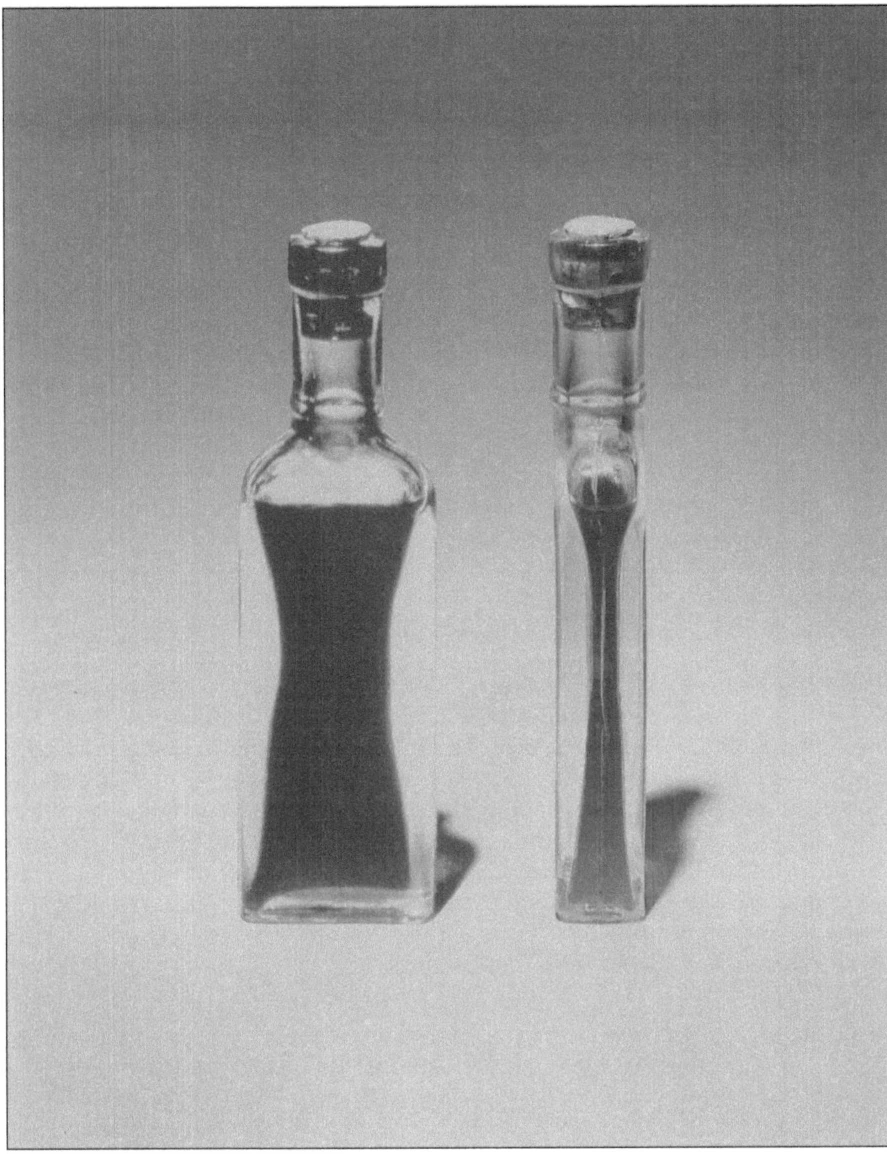

Figure 7.5. Extract bottles. Most women would have recognized this bottle by sight as a two-ounce bottle of flavoring extract. The thickened glass sides, however, reduced the capacity of the bottle to a single ounce, something that would have been obscured once the label was affixed. National Archives and Records Center, RG 88, Prints and Photographs.

Dr. Alsberg examined one of the small bottles. "'Of course, these panel bottles are made to deceive the public aren't they?' . . . The man hesitated and then smiled sheepishly. 'Yes, but the women insist on that size and shape, and on the fancy carton, and you insist on pure flavoring extracts until there is really no profit at all in the small size at ten cents. And now, if we are to be in trouble as to size and content . . .'" In response to Alsberg's suggestion that they talk to their glass manufacturer, Willsie reported that the man threw up his hands: "Glass factories and force! Why, doctor, the glass-blower's union is one of the strongest in the country. They turn out exactly the kind of bottles they want to. We complain to the factory owner and the factory owner goes to his blowers and they tell him to go to thunder."

Ending on a dramatic note, Willsie reports that Alsberg assured those present that "they would be dealt with fairly" and that the Bureau itself would look into bottle manufacturing, but in the end, they would have to comply with the law. "Contritely and "soberly," one of the men summed up their dilemma:

> I guess all of us here have been in business long enough to realize that the best good to the consumer ultimately works to the best good of the manufacturer. We've had to realize it, particularly of late! He looked meaningfully at Dr. Alsberg and his associates nodded. "We have to make good extract. We have to put it in honest containers. Now we have come to you to help us make it pay![79]

Bottle extract manufacturers, however, were not the only group under scrutiny as the Bureau began to consider how to enforce the amendment. Water, the weightiest adulterant, presented a constant short-weight challenge in fruit juices, canned vegetables, flour, vinegar, dried fruits, canned oysters, and milk. Many manufacturers had stopped marking packages and labels after 1906, since they were not required to do so, and the new mandatory markings greatly increased the need for net weight sampling.[80] Crackers, oats, and tea, for example, all stood accused of deceptive packaging practices, whether for selling five- and ten-cent sizes and then reducing their contents, short-filling containers, or making small reductions in standard-sized packages.[81]

Technical Studies and Commercial Ramifications

The key provision distinguishing the Gould amendment from its predecessors was a technical one: it allowed variations and tolerances as well as exemptions for small packages. Small packages were nearly exempted altogether owing to pressure from candy manufacturers, who argued it was too onerous a requirement to implement for packages selling for six cents or less.[82] Wiley had opposed any such allowance before he left office, offering his own variation proviso in 1912, and he railed against variations again in 1913, claiming that the mentioned variations "had reference to nothing but the legalization of on-the-average underweight packages."[83] Industry was allowed eighteen months to comply with the new law. The Bureau noted at the time that implementation presented practical difficulties related to measuring shrinkage, container variations, and errors in weighing, measuring, and counting by hand or by machinery, which had to be studied for a "vast variety of products."[84] Creating legally justifiable variations required tedious field studies and measurements that led to partnership with the National Bureau of Standards.[85] In 1915, the Bureau of Chemistry noted that an "abnormally large" number of imported products had been detained with net weight violations during the first year, owing to better supervision of Pacific ports and "abnormal trade conditions," for example, the First World War.[86] In 1917, the Bureau of Chemistry began educational efforts related to enforcement and began studying the accuracy of automatic weighing machines. Packages of tea, coffee, cocoa, spices, and other "free flowing" goods were studied with an eye to setting tolerances for filling packages.[87]

The short-weight problem was becoming larger than anyone had foreseen at the time the Gould amendment was enacted. In summarizing the Gould amendment in his case-law book, Mastin White editorialized that "despite its brevity, the enforcement of the 'net weight' amendment severely taxed administrative ingenuity. The investigations which it thrust upon the Bureau of Chemistry took years for the accumulation of the necessary facts upon which to base a policy to guide prosecution."[88] With such widespread support for the law, it was difficult to understand how the violations had become so flagrant by 1920 when the Bureau of Chemistry published in its annual report, a tally of regulatory actions of the past five years:

> Of all notices of judgment published . . . 307 or 9.2 percent, contain reference to violations of the net-weight amendment. Of these, 307 cases, 19 percent contain no other charge than violation of the net-weight amendment. Sixty two percent contain a charge of shortage in weight or volume. The average shortage in those cases prosecuted for that reason solely was 10.8 per cent. 125 seizures in which net weight violations were involved were made. . . . The products against which most of these notices of judgment have been published are, in order: olive oil, cottonseed meal, mineral water, tomato pulp, and evaporated apples.[89]

Container problems remained a source of deception. Consumers could not determine prior to opening a can whether it was properly filled or whether its net weight was as a result of too much liquid filler rather than solid product. By the time that the law's full force went into effect in 1915, Bureau inspectors discovered that important changes had taken place in machinery that allowed more precise fills for cans and a few other containers. In 1920 the Bureau announced that after investigations into the commercial canning of some thirty varieties of frequently canned fruits and vegetables, they had determined "what is the greatest amount of solid material, exclusive of liquid, which can be packed in cans of various sizes without causing any impairment of quality."[90] The Bureau followed up with circular letters making commercial canners aware of their results and the proper solid-to-liquid ratio that should be maintained. Slack fill containers, they reported, had been "very largely discontinued" as a result.

In addition to canning studies, the Bureau conducted studies of packaged and bottled goods.[91] In 1920 a report summarized the variations in net weight among packaged granular, solid, free-flowing food products including spices, coffee, sugar, and rice. The results of all of the technical studies were similar. In spite of the "complex manipulations" required in the packing of such products, the Bureau found evidence of a commonality in certain "methods of manipulation" that resulted in "a fairly definite range of variation in weight." Hand versus machine weighing and differences in the arm balances and size of the packages were responsible for some of the variability, but there were clearly "tricks of the trade" that were also responsible for some of the discrepancies. Bottled goods presented more of a challenge, since the studies had to address unique conditions posed by hand-blown glass bottles as well as semiautomatic and fully automatic bottle-making operations. Variations, however, separate for each type of manufactured bottle, were deemed both possible and achievable.

There were remarkably few legal challenges to the net weight regulations at the federal level, indicating that the precision required to meet the law's requirement was achievable and that the proscribed allowances and tolerances were acceptable. Meatpackers tried to escape regulation by arguing that fresh meats (not prepared by smoking, cooking, or curing) were not manufactured products and thus exempt from the law. The Solicitor of the Department of Agriculture refuted this, noting that all meat had to be "prepared" in some fashion prior to marketing.[92] In 1920, the Kenyon Amendment, enacted as a Senate rider to the Department Appropriations bill for 1920, addressed construction of the phrase "in package form" in the Gould amendment. Meatpackers had argued that wrapped hams and bacon delivered to the consumer and charged for on the basis of gross weights, including the wrapping, should be excluded from the Gould strictures. Congress disagreed and extended the word "package" to include "wrapped meats inclosed [*sic*] in papers or other materials as prepared by the manufacturers thereof for sale."[93]

One court held the "shrinkage defense" null and void—the fact that hot syrup cooled into less syrup gave no defense to the product label. "If the sirup was short in weight when shipped, it was misbranded," wrote the judge. In another suit, the judge ruled that the statute could not be held unconstitutional for any "uncertainty in describing the offense."[94] In 1932 the Supreme Court reaffirmed the lower court's decision and denied that the law was an "unconstitutional delegation of legislative power." The court upheld the FDA's interpretation accepting that the law "describes the offense with reasonable certainty and [therefore] is not invalid."[95]

Once upheld, the net weight provisions worked out under the Gould amendment were incorporated into the law that ultimately replaced the 1906 Act: the 1938 Food, Drug, and Cosmetic Act. It was the need to establish tolerances under the Gould amendment that ushered the FDA into the factory itself to observe the methodology and overall operations in order to help determine

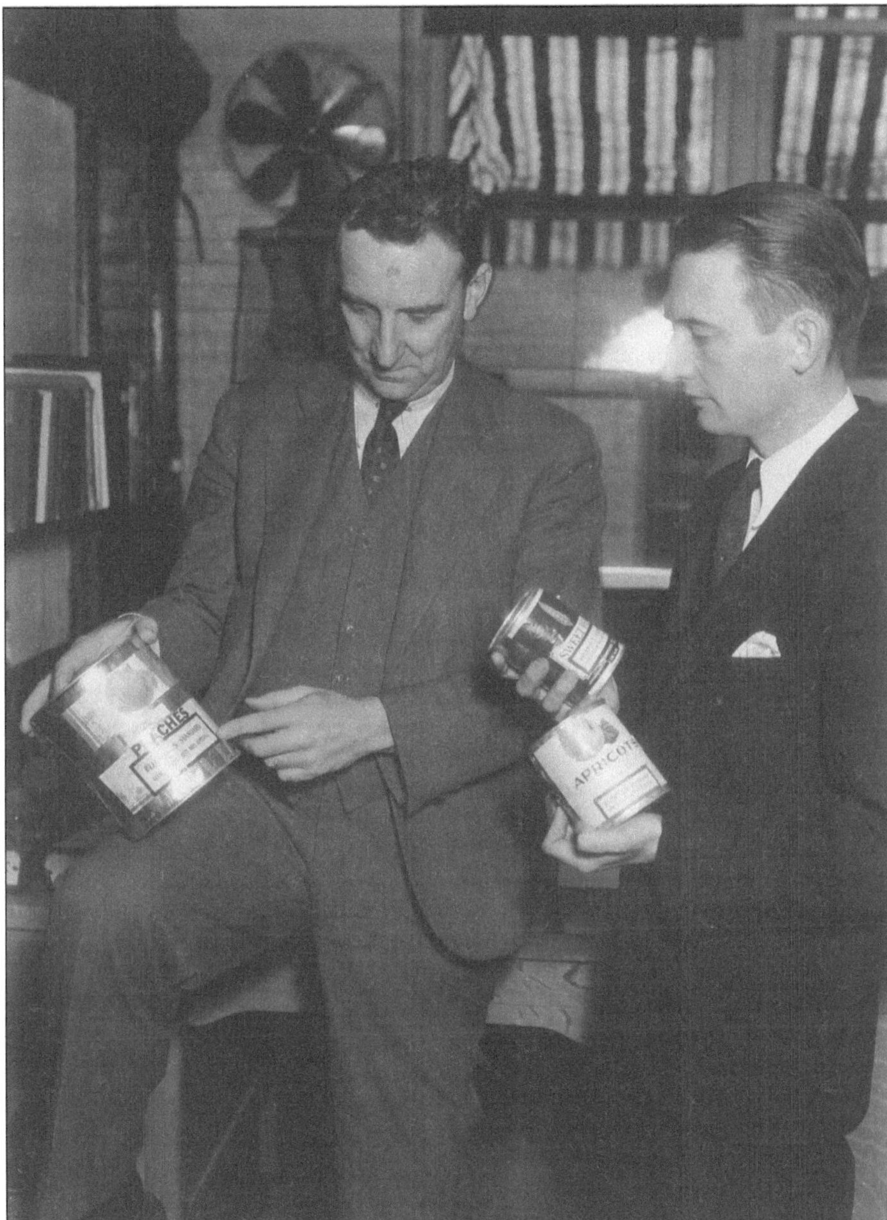

Figure 7.6. Federal food and drug inspector George Larrick (R) (later FDA Commissioner 1954–65) and another inspector (L) examining net weight statements on printed can labels to assure their compliance with the 1913 Gould Net Weight Amendment. National Archives and Records Center, RG 88, Prints and Photographs.

what was and was not possible in achieving uniform packaging for food products. Language in the 1938 law referring to "good manufacturing" and later "current good manufacturing" practices as well as tolerances for "unavoidable" problems all originated in or were related to research antecedent to implementing the Gould statute.

The net weight statement on packaged food products arguably encompasses requirements that comprise one of the most potent weapons in the consumer's arsenal against commercial fraud, and it served as an important first step in the transformation of the food label from solely a means of commercial identification and communication into a vehicle for the communication of more complex and increasingly personalized nutritional information. Changes in manufacturing processes, purchasing patterns, consumer demands, and retail structures were all important in making obvious the need to identify and curb patterns of container fraud, and in many ways the Gould Net Weight Amendment completed the circle of consumer protection initiated under the 1906 Pure Food and Drugs Act.

Conclusion

The 1906 Pure Food and Drugs Act, often referred to as the Wiley Act, was essentially a "truth in labeling" statute. What was stated on the label, whether it be the composition of a patent medicine or the net weight of a food product, had to be accurate and, in the words of the statute, could not be "false or misleading in any particular." The problem was that, with the lone exception of ten specified dangerous drug ingredients, nothing was positively required to be on the label to alert consumers to important facts about their increasingly packaged and processed foods. The 1913 Gould Net Weight Amendment provided that critical first step, a legal requirement that manufacturers reveal something specific about the content of their foods on the package label—the net weight.

In 1938, a replacement Food, Drug, and Cosmetic Act added the requirement that any artificial flavoring, coloring, or chemical preservative be listed on the product label. Until 1966, information on calories or sodium on a label marked a product "for special dietary uses." In 1973, however, new regulations allowed that nutrition information could be provided on the labels of all regulated foods so long as it included material facts both positive and negative: number of calories, grams of protein, carbohydrate, and fat, and the percent of US Recommended Dietary Allowance (RDA) for key nutrients. In 1992, the Nutrition Labeling and Education Act (NLEA) specified a specific format for nutrition labels—the now widely recognized Nutrition Facts graphic. Although the format is standardized, it was nonetheless expressly designed to allow consumers and regulators to adapt to the ever-changing landscape of nutritional knowledge.

Notes

Thank you for research assistance to Cindy Lachin in the FDA History Office, Terrence Gough, and to John Rees and Johnny Ho at the History of Medicine Division, National Library of Medicine. I am also grateful to Janet Golden, Peter Barton Hutt, Victoria Harden, David Smith, Dale Smith, and John Swann for their insightful comments.

1. 1990 Nutrition Labeling and Education Act, 104 STAT. 2353. The specific format for the Nutrition Facts label was issued in 1992 and the first such labels appeared in 1994.

2. Peter Barton Hutt, a legal history scholar and former FDA chief counsel cites the Gould amendment as one of his "top ten" turning points in food regulatory history. Peter B. Hutt, "Turning Points in FDA History," in *Perspectives on Risk and Regulation: The FDA at 100*, ed. Arthur Daemmrich and Joanna Radin (Philadelphia: Chemical Heritage Foundation, 2007), 17–18.

3. Louis A. Fischer, "Recent Developments in Weights and Measures in the U.S.," *Popular Science Monthly* 86 (April 1914): 24.

4. House of Representatives, Committee on Interstate and Foreign Commerce, *Net Weights and Contents of Packages*, 61st Congress, 3rd session, January 27, 1911, 4–5.

5. Richard O. Cummings, *The American and His Food* (Chicago: University of Chicago Press, 1940), 109–10.

6. L. Ethan Ellis, "James Robert Mann: Legislator Extraordinary," *Journal of the Illinois State Historical Society* 46, no. 1 (1952): 28–44, on 34. James Robert Mann, in *Dictionary of American Biographies*, ed. Dumas Malone (New York: Scribner and Son, 1933), 12: 244.

7. The Mann Act (1910) prohibited the transportation of women across state lines for immoral purposes, and the Mann-Elkins Act (1910) amended the Interstate Commerce clause of 1887.

8. Ellis, "James Robert Mann," 37.

9. House of Representatives, Hearings Before the Committee on Interstate and Foreign Commerce on the Pure Food Bills, 59th Congress, 1st session, February 26, 1906, 342–43.

10. Congressional Record, Senate, 59th Congress, 1st session, January 10, 1906, 897. It is worth noting that if HR6295 (January 1904 bill) had been enacted, providing that food would be adulterated "if it be labeled or branded so as to deceive the purchaser," the net weight issue could have been handled under this much more general provision. Cummings, *American and His Food*, 99.

11. House Committee on Interstate and Foreign Commerce, Report 2118 to Accompany S88 to the Committee of the Whole House, 59th Congress, 1st session, March 7, 1906, 3.

12. On March 14, 1906, Mr. Bartlett, from the CIFC submitted Rept. 2118, part 2, "Views of the Minority," to accompany S88.

13. Ibid., 3. House hearings, February 6, 1906, 15.

14. James P. Heaton, "Evading the Pure Food Law to 'Get Even with Wiley,'" *Saturday Evening Post*, May 4, 1912, 326. According to Heaton, "indifference disappeared" as a result of Fischer's investigation.

15. Lewis Judson, *Weights and Measures Standards of the United States: A Brief History* (Washington DC: US Dept. of Commerce, National Bureau of Standards, Special Publication 447, 1973 [updated 1976]), 20; Fischer, "Recent Developments in Weights and Measures," 24. In 1912 the only states with net weight provisions or statutes in place were Connecticut, Florida, New York City, North and South Dakota, Nebraska, Wyoming, and Nevada. Initiatives had been defeated in Massachusetts, Rhode Island, Vermont, New Jersey, Maryland, Virginia, South Carolina, Mississippi, Louisiana, Pennsylvania, Kentucky, and Illinois. Heaton, "Evading the Pure Food Law," 327; Department of Commerce and Labor, Bureau of Standards, *Second Annual Conference on the Weights and Measures of the US, Washington DC, April 12–13, 1906* (Washington, DC: GPO, 1906), 17. In subsequent meetings, they began drafting model state laws, but by 1914 most weights and measures activists had concluded that getting the various states to agree on uniform provisions was an "impossibility." They changed strategy, supporting instead a combination of state and local statutes and ordinances supplemented by federal laws governing interstate commerce.

16. Wiley to Mann, May 3, 1906, letters sent 1878–1907, vol. 184, 290–92, RG97, National Archives, Washington, DC.

17. Initially, the 1906 law allowed manufacturers to provide a "guaranty" stamped on goods shipped to retailers as a way of assuring them that their goods met the requirements of the Pure Food and Drugs Act. By 1913, however, the system was discontinued because, at least in part, consumers had come to view the guaranty as a guarantee of purity by the federal government itself.

18. Wiley to Mann, May 3, 1906, letters sent 1878–1907, vol. 184, 498.

19. House of Representatives, Committee on Interstate and Foreign Commerce, 9th Congress, 1st session, June 22, 1906, 8981, 8982.

20. Ibid., 9054, col 1.

21. Ibid.

22. Ibid., 9061. James D. Cox, Rio Grande Canning Co., NJ, to Honorable Benjamin F. Howell, April 2, 1906, File HR59A-H11.6, Committee on Interstate and Foreign Commerce, 59th Congress, Records of the US House of Representatives, RG233, National Archives. "Canned goods were originally put up in pint, quart, and gallon cans and were so called for years, but in some way they got to calling them no. 2., no. 3 and no 6. Next 2 lb, 3 lb, and 6 lb. The cans are still made the same in size and hold over one pint, quart, and gallon in liquid measure but do not weight 2 lbs., 3 lbs., and 6 lbs. though they are so called by the trade and they fill them as full as possible." As to fraud, Sherman simply assumed that containers themselves were beyond reproach. The Republican Senator Frederick C. Stevens opposed voluntary package net weight labeling for just this reason, arguing that it would not prohibit canners from short-filling standard-sized cans. In the end, he predicted, it would merely "offer a cover for swindling."

23. The lone exception is in the case of ten "dangerous" drug ingredients (including alcohol, cannabis, and opiates), which had to be labeled and labeled accurately under the 1906 statute.

24. Department of Commerce, Bureau of Standards, *Weights and Measures Fourth Annual Conference,* Washington, DC, December 17–18, 1908 (Washington, DC: GPO, 1914), 16.

25. House of Representatives, Committee on Interstate and Foreign Commerce, 59th Congress, 1st session, June 22, 1906, 9059.

26. Ibid., 8981–82.

27. Ibid., 9060–61.

28. Ibid., 9059, col 2.

29. Petitions, File HR 59A- H11.6, Committee on Interstate and Foreign Commerce, 59th Congress, Records of the US House of Representatives, RG 233, National Archives.

30. House of Representatives, Committee on Interstate and Foreign Commerce, 59th Congress, 1st session, February 26, 1906, Washington DC: GPO 1906, 97.

31. Fred B. Linton, "Federal Food and Drug Law Leaders," *Food, Drug, and Cosmetic Law Journal* 5, no. 2 (1950): 104–15. *Bureau of Chemistry Annual Report,* 1908 (Washington, DC: Government Printing Office, 1908), 47. T. F. Pappe, Chemist in Charge to Arthur W. MacMahon, Columbia University, January 7, 1921, 040.05, box 55, Records of the FDA, Federal Records Center, Suitland, MD.

32. James Harvey Young, "A Day in the Life of a Food and Drug Inspector," *Journal of the History of Medicine and Allied Sciences* 42 (1987): 30–53.

33. *FDA Annual Reports, 1909–1949* (Chicago: Commerce Clearing House, 1951), 170.

34. Honore Willsie, "Canning and the Cost of Living," *Harper's Weekly,* November 1, 1913, 8–9. Harvey Levenstein, *Revolution at the Table: The Transformation of the American Diet* (Oxford: Oxford University Press, 1987), 30, n 31.

35. Levenstein, *Revolution at the Table,* 37, n 19; Edward C. Hampe, Jr. and Merle Wittenberg, *The Lifeline of America* (New York: McGraw Hill, 1964), 119–23.

36. Department of Commerce and Labor, *Second Annual Conference of the Weight and Measures of the US,* 17.

37. Department of Commerce and Labor, Bureau of Standards, *Third Annual Conference on the Weight and Measures of the US,* May 16–17, 1907 (Washington DC: GPO, 1910), 13–14.

38. Ibid., 14, 21, 23, 24.

39. James Harvey Young, "Three Southern Food and Drug Cases," *Journal of Southern History* 49, no. 1 (1983): 3–19; Mark Pendergrast, *For God, Country, and Coca-Cola* (New York: MacMillan, 1993).

40. Oscar Anderson, *Health of a Nation* (Chicago: University of Chicago Press, 1958); Clayton Coppin and Jack High, *The Politics of Purity* (Ann Arbor: University of Michigan Press, 1999).

41. The statute left some room for disagreement over enforcement responsibilities. Anderson, *Health,* 199, 307, n 2.

42. *Administrative Procedure and Practice in the Department of Agriculture under the Federal Food, Drug, and Cosmetic Act of 1938,* ed. Mastin G. White, part 2, 125. Unpublished compilation dated 1940. FDA History Office, Silver Spring, MD.

43. Anderson, *Health of a Nation,* 204.

44. Pamela Walker Laird, *Advertising Progress: American Business and the Rise of Consumer Marketing* (Baltimore, MD: Johns Hopkins University Press, 1998); Susan Strasser, *Satisfaction Guaranteed: The Making of the American Mass Market* (New York: Pantheon Press, 1989).

45. Laird, *Advertising Progress,* 252.

46. Mitchell Okun, *Fair Play in the Marketplace* (DeKalb: Northern Illinois University Press, 1986).

47. James Harvey Young, *Pure Food* (Princeton, NJ: Princeton University Press, 1998), 4–6.

48. Lorine S. Goodwin, *Pure Food, Drug, and Drink Crusaders: 1879–1914* (Jefferson, NC: McFarland, 1999).

49. Goodwin, *Pure Food*, 37.

50. Mary I. Wood, *The History of the General Federation of Women's Clubs* (Norwood, MA: Norwood Press, 1912), 247, 59–60; Anderson, *Health of a Nation*, 169–70, 179.

51. Strasser, *Satisfaction Guaranteed*, 266.

52. US Department of Agriculture, Office of the Secretary, *Notice of Judgment, no. 542, Misbranding of Canned Tomatoes and Canned Corn*, vol. 3, September 6, 1910 (Silver Spring, MD: FDA History Office, 1910).

53. Levenstein, *Revolution at the Table*, 55.

54. Ibid., 62.

55. For example, see Andrew F. Smith, *Pure Ketchup: A History of America's National Condiment* (Columbia: University of South Carolina Press, 1996); Photo Series: "A Day in the Life of a Food and Drug Inspector" (Silver Spring, MD: FDA History Office, ca. 1912).

56. Strasser, *Satisfaction Guaranteed*, 35.

57. Levenstein notes that women's groups supported Wiley's efforts to regulate food additives and compel ingredient labeling (*Revolution at the Table*, 39), but fails to emphasize that Wiley was unsuccessful and neither he nor the women's groups became the subject of direct action in the 1906 statute.

58. Carolyn M. Goldstein, *Creating Consumers: Home Economists in Twentieth-Century America* (Chapel Hill: University of North Carolina Press, 2012).

59. As a rough indication of the growth in sales of packaged products, Strasser notes that between 1905 and 1906 alone, ten thousand new trademarks were registered as a means of protecting and asserting ownership of products, including food products. Strasser, *Satisfaction Guaranteed*, 45.

60. National Retail Grocers, National Wholesale Grocers Association, National Canner's Association, National Confectioner's Association, American Specialty Manufacturers' Association, Chocolate and Cocoa Manufacturer's Association, National Flavoring Extract Manufacturer's Association, Machine Bottle Manufacturer's Association, International Stewards' Association, Southern Hotel Men's Association, Georgia Hotel Men's Association, Atlanta Hotel Men's Association, Hotel Men's Association.

61. Senate Committee on Manufactures, *Amendment to Pure-Food Law*, Hearings on S.4727, 62nd Congress, 2nd session, 1913, 6–7.

62. Department of Commerce, Bureau of Standards, *Weights and Measures Eighth Annual Conference*, Washington, DC, May 14–17, 1913 (Washington DC: GPO, 1914), 16–17.

63. Strasser, *Satisfaction Guaranteed*, 30.

64. Ibid., 21.

65. "Gould, Samuel Wadsworth, (1852–1935)," *Biographical Directory of the United States Congress*, http://bioguide.congress.gov/scripts/biodisplay.pl?index=g000343 (accessed July 23, 2016).

66. Harvey Wiley, *The History of a Crime against the Food Law: The Amazing Story of the National Food and Drug Law Intended to Protect the Health of the People and Perverted to Protect Adulterators of Food and Drugs*, http://www.whale.to/a/wiley_b.html (accessed January 9, 2013).

67. "He Says He Will Be a Watchdog for the Nation's Housekeepers," *Good Housekeeping Magazine* 55 (1912): 252–53.

68. Ibid.

69. For example, see "False 'Ads' and Lying Labels," *Good Housekeeping* 57 (1913): 385–94.

70. Heaton, "Evading the Pure Food Law," 326.

71. Suzanne White, "Chemistry and Controversy: Regulating the Use of Chemicals in Foods, 1883–1959," unpublished diss., Emory University, 1994, 46–95.

72. Fred B. Linton, "Chief of the Bureau of Chemistry," in *Carl Alsberg, Scientist at Large*, ed. Joseph Davis (Stanford, CA: Stanford University Press, 1948), 37.

73. Alfred L. Kroeber, "The Making of the Man," in Davis, *Carl Alsberg*, 4–5.

74. Oral History, Robert P. Fischelis with James Harvey Young and Richard Hopkins, September 17–19, 1968, Ada, OH, 42–43; Oral History, Henry Lepper with Harvey Young and Harry Dowling, Silver Spring, MD, March 22, 1967, 94, http://www.fda.gov/AboutFDA/WhatWeDo/History/OralHistories/SelectedOralHistoryTranscripts/ucm258606.htm# (accessed September 23, 2013).

75. See the pepper shell case: F. B. Linton, "Reminiscences," *Food, Drug, and Cosmetic Law Journal* (April 1950): 111–12, 114.

76. Honore Willsie, "A Day in Dr. Alsberg's Office," *Harper's Weekly*, November 22, 1913, 6–8.

77. House of Representatives, 31st Congress, 3rd session, Committee on Interstate and Foreign Commerce, *Hearings on the Bills H.R. 29866 and 27275, Net Weights and Contents of Packages*, January 27, 1911, 29.

78. Willsie, "A Day in Dr. Alsberg's Office," 6.

79. The article's storybook ending editorialized: "The fruit extract man had gotten the point. And the situation was not without its pathetic as well as its humorous side. Men who had grown old in business were asking the young man of science to withhold the club until they had learned how to play the game with scientific integrity." Ibid., 8

80. House of Representatives, *Hearings on the Bills H.R. 29866 and 27275, Net Weights and Contents of Packages*, 39.

81. Ibid., 71, 76.

82. Conference Report No. 1579, 62nd Congress, 3rd session, 1913.

83. Wiley's proviso read: "Provided, however, that a slight or immaterial variation from the stated weight is permissible when the variations are made to appear as often above as below the stated weight or volume and to the same extent and proportion." Hearings before the House Committee on Interstate and Foreign Commerce, 62nd Congress, 2nd session (1912); Senate Report No. 1216, 62nd Congress, 3rd session (1913), 26–32. White, *Administrative Procedure and Practice*, part 1, 17.

84. *FDA Annual Report*, 1913, 312; *FDA Annual Report*, 1915, 195–96. Carl L. Alsberg, "The Net Weight Amendment to the National Food and Drugs Act," Department of Commerce, Bureau of Standards, *Ninth Annual Conference on Weights and Measures*, Washington, DC, May 26–29, 1914 (Washington, DC: GPO 1915), 18–22.

85. *FDA Annual Report,* 1913, 312.

86. *FDA Annual Report,* 1914, 339.

87. *FDA Annual Report,* 1917, 363.

88. White, *Administrative Procedure and Practice,* part 1, 37.

89. *FDA Annual Report,* 1920, 430.

90. Ibid.

91. H. Runkel, "Weight Variation of Packaged Foods," US Department of Agriculture, Bureau of Chemistry, *Bulletin 897,* November 15, 1920; H. Runkel, "Volume Variation of Bottled Foods," US Department of Agriculture, Bureau of Chemistry, *Bulletin 1009,* December 16, 1921.

92. Opinion of the Solicitor, No. 9481, dated April 7, 1920; 41 Stat. 234, 271, July 23, 1919, in White, *Administrative Procedure and Practice,* part 1, 39.

93. White, *Administrative Procedure and Practice,* part 1, 18, n 38.

94. US v. Scudder Syrup Co. (1913), NJ 2473, https://ceb.nlm.nih.gov/fdanj/ (accessed July 23, 2016).

95. Ibid. US v. Shreveport Grain and Elevator Co. (1933), NJ 18300; US v. Centralia Dairy Co. (1932), NJ 20139; US v. Rigney & Co. (1915), NJ 4057; US v. Trinidad Creamery Co. (1925), NJ 13365; US v. Barnet Creamery Association (1925), NJ 13707, https://ceb.nlm.nih.gov/fdanj/ (accessed July 23, 2016).

Chapter Eight

When Is a Famine Not a Famine?

Gauging Indian Hunger in Imperial and Cold War Contexts

Nick Cullather

Introduction

The World Food Programme predicted a famine would hit Niger in 2005. Even before the locusts came, drought had despoiled millet fields across the southern grasslands. As refugees began to collect around the town of Maradi, the international community mobilized. Doctors without Borders set up six emergency care centers, and the United Nations sent 7,000 tons of food.[1] Niger's prime minister, Hama Amadou, traveled to France to appeal for aid. Taking advantage of his absence, the president and Amadou's political rival, Mamadou Tandja, assembled the press corps to announce there was "no famine" and "the people of Niger look well-fed."[2] The denials split the aid community. The Swiss aid agency agreed that the crisis had been overplayed, finding "a big gap between the reality facing us on the ground and what the international community is saying."[3] The United States, which was arming and training Niger's military, disputed the United Nation's figures.[4] As the catastrophe unfolded, so did the debate. In 2008, social scientists were still working on models to determine whether a famine had occurred.[5]

Denials of this kind are not unusual. They predictably follow an international relief appeal that incorporates the word "famine." When international organizations raised concerns in 2008 about mass starvation in Ethiopia, the government of Meles Zanawi issued a statement affirming that "famine does not exist in Ethiopia. It is a story made up by the foreign media and aid organizations."[6]

Earthquakes, floods, and hurricanes provoke intense debates about environmental causes, the responsibility of governments, and the geography of need, and so it might be said that all disasters are politically constructed, but the narration of famine contains a further degree of subjectivity, a determination of whether an emergency exists at all. Decisions to declare or not declare may cost lives. Failure to announce a famine may delay a response until it is too late, but a premature or mistaken declaration invites a kind of collateral damage by causing thousands to gather at relief camps where they fall prey to disease. False claims touch off speculative runs on grain markets, sometimes turning an imaginary scarcity into a real one. But for leaders the stakes are even higher. In international politics famines are treated as recurring, even routine events, but also as anachronisms, as reminders of a chaotic premodern past. Famine signifies the state's and the system's failure to provide the most basic level of progress and, accordingly, imposes stern obligations on local governments and the international community. It strips legitimacy from a regime, elected or otherwise, and calls on all progressive countries to place the impotent state under international receivership. For a state, it is the ultimate loss of control and international standing.[7]

Despite these stakes (or maybe because of them) there never has been an agreed way to determine at what point routine scarcity turns into famine. In 1847 an Anglican pastor and pamphleteer, George Woollett, urged the British government to put an end to "false alarms of famine" by publishing "authentic statistical information as to the quantity of food available in the country."[8] But the prediction and measurement of hunger proved to be more than a technical problem. If famine were construed as the opposite of governmental efficacy, its definition would evolve along with the standards governments held themselves to. In 1913 the British economist Alexander Loveday observed that "the history of famines in India is largely the story of how the meaning of that word has been modified through the force of economic transition and the perfection of administrative organization."[9]

That evolution was gauged by statistics. Toward the end of the nineteenth century, social problems and their solutions came increasingly to be defined by new forms of quantification. Much like crime or health, famine came to be defined not by words but by figures. Statistics provided a defense and a justification for government policies, and imperial rulers reached for scientific-sounding interpretations of how much or how little could be done to alleviate food emergencies. It was in this context that dietary norms and standards were developed. Much of the pioneering work in nutritional measurement was designed not to show how much or what kind of food people ought to eat, but rather to determine how little food was needed to stave off mass deaths from starvation.[10] Not only did numerical standards themselves have powerful political effects, but a change in the system of numbering, just like a change in the vocabulary of public debate, also marked a significant shift in the global politics of hunger.

This essay examines a shift in this quantitative rhetoric that began around or just before the First World War and continues to guide the conceptualization of hunger as a social problem to the present day. In the nineteenth century, statisticians aimed to find patterns in human behavior that would restrain the state and bring it into conformity with underlying natural laws. But in the twentieth century, new statistical techniques, particularly the concept of "optimal values," authorized government interventions to bring human behavior into line with the dictates of social efficiency. The state, or at least the statistician, became the arbiter of how much we should eat or drink, how much we should pay, what we should learn, and a host of other intimate questions. But while these data authorized interventions in intimate realms of personal conduct, they paradoxically widened the reach of powerful nations to intervene in the affairs of distant countries in the name of humanitarianism. These old and new ways of reading the numbers clashed in an event called the Bihar famine of 1966.

The Famine Codes in Colonial India

The "scientific" study of famine emerged in a context of imperialism, economic liberalism, and faith in natural laws. This was no ideological straitjacket, but it had a sharply polarizing effect on opinion and the interpretation given to numbers. It was widely held, for instance, that under the free play of market forces famine was impossible. It was simultaneously believed by the demographer and economist Sir Thomas Malthus and his followers that famine was inevitable. Peter Gray, in his excellent book on the Irish famine, notes that official reaction, typified by Charles Trevelyan, a student of Malthus who was the British colonial official in charge of relief, clung to two moralistic claims, first that there was no famine, and second, that famine was good, a natural or divine retribution for Irish indolence or the "potato system." Statistics were available to substantiate both points: prices showed that food was both cheap and abundant in Irish markets, supporting the conclusion that there was no famine in the real sense. Measures of buying power, which might have shown the inability of millions to buy food at any price, had not yet been developed. Figures on mortality, workhouse entries, emigration, and land sales all showed Ireland was undergoing a thorough and probably beneficial transformation toward a new equilibrium at a lower level of population. Until the catastrophe reached its tragic climax in 1847, figures were used not to guide policy but to justify the absence of a policy.[11]

Following the same economic orthodoxies, colonial officials in India initially devised figures designed to minimize government obligation. In response to criticism that his relief allowances had been too generous, Sir Richard Temple, the governor of Bombay Presidency, initiated in 1877 his notorious experiments to find the minimum ration on which an Indian could survive. The ensuing argument between Temple and Surgeon-Major Robert Cornish indicated how things were beginning to change. Using Temple's own statistics and new scientific conceptions of nutrition, Cornish claimed that restricting aid to 1 pound of food grains (rice, wheat, or millet) per day per man produced longer-term effects in disease and debility. The cost to the government of relief works was small compared with losses in revenue and productivity from the weakening of the population. Knowing these effects, he argued, imposed responsibilities beyond reducing the death toll, and rather than striving to spend less, administrators should spend optimally.[12]

In India, unlike Ireland, the British were imperial successors, and they inherited from the Mughals obligations and procedures to forestall disorder and social collapse during subsistence crises. During the mass starvations of the 1870s and 1890s, they systematized and expanded these, through censuses, surveys, and administrative networks, creating what the historian Gyan Prakash has called an "elaborate grid of knowledges and practices that sought to produce a colonial complex of 'men and things.'"[13] Issues of land ownership, productivity, reproduction, and welfare came under government purview. The finding of the 1880 Famine Commission, a body constituted to develop policy for current and future emergencies, was that during times of crisis "the Government stands in the place of landlord to agriculturalists."[14]

The famine codes developed between 1883 and 1901 were both a system for measuring famine and a procedure for alleviating it. The designers of the codes were driven, first, by the embarrassment of recurring famine in a colony that was a large exporter of food. Cornelius Walford, a statistician and early innovator in the life insurance industry, concluded the first systematic study of famines in 1879. He found that contrary to Malthus, famines resulted "from the failure of human means and foresight" and that there had been a sudden increase in their number and severity since the advent of Company rule.[15] In 1896 the Indian National Congress passed two resolutions ascribing famine to the burden of British rule. Ten famines in forty years, with a combined toll of fifteen million deaths, Romesh Chunder Dutt, a regional magistrate and the only Indian in the Indian Civil Service, observed in an open letter to the viceroy, was "a melancholy phenomenon which is not presented today in any other country on earth enjoying a civilized administration."[16] George Hamilton, the secretary of state for India, acknowledged in 1901 that "if it could be shown that India has retrograded in material prosperity under our rule we stand self-condemned, and we ought no longer to be trusted with the control of the country."[17]

Second, colonial administrators needed to minimize their own responsibility without ceding it to private philanthropies, which were all too ready to jump into famine relief. The concept of "unrestricted charity" was anathema to Victorian principles. The 1878 Famine Commission warned against "the doctrine that in time of famine the poor are entitled to demand relief," which could only "lead to the doctrine that they are entitled to such relief at all times . . . which we cannot contemplate without serious apprehension."[18] The Indian government reserved the right to sanction fund drives and define "legitimate" relief activities, but, as graphic images of starvation filled the illustrated magazines, missionary societies, private corporations, and ad hoc groups grew too eager to intrude. British charities raised £1.7 million for relief in 1898 at public events that featured criticisms of official apathy and invidious comparisons with the sums spent on Queen Victoria's diamond jubilee.[19]

The codes were thus concerned less with alleviating famine than with representing it in a way that deflected censure or benevolence. "It is simply ridiculous to suppose that any charitable organization whatever can make headway against a calamity so vast," the *Spectator* assured its readers. "Only a great Government working full power, and pouring out resources from a national Treasury, can do anything effectual, and even that Government may be overstrained."[20]

Famine was also defined narrowly, to minimize public concern and to limit the scope of government responsibility. Under the codes, which evolved through the latter decades of the nineteenth century, a famine was, first, a spatially and temporally delimited event and not a symptom of widespread or persistent scarcity, and, second, a routine occurrence accounted for in the regular budget instead of an emergency requiring special appropriations. Officials reminded the British public of "the grim fact that famines have always occurred in India as far back as history can trace, and they probably always will, more or less severely."[21]

A model code was drafted by a commission and enacted provisionally in 1883. Separate provincial codes were adopted and refined by experience, with major revisions in 1893 and 1901. The timing is significant. Codes were in place before the invention of the calorie and modern statistical nutrition, and they made little use of the new knowledge of metabolism and later vitamins that would become common knowledge over the next few decades. Rather than optimizing nutrition for economic efficiency, they were a holdover from theories of political economy based on natural law. Famines and markets were believed to follow "natural" self-regulating cycles, and the official's primary obligation was to stay out of the way.[22]

They consisted of a set of indicators and reporting requirements for local magistrates and standing procedures for relief works. A 40 percent rise in food prices triggered "a period of observation and test" during which "the district officer should wait upon events and devote himself to careful observation." If prices continued to rise, he was to look for other signs—property sales, epidemics, increases in crime, emaciation, unusual rail traffic, or mass movements of flocks or people. A determination of famine did not incur a greater obligation, but only more detailed reporting. The relief works themselves were designed to gauge whether the visible distress was "real or deceptive" through a series of self-actuating tests. Victims were made to demonstrate the degree of their hunger by making choices, such as submitting to hard labor, sharing food with members of other castes, or working on holy days. The end result was a hard count of those in the absolute extremity of distress; officers were to expel anyone "found not to be at the end of their resources." Reports moved up the civil service hierarchy, allowing officials in New Delhi and, eventually, London to map the outbreak and schedule relief efforts.[23]

The end product of the famine codes was a set of maps and schedules that gave officials a counterrepresentation to the powerful visualization of famine in photographs. As the historian James Vernon points out, lurid images of starving Indians appearing in newspapers and lantern lectures threatened to upset the

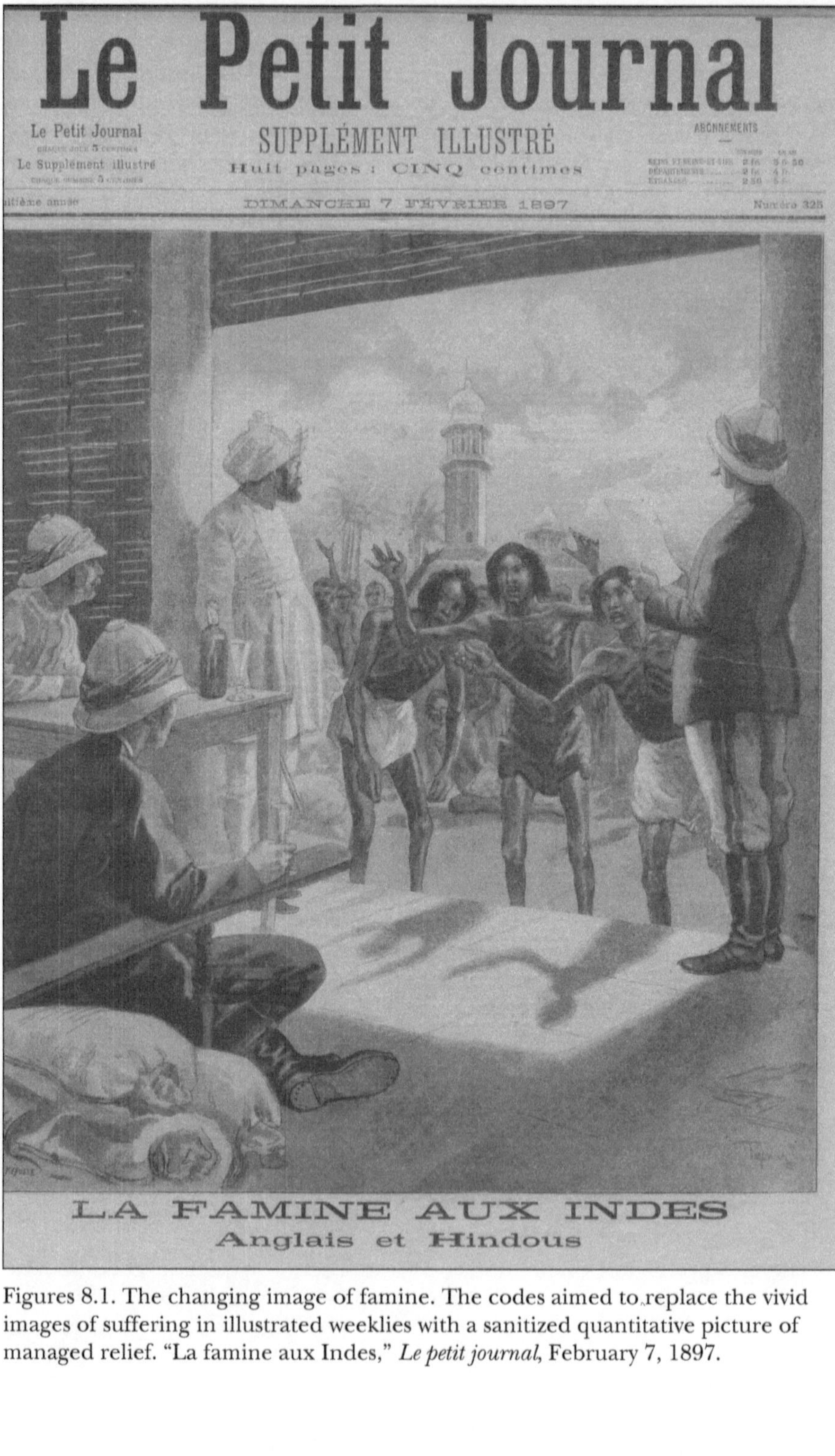

Le Petit Journal

Le Petit Journal
CHAQUE JOUR 5 CENTIMES
Le Supplément illustré
CHAQUE SEMAINE 5 CENTIMES

SUPPLÉMENT ILLUSTRÉ
Huit pages : CINQ centimes

ABONNEMENTS

DIMANCHE 7 FÉVRIER 1897

Numéro 325

LA FAMINE AUX INDES
Anglais et Hindous

Figures 8.1. The changing image of famine. The codes aimed to replace the vivid images of suffering in illustrated weeklies with a sanitized quantitative picture of managed relief. "La famine aux Indes," *Le petit journal*, February 7, 1897.

carefully nurtured illusion of colonial benevolence. One colonial governor complained that newspapers showed beggars and emaciated waifs, but "we never see photographs of tens of thousands of people tolerably comfortable, and certainly not hungry, busily earning bread from the State."[24] Images of distress were particularly jarring amid the spectacle of imperial power unfolding in celebrations of Victoria's diamond jubilee and the twentieth anniversary of her coronation as Empress of India. On June 22, 1897, a procession of fifty thousand native troops from Borneo, Trinidad, Sierra Leon, Canada, India, and Hong Kong passed through London. At Spithead a few days later, the Prince of Wales reviewed a thirty-mile-long column of warships. Edward Caird, master of Balliol College, delivering the jubilee lecture, declared Britain "has been, not a despotic mistress, but a fostering mother for those whom it has conquered."[25] Any contrary emotions aroused by photographs of the holocaust in Calcutta would be countered by the reassuring order of tables and timelines gazetted in the code reports, which promised that everything humanly possible was being done, and in the most efficient way.[26]

Caloric measurement was made practical by the American chemist Wilbur Olin Atwater, whose tables ranked various foods against the demands of various levels of physical exertion. The Atwater tables guided famine relief in Europe during the First World War and the Russian Revolution, but these never fully displaced the codes, which continued to be used in India well into the 1970s. Meanwhile, the calorie became both a popular and scientific measure of food needs by the 1920s. In the interwar period, the League of Nations promoted a new globalized understanding of food shortage based on a caloric balance between national supplies of food and demands, calculated by multiplying total national population against a standard minimum daily requirement. The new understanding was appropriate to a world market in which food crops and industrial crops were competing for land, and in which nutritional standards had become yet another arena for great power rivalry. Encoding a radical theory that all people, regardless of race, were entitled to an equal diet, the calorie faced considerable resistance from imperial authorities. In Britain, it provided a scientific basis for settling labor disputes over a minimum wage, but, using the accumulated research from famine studies, colonial officials insisted that Indians could subsist on less than the League's 2,500 calorie minimum. Anything higher than 1,500 calories would have highlighted the inadequacy of the famine codes.[27]

Codes and Balance Sheets in Postcolonial India

India, which became an independent country in 1947, inherited the famine codes intact. Despite the systemic collapse of the 1943 Bengal famine, Britain's last great imperial failure, in which between two and four million may have perished, the codes actually gained importance in independent India. The new government, led by the Congress Party and its leader Jawaharlal Nehru, launched a series of ambitious five-year plans to renovate the economy using tax and price policy to squeeze revenue out of the countryside for the industrial drive, and bring cultivators closer to a bare subsistence level. The codes continued to be refined into the 1960s, when their authority was challenged by a new concept devised by the Food and Agriculture Organization (FAO) and the United States Department of Agriculture (USDA). This method originated not as a gauge of famine but as a global food balance sheet broken down by country. Created in 1942, the FAO was a response to the global depression, when the chief problem of global agriculture was chronic surplus that could only be alleviated by matching superabundant food stocks in the United States, Europe, Canada, and Australia with consumer outlets in the postcolonial areas. In the late 1950s, the FAO's director was Binay Sen, the famine commissioner for Bengal during the 1943 catastrophe and a lifelong opponent of the famine codes.[28]

Beginning in February 1961, specialists at the USDA, including the agronomists Lester Brown and Wilhelm Anderson, aggregated Sen's country balance sheets into a "World Food Budget," an attempt to forecast total global food availability and need five years into the future. Although neither was an authority on economics, nutrition, or demography, Brown and Anderson's estimates would be widely influential within the US government because they provided a condensed and seemingly authoritative view of global food supply and demand. Because a complete survey of "the wide variety of foods people eat or would like to eat" would be "ponderously detailed," the compilers concentrated on a few key staples, and in the second edition on just one staple, wheat. After translating protein and carbohydrate into calories, Brown discovered, caloric measurements allowed all foods to be translated into bushels of wheat. Output of rice, maize, fish, and veal were thus rendered in units of wheat, and dietary needs—calculated by multiplying population figures against a caloric standard that varied by country but ranged from 2,000 per day for Pakistan to 3,220 for the United States—were also translated into wheat equivalent. The aim was to count all food supplies of whatever kind, and all food needs, regardless of location, in a single column so as to arrive at a positive or negative balance for each country.[29]

The choice of wheat as a standard unit had political value in dealing with the US Congress. The pattern of farm subsidies set by New Deal farm policies in the 1930s had overstimulated production of wheat so much that by 1962 the USDA was warehousing a surplus of over 34 million metric tons, more than the entire wheat consumption of Asia.[30] Making a virtue of necessity, the USDA's World Food Budget stressed the strategic importance of this reserve, particularly in Asia where food deficit areas aligned with US Cold War frontiers. It envisioned ramping up the Public Law 480, Food for Peace Program (generally known as P.L. 480), a scheme that had sent surplus US agricultural products, including food but also cotton and tobacco, abroad in the form of "aid" since 1959 in order to fund development and extend US influence. Although the food budget never used the word "famine," statistical deficit came to be seen as the same thing, and the statistical balance sheet was employed as a technique for forecasting famines worldwide. Like the famine codes, it encoded a narrative explaining the causes of famine, the duties of governments, and the limits on those obligations. The Bihar famine of 1966–67 resulted from a clash between these two fables.

The Construction of the Bihar Famine

The USDA's statistical models changed the nature of knowledge about famine in four ways. First, the flow of information was reversed. Under the colonial famine codes, awareness of a crisis moved from locality to the center, filtering up through the Indian bureaucracy from village outposts to provincial capitals, to Delhi, and eventually to London. In the Bengal famine, local officials appealed to New Delhi for weeks before the crisis was recognized. By contrast, the Bihar famine originated with forecasts made by Brown and other analysts in early December 1965 at USDA headquarters in Washington. To President Lyndon B. Johnson, contending with the Vietnam War abroad and the civil rights movement at home, this looked like one crisis that could be managed. First, he needed to persuade Indian officials that a crisis existed, and they in turn confronted the denials of local officials.

Second, the British method carefully avoided a theory of causation, casting famine as a recurring, natural calamity. Famine was seen as endemic to the Indian environment, a consequence of unreliable weather patterns. By contrast, USDA experts assumed causal relationships between drought, crop failure, population, and food availability. India's failure to manage food reserves, to assure functioning markets, and above all to check the reproductive urges of its people were at fault. These supposed "causes" were later discredited by Amartya Sen and other famine studies scholars in the 1980s, but the USDA team also discounted causes that could have been measured at the time, such as land tenure, wages, conflict, and trade patterns.[31] Moreover, their assumptions were built into the policy response; the USDA urged reforms consisting of a series of steps to improve the statistical indicators: population limitation, productivity, transport, and storage.[32]

Third, statistical projections afforded American forecasters substantially more latitude than imperial officials had in estimating (or overestimating) the gravity of a famine. Forecasts prepared by the Central Intelligence Agency (CIA) and the departments of agriculture and state were based on triangulations between figures denoting harvests, population, and nutritional needs, but in all three columns the numbers corresponded doubtfully with the realities they supposedly represented.[33] Ivan Bennett, Johnson's science adviser, explained to a Senate subcommittee on foreign aid in 1968 that an uncertainty principle precluded reliable calculations of food availability: the more central authorities needed to know, the more peasants and merchants were motivated to mislead them about the food inventory. Population figures and caloric requirements were guesstimates throwing in further margins of error of several hundred percent.[34] As the *Economist* observed, "Estimates of [India's] food gap represent, in these circumstances, a piece of political rather than economic arithmetic."[35] The White House had assessments from the Departments of Agriculture, State, the Agency for International Development (USAID), and CIA, giving President Lyndon Johnson a wide range to choose from, none more credible than the others.

Finally, the USDA forecasts were unspecific as to time and place. While the codes mapped and scheduled famines as precisely as a railway timetable, the USDA forecast a shortfall for the whole of India in annualized terms. It was up to Indian officials to guess where and when the crisis would hit. Nonetheless, famine came to be declared in a single province, Bihar, in April 1967. As Paul Brass has explained, assignment of that particular setting and timing was part of the famine's political script, which focused on Bihar, a state that had broken from the ruling Congress Party in the previous election. The famine provided an occasion to fight out a simmering conflict between state and central governments over the control of food and votes. State authorities used the disaster to level accusations of neglect against the central government, whereas New Delhi singled out Bihar to demonstrate the incompetence of its state administration.[36] US officials had their own reasons for narrating the crisis the same way.

Declaring a crisis, Johnson called for a worldwide rescue but sent American food aid only in small increments, one shipload at a time—a policy known as "short tether"—to force the liberalization of the Congress Party's socialist planning regime and steer it away from industry and toward agriculture. The policy began in May 1965 in response to the India-Pakistan border war, but on June 9 Johnson requested an interdepartmental review of aid to South Asia with an emphasis on "how to achieve more leverage for our money."[37] That summer, as drought struck across eastern India, the review grew to encompass the total foreign-aid budget and to focus on the problem of adapting foreign aid to the sudden lurches in domestic policy occurring in the 1960s. As a senator and president, Johnson's preferred style was to avoid taking on issues singly and, instead, to orchestrate policy ensembles that addressed numerous, seemingly unrelated problems in one movement.[38]

Three problems—seemingly unrelated to India or famine—were of primary concern to Johnson and his aides: First, a series of civil rights lawsuits had chipped away at the system for apportioning congressional seats that had historically given rural voters a level of political clout in the US House of Representatives entirely out of proportion to their actual numbers. Particularly in the South, voting districts had been drawn in such a way that urban votes counted for substantially less than rural votes. Beginning with the case of *Carr v. Baker* (1962) all that was about to change. One after another the Supreme Court threw out districting schemes, and with them the legislative power of the farm block.[39] Within a few election cycles food consumers would outvote producers, and the subsidies that kept prices high and built up the wheat surpluses would no longer be politically sustainable. But Johnson believed a reorientation of the global food market might provide a way out. Under the optimistic assumption that Asian countries could become self-sufficient in grain, Agriculture Secretary

Orville Freeman directed his economists to investigate the effects on the US farm economy and found that gains in Asian production might actually increase the demand for US food exports.[40] Higher standards of living and consumption would "spill out" into demand for imported food, including fats, oils, and processed foods that would be paid for in dollars.[41] Freeman suggested that a strategy based on increasing food output in underdeveloped countries would not only invigorate the US economy, but also convert some Congressional opponents of foreign aid.

Second, Johnson was apprehensive about Europe, where his relationships were frayed by opposition to the Vietnam War. A global rescue effort might allow him to reassert US leadership there. Finally, the administration had grave concerns about India, riven after Nehru's death by sectarian and linguistic factionalism. "The real threat to India is not invasion through the Himalayas," his aides concluded, but "disintegration and fragmentation of the as yet fragile Indian state." A collapse of the Congress government, a situation comparable to China's communist revolution in 1948, would most likely arise from a failure to meet popular demands for food and jobs. "Economic growth has become the test of political success," the State Department warned, and by that standard India "hasn't done well enough." Sharply restricted aid and a sense of urgency would provide "a new impulse toward unity" and turn "swords into plowshares" by channeling India's energies away from sectarian squabbles and toward agriculture. Even if the effort fell short, the push to achieve greater production in food would discipline India's politics and create "the kind of India we want."[42]

Johnson warmed to the idea of linking India aid to his farm policy. In July, he commiserated with the Indian ambassador B. K. Nehru (the deceased prime minister's nephew) about his congressional difficulties. Voting rights, Medicare, and Vietnam deployments had about exhausted his mandate, and he guessed he would "probably get licked" on the farm bill, the annual legislative renewal of federal subsidies for wheat, corn, rice, and other crops. He wanted Nehru's help in communicating a "food for famine" message to Congress and the public. The ambassador was taken aback. There was no famine. US food aid was a reciprocal deal; India helped the United States dispose of its "burdensome surplus" and, from the sale of the wheat, earned the revenue it needed for the five-year plan. Senators saw it differently, Johnson explained; they did not understand why India should be making steel instead of fertilizer. He "didn't want people to starve but he wanted the Congress to be in partnership on whatever we did."[43]

For Johnson, a famine could be useful for moving his domestic political agenda on agriculture and aid, and his foreign policy agenda in Europe and Asia. Reconfiguring food aid, farm policy, European alliances, and his congressional coalition in a single year could be justified only by international conditions. In the fall of 1965, Johnson developed the theme of a world food crisis brought on by runaway population growth. At a televised cabinet meeting on November 19, he declared a "world war against hunger" requiring a reorientation of global and domestic food policy. "Our strategy is to encourage rapid increase in food production in the underdeveloped countries themselves."[44]

Two weeks later, as Johnson prepared to present the new policy to Congress, the Department of Agriculture produced its first famine forecasts. On December 17, before the extent (or even the existence) of a crop failure could be confirmed, Johnson declared the existence of "near famine conditions . . . which may require a dramatic rescue operation."[45] A *Washington Post* article the previous week explained the domestic link: "A series of famines, such as that threatening India, may speed the evolutionary movement of U.S. farm policy." A "succession of such worldwide shortages" would propel "the transition from restriction to expansion of U.S. farm production."[46]

At this stage, Johnson chose the most dire assessments from among those available to him. Lester Brown's December 1965 prediction that India would need 18 million tons of grain above its standard P.L. 480 allotment in calendar year 1966 was countered by CIA estimates of a "minimal" requirement of only 3.5 million tons additional.[47] The CIA and State Department characterized India's food problem as a chronic dependency, whereas the USDA predicted a disaster larger than "the Bengal famine of 1943 by several fold."[48] Johnson's decision to continue doling out food aid in small amounts provoked resistance from his advisers, and the battle within the administration was fought over the wording of presidential statements and control of the statistics going to the president.[49]

Johnson's first and most difficult objective was to win acceptance of his claims, but the reality of the famine was persistently questioned by Indian officials and the Indian press. In February 1966, after Johnson referred again in a press conference to "the drought and the famine that exists there," Indian Food Minister Chidambara Subramaniam issued a denial and accused the press, and indirectly the United States, of "scaremongering."[50] The Indian Planning Commission, India's economic cabinet, defending the country's industrial sector, insisted that "the problem is not one of food supplies, but of providing adequate purchasing power."[51] Editorials described the American and even the lower Indian estimates as "grossly exaggerated."[52] The international press, too, had doubts. The US Ambassador to India, Chester Bowles, grew frustrated at reporters' requests to see actual starving Indians, which he could not produce.[53] Whereas the London *Times* appreciated the irony ("Food Ships Streaming into Famine-Free India," ran its headline), US newspapers swallowed the official version. The official National Security Council history of the crisis explained the press's willingness to go along: "It was an old story; Indians were always starving."[54]

But Johnson's statements had an effect. In February, Pope Paul VI, asserting that "people are literally dying of starvation," appealed for aid to India.[55] Subramaniam now applied to the United States for additional "emergency" food aid. Indian states imposed preemptive rationing, and in Kerala, Calcutta, and Punjab deadly food riots erupted. The moderate weekly *Eastern Economist* blamed the United States for exaggerating the food deficit, fostering a "psychology of scarcity."[56] The same thought occurred to William Gaud, director of USAID, and Freeman, the Secretary of Agriculture, who worried that Johnson's "loud international alarm about famine . . . could set off hoarding and price speculation, and make it even easier for the leftists to stir up food riots."[57] Ambassador

Nehru brought this point up directly with the president, urging a public reassurance to prevent disorder.[58]

The riots' separatist overtones set off alarms in Washington. Since the Kennedy administration, national security officials had warned that state separatism would be the vehicle for communist penetration of the subcontinent. The new prime minister, Indira Gandhi, appeared weak to Johnson's advisers, and her selection by powerful state political chiefs was further evidence that India was ready to "come apart at the seams." US officials also recognized that food policy was a flashpoint for separatist politics. The constitution gave the states full authority over agriculture, grain reserves, and prices, and in times of shortage, the gap in rations between states provided (literally) a visceral reminder of India's disunity.[59] The United States was pushing reforms that radically shifted power toward the center, establishing a national food budget, national grain reserves, and extending central authority into every rural village. "A successful national food policy," Freeman explained, "would further one of our political objectives for India—binding together the states with new ties of interdependence and strengthening the national government."[60] In this objective of consolidating power at the top, Indira Gandhi and Johnson found common ground.

During her state visit in March 1966, Gandhi and US officials jointly drafted a script for the famine. At a meeting on March 29, Dean Rusk, the secretary of state, began by noting "the dilemma concerning the public presentation on food. It shouldn't be such as to frighten people in India, but on the other hand the need must be seen to be real in the United States." Nehru agreed that "to get a response, the need must be somewhat overplayed." L. K. Jha, Prime Minister Gandhi's secretary, stressed that it should appear to be "a natural calamity" that was "averted." Gandhi, who had denied the existence of a famine up to this point, "suggested that the subject might be treated as a localized matter."[61] The famine that unfolded in Bihar later that year closely followed this sketch. Although the drought affected large areas of the country, the famine codes were invoked only in Bihar. The province was isolated, subjected to stringent rationing, and fed with supplies directly from the United States. Official statements claimed that no one died in Bihar, but half of the 2,353 "alleged starvation deaths" in India occurred in this one province.[62] The day after the Washington meeting, Gandhi referred to the crisis as a "famine" for the first time. The Indian press noted the rhetorical shift, but it brought no closure. State officials promptly issued a denial, and legislators denounced the ensuing "starvation controversy" as "part of the cold war between the Government and the Opposition."[63]

Conclusions

Where the famine codes had once absolved the government of responsibility and defeated efforts to internationalize the problem, famine forecasting based on nutritional standards and projections of population and crop production had the opposite effect, mobilizing a global campaign and justifying interventions that could serve a number of economic and political purposes. Johnson recorded in his memoirs that he had recognized the famine as an opportunity. "If we went about it the right way," he foresaw, "we could encourage increasingly far-reaching changes in India's economy and in the supporting actions of other nations."[64] His "we" did not include the Indian people or government.

The 1967 crisis might well have been the moment at which depoliticized, unaccountable, and undemocratic procedures for fighting hunger broke down under popular pressure, but instead it was the moment at which responsibility shifted from national governments to the international community, making famine policy even more remote from the needs of stricken people. A theoretical consensus has in recent years tended toward a depiction of famine as a complex political crisis, essentially idiosyncratic and local, but statistical representation has been in the opposite direction, toward denying its essential quality and representing it in simplified, standard, and increasingly global terms. Today, famine is forecast largely by use of "remote sensing" techniques such as satellite imagery.[65] The result may be that famine will be perceived only through automatic, unblinking eyes. Experts in multilateral agencies and aid ministries, viewing the crisis from their low orbital vantage point, will find it even harder to learn the causes.

Notes

1. M. Wines, "Niger's Anguish," *New York Times Upfront*, October 10, 2005, 18–19; E. Pape, "The Hunger Season," *Newsweek*, August 15, 2005, 30.

2. Olly Owen, "Details Emerge of Niger Famine Coverup," *Global Insight Daily Analysis*, August 12, 2005; Olly Owen, "Famine Row Provokes Split between President and Prime Minister," *Global Insight Daily Analysis*, August 30, 2005; BBC News, "Niger Famine Denial," August 12, 2005, http://newsvote.bbc.co.uk/mpapps/pagetools/print/news.bbc.co.uk/2/hi/talking_point/4134436.stm. (accessed May 26, 2015).

3. BBC Monitoring, "Swiss Play Down Reports of Niger Famine," August 11, 2005.

4. Robert D. Kaplan, "America's African Rifles," *Atlantic Monthly*, April 2005, 91–4.

5. Avid Reza, et al., "Retrospective Determination of Whether Famine Existed in Niger, 2005: Two Stage Cluster Survey," *British Medical Journal* 337, no. 7675 (2008): 915–18.

6. BBC Monitoring Africa, "Ethiopian Scholar Blames Government Policy for Food Shortages," August 9, 2011.

7. Jenny Edkins, *Whose Hunger? Concepts of Famine, Practices of Aid* (Minneapolis: University of Minnesota Press, 2000), 14.

8. George Woollett, *A Remedy against False Alarms of Famine and Real Scarcity* (London: Effingham Wilson, 1847), 17.

9. Alexander Loveday, *The History and Economics of Indian Famines* (London: G. Bell and Sons, 1914), vii.

10. Ian Hacking, *The Taming of Chance* (Cambridge: Cambridge University Press, 1990); Mary Poovey, *A History of the Modern Fact* (Chicago: University of Chicago Press, 1998); J. Adam Tooze, *Statistics and the Modern German State* (Cambridge: Cambridge

University Press, 2001); Silvana Patriarca, *Numbers and Nationhood* (Cambridge: Cambridge University Press, 1996).

11. Peter Gray, *Famine, Land, and Politics: British Government and Irish Society, 1843–1850* (Dublin: Irish Academic Press, 1999).

12. David Hall-Matthews, "Inaccurate Conceptions: Disputed Measures of Nutritional Needs and Famine Deaths in Colonial India," *Modern Asian Studies* 42, no. 6 (2008): 1189–1212.

13. Gyan Prakash, *Another Reason: Science and the Imagination of Modern India* (Princeton, NJ: Princeton University Press, 1999).

14. Sunil S. Amrith, "Food and Welfare in India, c. 1900–1950," *Comparative Studies in Society and History* 50, no. 4 (2008): 1013.

15. Cornelius Walford, *The Famines of the World: Past and Present* (London: E. Stanford, 1879), 2, 89–90.

16. Romesh Chunder Dutt, *Open Letters to Lord Curzon on Famines and Land Assessments in India* (London: K. Paul, Trench, 1900), 16.

17. Quoted in James Vernon, *Hunger: A Modern History* (Cambridge, MA: Harvard University Press, 2007), 50.

18. Quoted in Vivek Chibber, "The Good Empire," *Boston Review* 30 (January 2005): 1.

19. Georgina Brewis, "'Fill Full the Mouth of Famine': Voluntary Action in Famine Relief in India 1896–1901," *Modern Asian Studies* 44, no. 4 (2010): 897–99.

20. "Pestilence and Famine in India," *The Spectator*, January 16, 1897, 81.

21. G. Bradshaw, "Indian Famines," *Longman's Magazine*, November 1900, 51.

22. Madras Presidency, *Famine Relief Code* (Madras, 1884); Bengal, *Bengal Famine Code, Revised Edition of December 1895* (Calcutta, 1897); House of Commons, *Papers regarding the Famine and the Relief Operations in India during the Year 1896 with Copy of the Famine Code the North-West Provinces and Oudh* (London: HMSO, 1897).

23. Bombay Presidency, *Famine Relief Code* (Bombay: Presidency Secretariat, 1904), 22; Bengal, *Bengal Famine Code, Revised Edition of 1913* (Calcutta: Bengal Secretariat Book Depot, 1913); Bengal, *Bengal Famine Code* (Calcutta: Bengal Secretariat Book Depot, 1908), 14; *The Bihar and Orissa Famine Code 1930* (Patna: Superintendent Government Printing, 1930), 2, 11, 15.

24. Vernon, *Hunger*, 34.

25. Edward Caird, *Lay Sermons and Addresses Delivered in the Hall of Balliol College, Oxford* (London: J. MacLehose, 1907), 91.

26. Edward W. Ellsworth, "Victoria's Diamond Jubilee and the British Press," *Social Studies* 56, no. 5 (1965): 173.

27. Nick Cullather, "The Foreign Policy of the Calorie," *American Historical Review* 112, no. 2 (2007): 337–64.

28. On the origins of the FAO, see Amy L. S. Staples, *The Birth of Development: How the World Bank, Food and Agriculture Organization, and World Health Organization Changed the World* (Kent, OH: Kent State University Press, 2006), 64–81; Binay R. Sen, *Towards a Newer World* (Dublin: Tycooly, 1982).

29. Economic Research Service, *The World Food Budget 1962 and 1966* (Washington, DC: USDA, 1961); Lester Brown, *Man, Land and Food: Looking Ahead at World Food Needs* (Washington, DC: USDA, 1963).

30. Richard Orr, "Surplus of Wheat Still Growing," *Chicago Tribune*, May 10, 1961, A8.

31. Amartya Sen, *Poverty and Famines: An Essay on Entitlement and Deprivation* (New York: Oxford University Press, 1981).

32. Carolyn Castore, "The United States and India: The Use of Food to Apply Economic Pressure, 1965–1967," in *Economic Coercion and U.S. Foreign Policy: Implications of Case Studies from the Johnson Administration*, ed. Sidney Weintraub (Boulder, CO: Westview, 1982), 130–46.

33. Port capacity figures varied widely, and although Johnson dispatched the agriculture secretary Orville Freeman, the national security adviser Robert Komer, and Senator Bob Dole on missions to inspect the ports, he remained unsatisfied. The National Security Council estimated port capacity at 600,000 tons monthly, while Freeman put the figure at 1 million tons. Harold H. Saunders to McGeorge Bundy, "Indian Food Crisis," December 2, 1965, box 24, Robert W. Komer Papers, National Security Files (NSF), Lyndon Baines Johnson Library (LBJL), Austin, TX; Freeman to LBJ, "Talks with the Indian Minister of Food and Agriculture," December 23, 1965, Indian Famine, vol. 1, box 25, NSF, NSC History, LBJL.

34. Senate Subcommittee on Foreign Aid, *Population Crisis*, 90th Congress, 2nd session, pt. 2, 1968, 312; Barbara Tufty, "Analysis of Famine," *Science News*, July 30, 1966, 74–75.

35. "Food Is Politics," *Economist*, February 5, 1966, 503.

36. Paul R. Brass, "The Political Uses of Crisis: The Bihar Famine of 1966–1967," *Journal of Asian Studies* 45, no. 2 (1986): 245–67.

37. Bundy to Rusk and McNamara, "Presidential Decisions on Aid to India/Pakistan," June 9, 1965, *Foreign Relations of the United States, 1964–1968* (Washington, DC: USGPO, 1997), 25: 274 (hereafter FRUS).

38. Philip Geyelin, *Lyndon B. Johnson and the World* (New York: F. A. Praeger, 1966), 157.

39. In a series of landmark decisions, beginning with *Baker v. Carr* (1962) and culminating with *Westberry v. Sanders* and *Reynolds v. Sims* (1964), the Warren court struck down systems of apportionment that favored rural voters.

40. P.L. 480 had been designed on the opposite assumption, that donations would expand foreign markets for US grain. Vernon W. Ruttan, ed., *Why Food Aid?* (Baltimore, MD: Johns Hopkins University Press, 1993), 88.

41. "Johnson May Revise Food Aid Policy," *New York Times*, November 8, 1965, 1, 39.

42. Department of State, "A United States Assistance Strategy for India," November 8, 1965, Indian Famine, vol. 2, tab 4, NSF, NSC History, LBJL; Rusk to Bowles, November 10, 1965, *FRUS*, 25: 461.

43. Komer, "President's Talk with Ambassador B. K. Nehru," July 16, 1965, Indian Famine, vol. 1, box 25, NSF, NSC History, LBJL; B. K. Nehru, *Nice Guys Finish Second* (Delhi: Viking, 1997), 430–31.

44. "Cabinet Agenda," November 19, 1965, Cabinet Papers, Meeting 11/19/65, box 4, LBJL.

45. LBJ to Freeman, "Critical Indian Food Situation," NSAM 339, December 17, 1965, *FRUS*, 25: 513–14.

46. Thomas J. Foley, "Famines May Alter Farm Policy," *Washington Post*, December 12, 1965, R5. The article went on to observe that "the actual turnaround in U.S. output is still some years away and that only a series of 'India' crises could bring it closer."

47. Brown memorandum of December 6, 1965, quoted in Castore, "United States and India," 137; CIA, "India's New Prime Minister," January 20, 1966, *Declassified Documents Reference System*, 1977–270A; at a February 5 press conference, LBJ cited the figure of 19 million tons: "Transcript of President's Press Conference on Indian Famine," *New York Times*, February 5, 1966, 8. The Indian food ministry estimated the shortfall at between 3 and 8 million tons, whereas adding up state estimates produced a figure of 14 million tons. "With Only P.L. 480," *Economic Weekly*, December 11, 1965, 1807.

48. Thomas L. Hughes to Rusk, "Some Political Implications of the Indian Food Shortage," December 21, 1965, Files of Robert Komer, India—Food 1964–65, box 24, NSF, LBJL; CIA, "Indo-Pakistani Reactions to Certain US Courses of Action," December 7, 1965, SNIE 31–32–65, *FRUS*, 25: 489–90; Castore, "United States and India," 137.

49. Bowles, who considered his embassy's estimates "remarkably accurate," fiercely resisted the Department of Agriculture's claims to expertise. Bowles, *Promises to Keep* (New York: Harper and Row, 1971), 526–27.

50. "Transcript of President's Press Conference on Indian Famine," *New York Times*, February 5, 1966, 8; "Food Ships Streaming into Famine-Free India," *Times* (London), February 22, 1966, 8.

51. February planning commission report quoted in "Shortage Not of Food but of Money," *Yojana*, May 29, 1966, 2.

52. "Food Deficit in Southern States," *Eastern Economist*, March 4, 1966, 366. *Yojana* observed that "the Prime Minister is very correct in saying there is no famine in the country." "Food, 1966," *Yojana*, March 20, 1966, 1.

53. Bowles, *Promises to Keep*, 530; Kingsley Martin, "A Famine in India?" *New Statesman*, March 4, 1966, 286. A British reporter noted that much of the foreign press corps wondered "if the Indian government hadn't been bleating unnecessarily." Chanchal Sarkar, "Below the Wheatline," *Spectator*, March 4, 1966, 255–56.

54. NSC, "India's Food Crisis, 1965–67," vol. 5, NSF, NSC History, LBJL.

55. "Pope Asks World Give Famine Aid," *New York Times*, February 10, 1966, 26.

56. "Riceless in Kerala," *Eastern Economist*, February 11, 1966, 211.

57. Quoted in Kristin Ahlberg, *Transplanting the Great Society: Lyndon Johnson and Food for Peace* (Columbia: University of Missouri Press, 2008), 230–31. Gaud to Califano, "Proposed Message on India's Food Needs," March 25, 1966, White House Aides, box 10, Bob Hardesty file, LBJL.

58. R. W. Komer, "President's Meeting with Indian Ambassador Nehru," February 3, 1966, NSC History, vol. 1, box 25, NSF, LBJL.

59. And through press accounts too. Joseph Lelyveld wrote that "the crux of the food problem is in the difficult negotiations between New Delhi and the state governments." "India," *The Atlantic*, February 1968, 14. See also "Why Hunger Still Stalks India," *Newsweek*, April 4, 1966, 44.

60. Freeman and Gaud to LBJ, "Food Aid for India in 1968," October 10, 1967, NSC Meeting, 1/11/67, box 2, NSF, LBJL; the "adversity" caused by short tether,

Freeman argued, would "provide new impulse toward unity." Rusk, "A United States Assistance Strategy for India," November 8, 1965, NSC History, Indian Famine, vol. 2, box 25, NSF, LBJL.

61. "Indo-U.S. Talks: Food, Disarmament and Nuclear Policy," *FRUS,* 25: 599. Significantly, public presentation was the only aspect of the famine discussed.

62. Jean Drèze, *The Political Economy of Hunger: Selected Essays* (Oxford: Oxford University Press, 1995), 59.

63. "Death in Orissa," *Himmat,* April 8, 1966, 3; G. S. Bhargava, "Starvation vs. Malnutrition," *Yojana,* May 15, 1966, 27.

64. Lyndon B. Johnson, *The Vantage Point* (New York: Norton, 1971), 228.

65. Meg Marquardt, "An Eye on Africa," *Earth,* March 2011, 28–33.

Selected Bibliography

The following bibliography contains a selection of secondary literature and published primary sources. The works listed here were chosen for their central position in the historical narratives presented in the essays and for their broader significance for the history of debates on nutritional and dietary standards. Included are a number of more general historical works that provide a context for interpreting these debates and concerns for nutrition and diet within the periods under discussion. Whereas edited volumes on the history of nutrition science are contained in this bibliography, individual essays in these volumes are not listed separately.

Amrith, Sunil S. "Food and Welfare in India, c. 1900–1950." *Comparative Studies in Society and History* 50 (2008): 1010–35.

Anderson, Oscar. *Health of a Nation.* Chicago: University of Chicago Press, 1958.

Apple, Rima Dombrow. *Vitamania: Vitamins in American Culture.* New Brunswick, NJ: Rutgers University Press, 1996.

Aronson, Naomi. "The Discovery of Resistance: Historical Accounts and Scientific Careers." *Isis* 77 (1986): 286–306.

———. "Nutrition as a Social Problem: A Case Study of Entrepreneurial Strategy in Science." *Social Problems* 29 (1982): 474–87.

———. "Social Definitions of Entitlement: Food Needs, 1885–1920." *Media, Culture, and Society* 4 (1982): 51–61.

Atkins, Peter J., Peter Lummel, and Derek J. Oddy, eds. *Food and the City in Europe to 1800.* Aldershot: Ashgate, 2007.

Atwater, Wilbur Olin. "American and European Dietaries and Dietary Standards." *Fourth Annual Report of the Storrs Agricultural Experiment Station* (1891): 106–61.

———. "Pecuniary Economy of Food: The Chemistry of Foods and Nutrition. V." *Century Magazine* 35 (1887–88): 437–46.

Bächi, Beat. *Vitamin C für alle! Pharmazeutische Produktion, Vermarktung und Gesundheitspolitik (1933–1953).* Zürich: Chronos, 2009.

Baltzer, Eduard. *Die natürliche Lebensweise.* 4 vols. Nordhausen: Förstemann, 1867–72.

Barona, Josep. *The Problem of Nutrition: Experimental Science, Public Health and Economy in Europe, 1914–1945.* Brussels: Peter Lang, 2010.

Benedict, Francis Gano, Walter Richard Miles, Paul Roth, and Henry Monmouth Smith. *Human Vitality and Efficiency under Prolonged Restricted Diet.* Washington, DC: Government Printing Office, 1919.

Biltekoff, Charlotte. *Eating Right in America: The Cultural Politics of Food and Health.* Durham, NC: Duke University Press, 2013.

Bonah, Christian, David Cantor, and Matthias Doerries, eds. *Meat, Medicine, and Human Health in the Twentieth Century.* London: Pickering and Chatto, 2010.

Bowie, Hamilton C. "Ueber den Eiweissbedarf eines mittleren Arbeiters." *Zeitschrift für Biologie* 15 (1879): 459–84.

Bowles, Chester. *Promises to Keep.* New York: Harper and Row, 1971.

Brass, Paul R. "The Political Uses of Crisis: The Bihar Famine of 1966–1967." *Journal of Asian Studies* 45 (1986): 245–67.

Canguilhem, Georges. *The Normal and the Pathological.* New York: Zone Books, 1991.

Carpenter, Kenneth John. *Protein and Energy.* Cambridge: Cambridge University Press, 1994.

Caspari, Wilhelm, and Karl Glaessner. "Ein Stoffwechselversuch an Vegetariern." *Zeitschrift für diätetische und physikalische Therapie* 7 (1903): 475–85.

Chittenden, Russell Henry. *The Nutrition of Man.* New York: Frederick A. Stokes, 1907.

———. *Physiological Economy in Nutrition.* New York: Frederick A. Stokes, 1904.

Coppin, Clayton, and Jack High. *The Politics of Purity.* Ann Arbor: University of Michigan Press, 1999.

Coveney, John. *Food, Morals and Meaning: The Pleasure and Anxiety of Eating.* New York: Routledge, 2000.

Cullather, Nick. "The Foreign Policy of the Calorie." *American Historical Review* 112 (2007): 337–64.

———. *The Hungry World: America's Cold War Battle against Poverty in Asia.* Cambridge, MA: Harvard University Press, 2010.

Cummings, Richard O. *The American and His Food.* Chicago: University of Chicago Press, 1940.

Dally, Ann. *Fantasy Surgery, 1880–1930: With Special Reference to Sir William Arbuthnot Lane.* Amsterdam: Rodopi, 1996.

Dopter, Charles, and Jean Rouget. *Hygiène alimentaire.* Paris: Baillière et fils, 1906.

Engel, Ernst. "Die Productions- und Consumtionsverhältnisse des Königreichs Sachsen." Appendix 1 to Ernst Engel, "Lebenskosten belgischer Arbeiterfamilien früher und jetzt." *Bulletin de l'Institut International de Statistique* 9 (1895): 1–54.

Food and Drugs Administration. *Annual Reports, 1909–1949.* Chicago: Commerce Clearing House, 1951.

Gautier, Armand. *L'Alimentation et les régimes chez l'homme sain ou malade.* 3rd ed. Paris: Masson, 1908.

Goldstein, Carolyn M. *Creating Consumers: Home Economists in Twentieth-Century America.* Chapel Hill: University of North Carolina Press, 2012.

Goodwin, Lorine S. *Pure Food, Drug, and Drink Crusaders: 1879–1914.* Jefferson, NC: McFarland and Company, 1999.

Gould, Elgin Ralston Lovell. *The Social Condition of Labor.* Baltimore, MD: Johns Hopkins University Press, 1893.

Hacking, Ian. *The Taming of Chance.* Cambridge: Cambridge University Press, 1990.

Hahn, Theodor. *Die naturgemässe Diät, die Diät der Zukunft: Nach Erfahrung und Wissenschaft aller Zeiten und Völker.* Cöthen: Paul Schettler, 1859.

Heischkelt-Artelt, Edith, ed. *Ernährung und Ernährungslehre im 19. Jahrhundert.* Göttingen: Vandenhoeck and Ruprecht, 1976.

Hildesheim, Wilhelm. *Die Normal-Diät: Physiologisch-chemischer Versuch zur Ermittelung des normalen Nahrungsbedürfnisses des Menschen behufs Aufstellung einer Normal-Diät. Mit besonderer Rücksicht auf das Diät-Regulativ des neuen Reglements für die Friedens-Garnisons-Lazarethe und die Natural-Verpflegung der Soldaten sowie auf die Verpflegung der Armen.* Berlin: Hirschwald, 1856.

Holmes, Frederic L. "Carl Voit and the Quantitative Tradition in Biology." In *Transformations and Tradition in the Sciences: Essays in Honour of I. Bernard Cohen,* edited by Everett Mendelsohn, 455–70. Cambridge: Cambridge University Press, 1984.

———. "The Formation of the Munich School of Metabolism." In *The Investigative Enterprise: Experimental Physiology in Nineteenth-Century Medicine,* edited by William Coleman and Frederic L. Holmes, 179–210. Berkeley: University of California Press, 1988.

———. "The Intake-Output Method in Physiology." *Historical Studies in the Physical and Biological Sciences* 17 (1987): 245–70.

Hopkins, Frederick Gowland. "The Analyst and the Medical Man." *Analyst* 31 (1906): 385–97.

———. "Feeding Experiments Illustrating the Importance of Accessory Food Factors in Normal Dietaries." *Journal of Physiology* 44 (1912): 425–60.

House of Commons. *Papers regarding the Famine and the Relief Operations in India during the Year 1896 with Copy of the Famine Code the North-West Provinces and Oudh.* London: Her Majesty's Stationery Office, 1897.

Kamminga, Harmke, and Andrew Cunningham, eds. *The Science and Culture of Nutrition, 1840s–1940s.* Amsterdam: Rodopi, 1995.

Kellner, Oskar Johann, and Y. Mori. "Untersuchungen über die Ernährung der Japaner." *Zeitschrift für Biologie* 25 (1889): 102–21.

Klencke, Hermann. *Die Nahrungsmittelfrage in Deutschland oder: Welches sind die Naturanforderungen menschlicher Ernährung, wie müssen sie durch die deutsche Küche erfüllt und wie dann dem Unbemittelten eine billige und kräftige Nahrung geboten werden? Vom Standpunkte der praktischen Naturwissenschaft beantwortet.* Leipzig: Eduard Kummer, 1855.

Kumagawa, Muneo. "Vergleichende Untersuchungen über die Ernährung mit gemischter und rein vegetabilischer Kost mit Berücksichtigung des Eiweissbedarfs." *Virchows Archiv* 116 (1889): 370–431.

Landouzy, Louis, Henri Labbé, and Marcel Labbé. *Enquête sur l'alimentation d'une centaine d'ouvriers et d'employés parisiens.* Paris: Masson, 1905.

League of Nations Mixed Committee on the Problem of Nutrition. *The Problem of Nutrition,* vol. 1. Geneva: League of Nations Publications Department, 1936.

League of Nations. *Report on the Physiological Basis of Nutrition.* Geneva: League of Nations Publications Department, 1935.

Levenstein, Harvey. *Revolution at the Table: The Transformation of the American Diet.* Berkeley: University of California Press, 2003.

Levine, Susan. *School Lunch Politics: The Surprising History of American's Favorite Welfare Program.* Princeton, NJ: Princeton University Press, 2008.

Liebig, Justus. *Die Thier-Chemie oder die organische Chemie in ihrer Anwendung auf Physiologie und Pathologie.* Braunschweig: Vieweg und Sohn, 1843.

Loveday, Alexander. *The History and Economics of Indian Famines.* London: G. Bell and Sons, 1914.

Magendie, François. "Rapport fait à l'Académie des Sciences au nom de la Commission dite de la gélatine." *Comte rendu des séances de l'Académie des science* (1841): 237–95.

Maurer, Donna, and Jeffrey Sobal, eds. *Food, Eating, and Nutrition as Social Problems: Constructivist Perspectives.* New York: Transaction, 1995.

McCance, Robert Alexander, and Robert Daniel Lawrence. *The Carbohydrate Content of Foods.* Medical Research Council Special Reports 135. London: His Majesty's Stationery Office, 1929.

McCollum, Elmer Verner. *A History of Nutrition: The Sequence of Ideas in Nutrition Investigations.* Boston: Houghton Mifflin, 1957.

Meinert, Carl A. *Armee- und Volksernährung: Ein Versuch Professor C. von Voit Ernährungstheorie für die Praxis zu verwerthen.* 2 vols. Berlin: Mittler und Sohn, 1880.

Mellanby, Edward. "Diet and Health." *British Medical Journal Supplement* 21 (March 1931): 85–92.

———. "Duties of the State in Relation to the Nation's Food Supply." *British Medical Journal* 2 (1927): 633–36.

Moleschott, Jacob. *Lehre der Nahrungsmittel, für das Volk.* Erlangen: Ferdinand Enke, 1850.

Mudry, Jessica. *Measured Meals: Nutrition in America.* Albany: State University of New York Press, 2009.

Nakahama, T[oichiri]. "Ueber den Eiweissbedarf des Erwachsenen mit Berücksichtigung der Beköstigung in Japan." *Archiv für Hygiene* 5 (1888): 78–104.

Neill, Deborah. "Finding the 'Ideal Diet': Nutrition, Culture and Dietary Practices in France and French Equatorial Africa, c. 1890s to 1920s." *Food and Foodways* 17 (2009): 1–28.

Nitti, Francesco S. "Food and the Labour-Power of Nations." *Economic Journal* 6 (1896): 30–63.

Nordau, Max. *Degeneration.* London: William Heinemann, [1892] 1895.

Oddy, Derek J., Peter J. Atkins, and Virginie Amilien, eds. *The Rise of Obesity in Europe: A Twentieth-Century Food History.* Aldershot: Ashgate, 2009.

Orr, John Boyd. *Food, Health and Income: A Report on a Survey of Adequacy of Diet in Relation to Income.* London: Macmillan, 1936.

———. *The National Food Supply and Its influence on Public Health.* London: Chadwick Trust, 1934.

Orr, John Boyd, and J. L. Gilks. *The Physique and Health of Two African Tribes.* Medical Research Council Special Reports 155. London: His Majesty's Stationery Office, 1931.

Pettenkofer, Max, and Carl Voit. "Untersuchungen über den Stoffverbrauch des normalen Menschen." *Zeitschrift für Biologie* 2 (1866): 459–573.

Pickstone, John. "Production, Community and Consumption: The Political Economy of Twentieth-Century Medicine." In *Companion to Medicine in the Twentieth Century,* edited by Roger Cooter and John Pickstone, 1–20. London: Routledge, 2003.

Plagge, Wenzeslaus, and Georg Lebbin. *Untersuchungen über das Soldatenbrot: Im Auftrage des Königlichen Kriegsministeriums (Medizinal-Abtheilung).* Berlin: Verlag von August Hirschwald, 1897.

Polin, Louis Henri August Marie, and Henri Joseph Jules Pierre Labi. *L'hygiène alimentaire.* Paris: Rueff, 1893.

Pollan, Michael. *Food Rules: An Eater's Manual.* New York: Penguin Press, 2009.

———. *Omnivore's Dilemma: A Natural History of Four Meals.* New York: Penguin Press, 2006.

Rabinbach, Anson. *The Human Motor: Energy, Fatigue, and the Origins of Modernity.* Berkeley: University of California Press, 1992.

Rubner, Max. *Volksernährungsfragen.* Leipzig: Akademische Verlagsgesellschaft, 1908.

Schneider, William. *Quality and Quantity: The Quest for Biological Regeneration in Twentieth-Century France.* Cambridge: Cambridge University Press, 1990.

Schumburg, Wilhelm. "Hygiene der Einzelernährung und Massenernährung." In *Handbuch der Hygiene,* edited by Theodor Weil. Vol. 3, part 3. 2nd ed. Leipzig: Johann Ambrosius Barth, 1913.

Scrinis, Gyorgy. *Nutritionism: The Science and Politics of Dietary Advice.* New York: Columbia University Press, 2013.

Semba, Richard D. "Vitamin A as 'Anti-infective' Therapy, 1920–1940." *Journal of Nutrition* 129 (1999): 783–91.

———. *The Vitamin A Story—Lifting the Shadow of Death.* Basel: Karger, 2012.

Sen, Amartya. *Poverty and Famines: An Essay on Entitlement and Deprivation.* New York: Oxford University Press, 1981.

Sir William Arbuthnot Lane. *The Prevention of Diseases Peculiar to Civilization.* London: Faber and Faber, 1929.

Siven, V. O. "Ueber das Stickstoffgleichgewicht beim erwachsenen Menschen." *Skandinavisches Archiv für Physiologie* 10 (1900): 91–148.

Smith, David Frederick, ed. *Nutrition in Britain: Science, Scientists and Politics in the Twentieth Century.* London: Routledge, 1997.

Smith, David Frederick, and Malcolm Nicolson. "The 'Glasgow School' of Paton, Findlay and Cathcart: Conservative Thought in Chemical Physiology, Nutrition and Public Health." *Social Studies of Science* 19 (1989): 195–238.

Smith, David Frederick, and Jim Phillips, eds. *Food, Science, Policy and Regulation in the Twentieth Century: International and Comparative Perspectives.* London: Routledge, 2000.

Staples, Amy L. S. *The Birth of Development: How the World Bank, Food and Agriculture Organization, and World Health Organization Changed the World.* Kent, OH: Kent State University Press, 2006.

Tanner, Jakob. *Fabrikmahlzeit: Ernährungswissenschaft, Industriearbeit and Volksernährung in der Schweiz 1890–1950.* Zürich: Chronos, 1999.

Thompson, Benjamin. "Of Food; and Particularly of Feeding the Poor." In *The Complete Works of Count Rumford,* vol. 4, 397–490. Boston: American Academy of Arts and Sciences, 1875.

Thoms, Ulrike. *Anstaltskost in Rationalisierungsprozeß: Die Ernährung in Krankenhäusern und Gefängnissen im 18. und 19. Jahrhundert.* Stuttgart: Frank Steiner Verlag, 2005.

———. "'Vitaminfragen—kein Vitaminrummel?' Die deutsche Vitaminforschung in der ersten Hälfte des 20. Jahrhunderts und ihr Verhältnis zur Öffentlichkeit." In *Wissenschaft und Öffentlichkeit als Ressource füreinander,* edited by Sybilla Nikolow and Arne Schirrmacher, 75–96. Bielefeld: Transcript, 2007.

Trentmann, Frank, and Flemming Just, eds. *Food and Conflict in Europe in the Age of the Two World Wars.* Basingstoke, England: Palgrave Macmillan, 2006.

Turner, Bryan S. "The Government of the Body: Medical Regimens and the Rationalization of Diet." *British Journal of Sociology* 33 (1982): 254–69.

Turner, Katherine Leonard. *How the Other Half Ate: A History of Working-Class Meals at the Turn of the Century.* Berkeley: University of California Press, 2014.

Veit, Helen Zoe. *Modern Food, Moral Food: Self-control, Science, and the Rise of Modern American Eating in the Early Twentieth Century.* Chapel Hill: University of North Carolina Press, 2013.

Vernon, James. *Hunger: A Modern History.* Cambridge, MA: Belknap Press, 2007.

Voit, Carl. "Anforderungen der Gesundheitspflege an die Kost in Waisenhäusern, Casernen, Gefangenen- und Altersversorgungsanstalten, sowie in Volksküchen: Bericht des Ausschussses über die dritte Versammlung des öffentlichen Vereins für Gesundheitspflege zu München." *Deutsche Vierteljahresschrift für öffentliche Gesundheitspflege* 8 (1876): 7–57.

———. "Physiologie des allgemeinen Stoffwechsels und die Ernährung." *Handbuch der Physiologie,* vol. 6, part 1, edited by L. Hermann. Leipzig: F. C. W. Vogel, 1881.

———. "Ueber die Kost eines Vegetariers." *Zeitschrift für Biologie* 25 (1889): 232–36, 255–88.

———. *Ueber die Kost in öffentlichen Anstalten.* Munich: Oldenbourg, 1876.

———, ed. *Untersuchung der Kost in einigen öffentlichen Anstalten.* Munich: Oldenbourg, 1877.

White, Mastin G., and Otis H. Gates. *Decisions of Courts in Cases under the Federal Food and Drugs Act.* Washington, DC: Government Printing Office, 1934.

Whorton, James C. *Inner Hygiene: Constipation and the Pursuit of Health in Modern Society.* New York: Oxford University Press, 2000.

Wiley, Harvey. *The History of a Crime against the Food Law: The Amazing Story of the National Food and Drug Law Intended to Protect the Health of the People and Perverted to Protect Adulterators of Food and Drugs.* Washington, DC: Harvey Wiley, 1929. http://www.whale.to/a/wiley_b.html. Accessed January 9, 2013.

Wright, Carroll D. [and W. O. Atwater]. "Food Consumption: Quantities, Costs, and Nutrients of Food-Materials." In *17th Annual Report of the Bureau of Statistics of Labor.* Boston: Wright and Potter, 1886, 237–326.

Ziegelmayer, Wilhelm. "Die Wehrmacht als Erzieher zur richtigen Verbrauchslenkung und gesunden Ernährung." *Zeitschrift für Volksernährung* 12 (1937): 13–15.

Zweiniger-Bargielowska, Ina. *Managing the Body: Beauty, Health, and Fitness in Britain, 1880–1939.* Oxford: Oxford University Press, 2010.

Zweiniger-Bargielowska, Ina, Rachel Duffett, and Alain Drouard, eds. *Food and War in Twentieth-Century Europe.* Burlington: Ashgate, 2011.

Contributors

NICK CULLATHER is professor of history and international studies at Indiana University, with a research focus on US foreign policy and intelligence services. He is the author of *Illusions of Influence* (1994), *Secret History: The CIA's Classified Account of Its Operations in Guatemala, 1952–1954* (2006), and *The Hungry World: America's Cold War Battle against Poverty in Asia* (2010).

SUZANNE JUNOD received her MA and PhD from Emory University in the history of medicine. She came to the FDA History Office in 1984 as its first professional historian. In 1994–95, she served as FDA liaison and historical consultant for President Clinton's Advisory Committee on Human Radiation Experiments (ACHRE). She serves on the editorial board of the *Journal of the History of Medicine and Allied Sciences.* She has received numerous awards for her work, including the Food and Drug Law Institute's Outstanding Service Award and the FDA's Award of Merit. She has wide-ranging publications in the history of medicine, public health, women's health, clinical trials, the Progressive Era, and food additive regulation.

DEBORAH NEILL is associate professor of history at York University in Toronto. Her research focuses on the histories of globalization and European colonial expansion into sub-Saharan Africa in the late nineteenth and early twentieth centuries. She is particularly interested in the development of transnational connections in the areas of science, humanitarianism, and trade across French, German, and British colonies. Her book, *Networks in Tropical Medicine: Internationalism, Colonialism, and the Rise of a Medical Specialty, 1890–1930,* was published by Stanford University Press in 2012.

ELIZABETH NESWALD is associate professor in the Department of History at Brock University. Before coming to Brock in 2006, she spent time at the University of Aberdeen, the National University of Ireland at Galway, and the Humboldt University in Berlin. She is the author of *Thermodynamik als kultureller Kampfplatz: Eine Faszinationsgeschichte der Entropie, 1850–1915* (2006) and *Medien-Philosophie: Das Werk Vilém Flussers* (1998). Her current work focuses on the history of metabolism research, nutritional physiology, and dietary standards in the nineteenth and early twentieth centuries.

DAVID F. SMITH is honorary senior lecturer in the history of medicine at the University of Aberdeen. He is the editor of *Nutrition in Britain: Science, Scientists and Politics in the Twentieth Century* (1997), joint editor of *Food, Science, Policy and Regulation in the Twentieth Century: International and Comparative Perspectives* (2000), and leading author of *Food Poisoning, Policy and Politics: Corned Beef and Typhoid in Britain in the 1960s* (2005).

ULRIKE THOMS studied economic and social history before moving into the history of science. She has numerous publications in the history of the nutritional sciences, clinical trials, and pharmaceuticals. She is currently researching the social history of the Max Planck Society and its relations to the public at the Max Planck Institute for the History of Science. Her publications on the history of nutrition and medicine include *Anstaltskost im Rationalisierungsprozess: Die Ernährung in Krankenhäusern und Gefängnissen im 18. und 19. Jahrhundert* (2005), and is coeditor (with Jean-Paul Gaudillière) of *The Birth of Scientific Marketing in the Twentieth Century: Research for Sales in the Pharmaceutical Industry* (2015).

CORINNA TREITEL is associate professor in the Department of History at Washington University in St. Louis. She is a German historian interested in the intersection of science, medicine, and culture since the late eighteenth century. Her first book, *A Science for the Soul: Occultism and the Genesis of the German Modern* (2004), examined the German occult movement as an aspect of European modernism. Her current research concerns the history of food and nutrition. She is finishing a second book on the history of natural foods and farming in German-speaking Europe from the early nineteenth century to the present.

INA ZWEINIGER-BARGIELOWSKA is professor of modern British history at the University of Illinois, Chicago. She has published widely on modern British history. She is author of *Austerity in Britain: Rationing, Controls and Consumption, 1939–1955* (2000). Her most recent books are *Managing the Body: Beauty, Health and Fitness in Britain, 1880s–1939* (2010) and the coedited collection *Food and War in Twentieth-Century Europe* (2011).

Index

www.ingramcontent.com/pod-product-compliance
Lightning Source LLC
Chambersburg PA
CBHW051256200926
51612CB00002B/65
* 9 7 8 1 5 8 0 4 6 5 7 6 2 *